Health Policy and Politics
A Nurse's Guide

Third Edition

Jeri A. Milstead, PhD, RN, FAAN
Dean and Professor
College of Nursing
University of Toledo
Toledo, Ohio

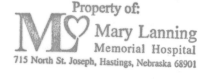
JONES AND BARTLETT PUBLISHERS
Sudbury, Massachusetts
BOSTON   TORONTO   LONDON   SINGAPORE

World Headquarters
Jones and Bartlett Publishers
40 Tall Pine Drive
Sudbury, MA 01776
978-443-5000
info@jbpub.com
www.jbpub.com

Jones and Bartlett Publishers
Canada
6339 Ormindale Way
Mississauga, Ontario L5V 1J2
CANADA

Jones and Bartlett Publishers
International
Barb House, Barb Mews
London W6 7PA
United Kingdom

Jones and Bartlett's books and products are available through most bookstores and online booksellers. To contact Jones and Bartlett Publishers directly, call 800-832-0034, fax 978-443-8000, or visit our website www.jbpub.com.

Substantial discounts on bulk quantities of Jones and Bartlett's publications are available to corporations, professional associations, and other qualified organizations. For details and specific discount information, contact the special sales department at Jones and Bartlett via the above contact information or send an email to specialsales@jbpub.com.

The authors, editor, and publisher have made every effort to provide accurate information. However, they are not responsible for errors, omissions, or for any outcomes related to the use of the contents of this book and take no responsibility for the use of the products and procedures described. Treatments and side effects described in this book may not be applicable to all people; likewise, some people may require a dose or experience a side effect that is not described herein. Drugs and medical devices are discussed that may have limited availability or are controlled by the Food and Drug Administration (FDA) for use only in a research study or clinical trial. Research, clinical practice, and government regulations often change the accepted standard in this field. When consideration is being given to use of any drug in the clinical setting, the healthcare provider or reader is responsible for determining FDA status of the drug, reading the package insert, and reviewing prescribing information for the most up-to-date recommendations on dose, precautions, and contraindications, and determining the appropriate usage for the product. This is especially important in the case of drugs that are new or seldom used.

Production Credits
Executive Editor: Kevin Sullivan
Acquisitions Editor: Emily Ekle
Associate Editor: Amy Sibley
Editorial Assistant: Patricia Donnelly
Production Director: Amy Rose
Associate Production Editor: Wendy Swanson
Senior Marketing Manager: Katrina Gosek
Associate Marketing Manager: Rebecca Wasley
Manufacturing and Inventory Coordinator: Amy Bacus
Text Design: Auburn Associates, Inc.
Composition: Auburn Associates, Inc.
Cover Design: Kate Ternullo
Cover Image: ©Eddie Lepp/ShutterStock, Inc.
Printing and Binding: Malloy, Inc.
Cover Printing: Malloy, Inc.

Library of Congress Cataloging-in-Publication Data

Health policy and politics : a nurse's guide / [edited by] Jeri A. Milstead. — 3rd ed.
  p. ; cm.
  Includes bibliographical references and index.
  ISBN-13: 978-0-7637-5127-2 (casebound : alk. paper)
  ISBN-10: 0-7637-5127-8 (casebound : alk. paper) 1. Nurses—United States—Political activity. 2. Nursing—Political aspects—United States. 3. Medical policy—United States. 4. Medical care—Political aspects—United States. I. Milstead, Jeri A.
  [DNLM: 1. Legislation, Nursing—United States. 2. Health Policy—United States. 3. Politics—United States. WY 33 AA1 H399 2008]
  RT86.5.M54 2008
  362.17'30973—dc22

                                                            2007019298

6048
Printed in the United States of America
11 10 09 08 07   10 9 8 7 6 5 4 3 2 1

Contents

Contributors vii

Preface ix

Acknowledgments xvii

Chapter 1 Advanced Practice Nurses and
Public Policy, Naturally 1
Jeri A. Milstead, PhD, RN, FAAN

Introduction 2
Changes in the Practice of Nursing 2
The Emerging Political Role of Nurses 5
Finding a Foundation in Theory and Research 8
A New Organizational Paradigm 10
The Changing Paradigm in Health Care 12
What Is Public Policy? 15
An Overview of the Policy Process 21
A Bright Future 25
Conclusion 32

Chapter 2 Agenda Setting 41
Elizabeth Ann Furlong, JD, PhD, RN

Introduction 42
The Nebraska Humane Care Amendment 43
The National Center for Nursing Research Amendment 46
Overview of Models 48
Kingdon Model 48
Importance of Contextual Dimensions 52
Schneider and Ingram Model 58
Conclusion 60

Chapter 3 Government Response: Legislation 65
Mary K. Wakefield, PhD, RN, FAAN

Introduction 66
The Players 66
The Process 78
Research 81
Putting Issues in Context 81
Visibility 82
Effective Communication 83
Eleven Lessons Learned from Nine Years on Capitol Hill 85
Conclusion 88

Chapter 4 Government Regulation: Parallel and Powerful 91
Jacqueline M. Loversidge, MS, RN, C

Introduction 92
Regulation Versus Legislation 92
Health Professions Regulation and Licensing 94
Methods of Professional Credentialing 97
The State Regulatory Process 101
The Federal Regulatory Process 107
Emergency Regulations 110
Locating Information 111
Providing Public Comment 114
Lobbying and Political Decision Making 115
Strengths and Weaknesses of the Regulatory Process 116
Current Issues in Regulation and Licensure 117
The Future of Advanced Practice Nurse Regulation 121
Conclusion 125

Chapter 5 Policy Design 129

Patricia Smart, PhD, RN, FNP-BC

Introduction 129
The Policy Process 131
Review of Policy Research 131
The Design Issue 134
Policy Instruments 136
Policy Design Model 138
Behavioral Dimensions 139
Conclusion 141
Case Study in Policy Design 141

Chapter 6 Policy Implementation 157

Marlene Wilken, PhD, RN

Introduction 158
Policy Implementation Players 159
Conclusion 161
Case Study: Advanced Practice Nurses and
Pain Management 161
Case Study: Lead Poisoning in Children 163
Case Study: Back to Sleep and Nothing But Baby Campaigns . . . 164

Chapter 7 Program Evaluation 171

Ardith L. Sudduth, PhD, RN, APRN-BC, FNP

Introduction 172
Policy, Public Policy, and Social Programs 173
Program Evaluation 176
Accountability in Program Evaluation 179
Theory: A Valuable Tool in Evaluation 181
Ethics and Evaluation 182
Suggestions to Reduce Ethical Dilemmas in
Program Evaluation 186
Program Evaluation Design Options 188
Evaluation Reports: Sharing the Findings 190
Conclusion 193

Chapter 8 The Internet and Healthcare Policy Information 197

Ramona Nelson, PhD, RN-BC, FAAN

Introduction 198
Information Literacy and Health Policy 199
Key Health Policy–Related Sites on the Internet 210
Impact of the Internet on the Process of
Developing Health Policy 215
Conclusion 216

Chapter 9 Policy Nurses Advance Policy Agendas in
Many Arenas 221
Nancy J. Sharp, MSN, RN, FAAN

Introduction 222
Policy Nurses in Nursing Associations 222
Nurse in Washington Roundtable 223
Nursing Specialties Advocacy 223
Nurses in Washington Internship 224
Advanced Practice Nurse Organizations' Advocacy 225
The Nurse's Directory of Capitol Connections 226
University Policy Courses 227
Nightingale Policy Institute 227
Conclusion 229

Chapter 10 Applied Healthcare Economics for the
Noneconomics Major 231
Nancy Munn Short, DrPH, MBA, RN

Introduction 232
How Do Markets Work and What Is the Healthcare Market? . . . 232
Nurse Shortages 233
Economic Rationality 234
Information Economics 234
Adverse Selection and Moral Hazard 236
Externalities 236
Opportunity Costs 237
What Makes the U.S. Healthcare System and Economy Strong? . . 238
Web Sites of Interest 238
Case Study: The Economics of End-Stage Renal Disease 240

Chapter 11 Global Connections 245
Jeri A. Milstead, PhD, RN, FAAN

Introduction 246
Global Issues 246
Case Study: Implementation of Three Needle-
    Exchange Programs 250
Case Study: Implementation of Three Needle-Exchange
    Programs through Application of the Milstead Model 253
Conclusion 264

Contributors

Elizabeth Ann Furlong, JD, PhD, RN
Associate Professor
School of Nursing
Creighton University
Omaha, Nebraska

Jacqueline M. Loversidge, MS, RN, C
Assistant Professor
Capital University
Columbus, Ohio

Jeri A. Milstead, PhD, RN, FAAN
Dean and Professor
College of Nursing
University of Toledo
Toledo, Ohio

Ramona Nelson, PhD, RN-BC, FAAN
Professor and Co-Director of Health Care
  Informatics Program
College of Health and Human Services
Slippery Rock University of
  Pennsylvania
Slippery Rock, Pennsylvania

Nancy J. Sharp, MSN, RN, FAAN
Vice President Communications/
  Capitol Connections
Nightingale Policy Institute
Bethesda, Maryland

Patricia Smart, PhD, RN, FNP-BC
Professor and Faculty Assistant to the Provost and
  Assistant to the President
Clemson University
Clemson, South Carolina

Nancy Munn Short, DrPH, MBA, RN
Assistant Professor and Senior Research Fellow
Duke University School of Nursing
Durham, North Carolina

**Ardith L. Sudduth, PhD, RN,
  APRN-BC, FNP**
Assistant Professor
School of Nursing
University of Louisiana at Lafayette
Lafayette, Louisiana

Mary K. Wakefield, PhD, RN, FAAN
Director, Center for Rural Health
University of North Dakota
Grand Forks, North Dakota

Marlene Wilken, PhD, RN
Assistant Professor
School of Nursing
Creighton University
Omaha, Nebraska

Preface

This book is a contributed text for advanced practice nurses (APNs) that is based on research conducted by the contributors and experience in real-world policy making and political action. The scope of the content covers the whole process of making public policy. Components of the process are addressed within broad categories of agenda setting; government response; and program design, implementation, and evaluation. The primary focus is at the federal and state levels, although the reader can adapt concepts to the global or local level.

Some nurses are sophisticated in their political activity. They have served as Senate or congressional district coordinators for the American Nurses Association, worked as campaign managers for elected officials, or presented testimony at congressional or state hearings. However, even these nurses often think "legislation" when they hear policy. Few know the reality of how a bill becomes a law, where ideas for those bills are derived, or how the decisions to create one program rather than another are made.

This book addresses the policy process as a broad range of decision points, strategies, activities, and outcomes that involve elected and appointed government officials and their staffs, bureaucratic agencies, private citizens, and interest groups. The process is dynamic, convoluted, and ongoing; not static, linear, or concise. Knowledgeable nurses in advanced practice must demonstrate their commitment to action by being a part of relevant decisions that will ensure the delivery of quality health care by appropriate providers in a cost-effective manner.

Nursing as a practice profession is based on theory and evidence. For many years that practice has been interpreted as direct, hands-on care of individuals. Although this still is true, the profession has matured to the point where the provision of expert, direct care is not enough. Nurses of the third millennium can stand tall in their multiple roles of provider of care, educator, administrator, consultant, researcher, political activist, and policymaker. The question of how much a nurse in advanced practice can or should take on may be raised. The Information Age continues to present new knowledge exponentially. Nurses have added more and more tasks that seem important to professional nurses and essential for the provision of safe care to the client. Is political activism necessary? All health professionals are expected to do more with fewer resources. Realistically, how much can a specialist do?

Drucker (1995), in addressing the need for more general-practitioner physicians rather than specialists, redefines the generalist of today as one who puts multiple specialties together rapidly. Nursing can benefit from that thought. In Drucker's definition, the APN must be a multidimensional generalist/specialist. This means that the APN combines knowledge and skills from a variety of fields or subspecialties to function effectively to design the new paradigm of healthcare delivery. This also means that the APN must demonstrate competence in the multiple roles in which he or she operates. To function effectively in the role of political activist, the APN must realize the scope of the whole policy process, and the process is much broader than how a bill becomes a law.

It is natural for nurses to talk with bureaucrats, agency staff, legislators, and others in public service about what nurses do, what nurses need, and the extent of their cost-effectiveness and long-term impact on health care in this country. For too long, nurses talked to each other. Each knew their value; each told great stories; they "preached to the choir" of other nurses instead of sharing their wisdom with those who could help change the healthcare system for the better.

Today's nurses, especially those in advanced practice who have a solid foundation of focused education and competent experience, know how to market themselves and their talents and know how to harness their irritations and direct them toward positive resolution. As nurses, each must embrace the whole range of options available in the various parts of the policy process. The opportunity to sustain an ongoing, meaningful dialogue with those who represent the districts and states and those who administer public programs is theirs to initiate. Nurses must become indispensable to elected and appointed officials. APNs must demonstrate leadership by becoming those officials and by participating with others in planning and decision making.

Why a Third Edition?

The First Edition was well received and has been used by nurses in at least five countries. When the original publisher changed focus from health, education, and criminal justice to law and business, Jones and Bartlett picked up the option for this book and encouraged us to write a Second Edition. The contributors were enthusiastic and agreed that it was time. The Information Age was upon us and everyone struggled to stay current.

The Third Edition finds us in a different place. We now live in a world of uncertainty. The United States has lost its place as the benevolent, wise-for-our-age country where world leadership was a given. Other countries have lost confidence in our vision of economics, the environment, education, health care, and politics. We have been thrust into the world spotlight not because of our successes but because of our failures. The United States can no longer justify using so many of the environmental resources available, can no longer justify rearing a generation (or more) of children who cannot read or compute and who are prone to violence, can no longer justify an economic system where the rich really are getting richer and the poor really are getting poorer and the middle class is beginning to diminish.

We are the generation in charge now. We must harness our will, gather our best minds and spirits, and employ the widest range of technology to make our earth sustainable, beautiful, and safe. The ability to work with other governments requires exquisite political leadership. We must use our communications skills and our knowledge of policymaking to forge change that will make our country and the world better. We can start by educating ourselves about the full range of the policy process.

Each chapter in this edition has been written or updated with current thought and references. Beth Furlong, in Chapter 2, includes a new approach to agenda setting through case scenarios. Beth has retained the wonderful story about how an army nurse, Diane Carlson Evans, created the Vietnam Women's Memorial. Dr. Furlong also updated how the National Institute of Nursing Research (NINR) contributes to the profession of nursing and added more practice implications for APNs. Dr. Mary Wakefield continues to share the down-to-earth yet sophisticated wisdom she developed through years as a Washington, DC insider. Renatta Loquist, who wrote the original chapter on government regulation, has retired and is very involved in congregational nursing. She and I have known Jackie Loversidge for many years and have great respect for Jackie's working knowledge of the regulatory process. Although Jackie is deeply immersed in her doctoral study, she made time to add her own flavor to a topic with which many nurses are not familiar in Chapter 4, even though we are subject to regulatory practices every day. Dr. Pat Smart continues with her discussion of policy tools in her updated Chapter 5 on policy design. The idea of "tools" is a wonderful way to conceptualize how programs and policies are put together. Dr. Marty Wilken has included several case studies in Chapter 6 as she helps the reader understand the intricacies of policy and program implementation. Ardie Sudduth takes a fresh look at program evaluation in Chapter 7. Dr. Sudduth presents rational arguments as to why APNs should become involved in the process of evaluating programs and offers practical and helpful suggestions in weaving through the process. She also broadens the discussion of outcome-based evaluation and the ethics of program evaluation.

In Chapter 8, Dr. Ramona Nelson updated and revised all Internet sources and links—a formidable task in the fast-changing world of information technology. Dr. Nelson discusses the impact of the Internet on all steps of health policy development. Chapter 9 brings a fresh face to the book, although Nancy Sharp has been a recognized leader in policy and politics for many years. Nancy's background as a lobbyist and her exceptional energy as a motivator and doer is reflected in her discussion of nurse organizations and how they are positioned in the political world. Dr. Nancy Short also brings a new perspective to the book in Chapter 10 as she presents a primer on the economics of health care, a topic many nurses are not familiar with but recognize a need to know. Chapter 11 presents a section on current health issues around the world with a plea to consider all health care in a global context. The research on needle-exchange programs has been shortened to a case study discussion within the Milstead Model, a comprehensive framework for studying nursing and health policy across countries and cultures. The model integrates policy components and the role of the advanced practice nurse.

Finally, most colleagues with whom I have spoken were not aware that there was an Instructor's Manual that was developed with the original edition. The handbook was designed to offer activities for learners and to suggest ideas for discussion that would enhance the content of the text. Because there seems to have been limited use, we have incorporated many of the items from the manual into the Third Edition. We hope you take advantage of the creative suggestions!

We hope you like the changes and will continue to contact us if you have questions or want further information.

Target Audience

This book is intended for several audiences:

- Nurses who work in advanced practice in clinical, education, administrative, research, or consultative settings can use this book as a guide for understanding the full range of the policy components that they did not learn in graduate school. Components are presented with theoretical foundations and are brought to life through actual nursing research and nurses' experiences. This book will help the nurse who is searching for knowledge of how leaders of today influence public policy toward better health care for the future. Nurses in leadership positions clearly articulate nursing's societal mission. Nurses, as the largest group of healthcare workers in the country, realize that the way to make a permanent impact on the delivery of health care is to be a part of the decision making that occurs at every step of the healthcare policy process.
- Graduate and doctoral students in nursing can use this text for in-depth study of the full policy process. Works of scholars in each segment provide a solid foundation for examining each component. This book goes beyond the narrow elementary explanation of legislation and bridges the gap toward understanding of a broader policy process in which multiple opportunities for involvement exist.
- Faculty in graduate programs and other current nurse leaders can use this book as a reference for their own policy activity. Faculty and other leaders should be mentors for those they teach and for other nurses throughout the profession. Because the whole policy process is so broad, these leaders can track their own experiences through the policy process by referring to the components described in this book.
- Other healthcare professionals who are interested in the area of healthcare policy will find this book useful in directing their thoughts and actions toward the complex issues of both healthcare policy and public policy. Physicians, pharmacists, psychologists, occupational and physical therapists, physicians' assistants, and others will discover parallels with their own practices as they examine case studies and other research. Nurses cannot change huge systems alone. APNs can use this book as a vehicle to educate other professionals so that, together, everyone in the healthcare profession can influence policymakers.
- Those professionals who do not provide health care directly but who are involved in areas of the environment that produce

actual and potential threats to personal and community health and safety will find this book a valuable resource regarding how a problem becomes known, who decides what to do about it, and what type of governmental response might result. Environmental scientists, public health officials, sociologists, political scientists, psychologists, and other professionals involved with health problems in the public interest will benefit from the ideas generated in this book.

- Interest groups can use this book as a tool to consider opportunities to become involved in public policymaking. Interest groups can be extremely helpful in changing systems because the passion for their causes energizes them to act. Interest groups can become partners in the political activity of nurses by knowing how and when to use their influence to assist APNs at junctures in the policy process.
- Corporate leaders can use this book to gain an understanding of the broad roles within which nurses function. Chief executive officers (CEOs) and other top business administrators must learn that nurses are articulate, assertive, and intelligent experts in health care who have a solid knowledge base and a political agenda. The wise CEO and colleagues will seek out APNs for counsel and collaboration when moving policy ideas forward.

Using This Book

Each chapter is freestanding; that is, chapters do not rely, or necessarily build, on one another. The sequence of the chapters is presented in a linear fashion, but readers will note immediately that the policy process is not linear. For example, readers of the policy implementation chapter will find reference to scholars and concepts featured in the agenda setting and policy design chapters. Such is the nature of the public process of making decisions. The material covered is a small portion of the existing research, argument, and considered thought about policymaking and the broader political, economic, and social concepts and issues. Therefore, readers should use this book as a starting point for their own scholarly inquiry.

This book can be used to initiate discussions about issues of policy and nurses' opportunities and responsibilities throughout the process. The research studies that are presented should raise some questions about what should have happened or why something else did not happen. In this way, the book can serve as a guide through what some think of as a maze of activity with no direction but which is actually a rational, albeit chaotic, system.

The Discussion Points and Activities at the end of the each chapter are ideal for planning a class or addressing an audience. Many activities are presented, and I hope that they serve to stimulate the readers' own creative thoughts about how to engage others. Gone are the days of the "sage on stage"—the teacher who had all the answers and lectured to students who had no questions. Good teachers always have learned from students and vice versa. Today's teachers/learners are interactive, technically savvy, curious and questioning, and capable of helping learners integrate large amounts of data and information. The manual can serve as a guide and a beginning.

Reference

Drucker, P. F. (1995, February). The age of social transformation. *Quality Digest*, 36, 39.

Acknowledgments

Only a few nurses in the United States with master's degrees in nursing also hold earned doctorates in political science. When I discovered that each of these nurses had researched a different component of the policy process, a book immediately came to mind. The authors realize that there is much more to public decision making than the process of writing laws and that this knowledge affords them the opportunity and responsibility for contributing seriously to public policy. When I approached these nurses about contributing to this book, each agreed enthusiastically. Therefore, special thanks must go to Dr. Beth Furlong, Dr. Patricia Smart, Dr. Ardith Sudduth, and Dr. Marlene Wilken for their scholarly contributions. The two chapters on government response are a welcome addition because of the importance of the content. Dr. Mary Wakefield served as chief of staff for North Dakota Senators Quentin Burdick and Kent Conrad for several years. She has "been there, done that" and can explain just how a bill really does become a law. She adds the strong dimension of informal communication and negotiation that occurs as ideas are formalized into laws. Jackie Loversidge, former education consultant for the Ohio Board of Nursing and active participant in committees of the National Council of State Boards of Nursing, possesses down-to-earth knowledge and experience about the regulatory process. In many ways a parallel process to legislation, the course of devising and approving regulations, often is not recognized by nurses as important or as an opportunity for nursing input. Nancy Sharp's approach to nursing is so positive and full of life. She always brings a sense of hope and action to others through her writing. Dr. Nancy Short deals with very serious content in a very knowledgeable way. She has the ability to link important material to issues that are very dear to nurses. We welcome both Nancys as contributors. Dr. Ramona Nelson's experience brings the nurse in advanced practice well into the 21st century by identifying electronic resources that can assist the advanced practice nurse in preparing material, studying issues, and locating assets. There is a plethora of data that nurses can share with colleagues and officials. Dr. Nelson helps the reader figure out what is useful and what is not.

I must thank Jones and Bartlett Publishers for their encouragement and guidance in writing the *Third Edition*. Their confidence in all of the contributors and me has been consistent and unwavering. I also thank the readers of this book for their interest in the policy process. For those of you who have integrated these components and concepts into your nursing careers, I applaud you. You will continue to contribute to the profession and to the broader society. For those readers who are struggling with how to incorporate one more piece of anything into your role as an advanced practice nurse, remember that you are advancing the cause of your own personal work, the profession, and healthcare delivery in this country and throughout the world every time you use the concepts in this book. Nurses are a powerful force and can exercise their many talents to further good public policy, which, ultimately, must improve health care for patients, consumers, and families.

Finally, I acknowledge my forever-cheering section—my four children, their spouses and significant others, and three grandchildren. They are always there for me and provide continuous support, encouragement, and unconditional love. I love you, Kerrin, George, Sunny, and George Biddle; Joan Milstead; Kevin Milstead and Gregg Peace; Sara, Steve, and Matthew Lott. You are a fun bunch and you make me smile.

Jeri A. Milstead

Advanced Practice Nurses and Public Policy, Naturally

Jeri A. Milstead, PhD, RN, FAAN

Key Terms

- ➤ **Advanced practice nurse (APN)** A registered nurse with a master's or doctoral degree in nursing, who demonstrates expert knowledge, skills, and attitudes in the practice of nursing.
- ➤ **New organizational paradigm** Conceptual approach to the arrangement of work from the traditional hierarchical bureaucracy to systems appropriate to the current information age.
- ➤ **Nursing's agenda for health** Policy expectations of a vision for nursing practice that includes prevention of illness, promotion of health, empowerment of individuals to assume responsibility for the state of their own health, expertise in the provision of direct nursing care, delegation and supervision of selected care to appropriate individuals, and the political influence to accomplish these goals.
- ➤ **Policy process** The course of bringing problems to government and obtaining a reply. The process includes agenda setting, design, government response, implementation, and evaluation.
- ➤ **Public policy** Actual directives that document government decisions; also, the process of taking problems to government agents and obtaining a decision or reply in the form of a program, law, or regulation.

Introduction

The **advanced practice nurse (APN)** of the third millennium must be technically competent, use critical thinking and decision models, possess vision that is shared with colleagues and consumers, and function in a vast array of roles. One of these roles is policy expert. Despite the influence of Florence Nightingale in the 19th century, nurses in the 20th century nearly lost the role of the nurse in the political arena. Only at the end of the 1990s was this aspect of the role becoming integrated into the scope of practice of the advanced practice nurse. Policy and politics is a natural domain for nurses, and the full integration into practice chronicles nursing's heritage and the evolution of the profession and the healthcare system. Major changes in the profession and society mirror the evolution: changes in the practice of nursing, the emerging political role of nurses, finding a foundation in theory, and a **new organizational paradigm**.

Changes in the Practice of Nursing

The changing paradigm in the delivery of health care of the late 20th century is reflected in changes in the practice of nursing. In the early 1900s, when nurses traditionally worked in homes or did home visits through an organized nursing service, nurses focused on personal care of individuals who were sick. As hospitals took on the function of workshops for physicians, nurses were employed to provide care to many individuals in one site. Just as organizational theorists were trying to establish the structure and function of institutional arrangements that developed with the industrial age, nurses were trying to establish the roles and functions of organizational employees in a system that was becoming very complex. Nurses categorized patients as those with primarily medical or primarily surgical problems, which led to the early differentiation of types of "floors" or areas in which nurses worked and which also differentiated nursing expertise in specific areas. Some nurses became organizational experts as they managed nursing units and whole hospitals.

As early as the 1940s, nurses were creating typographies of areas of nursing. Psychiatric, pediatric, obstetrical, medical, and surgical nursing were considered distinct clinical areas that were required for basic practice and, as such, were tested in early examinations for licensure. By the 1950s, nursing programs long had recognized the teaching of nursing as an area that required knowledge beyond the traditional baccalaureate degree. Bachelor of science degrees in nursing education (BSNE) had been offered at the undergraduate level to prepare nurses to teach in diploma schools of nursing. BSNE programs were phased out as specialization in all areas of nursing education took place, and clinical practice was ascribed to the master's level.

After World War II, veterans (including nurses) pursued college degrees through the GI bill. With the dearth of advanced nursing education programs, many nurses enrolled in education majors. Students and faculty in many areas were struggling with the impact of an explosion of knowledge and questioned whether their fields were "science" and whether the discipline fit the definition and expectations of a profession. For example, the discipline of political economy changed its name to political science and many nursing programs became "nursing science" programs. Practitioners of nursing adopted the scientific process and embraced the scientific theory of assessing, planning, implementing, and evaluating what nurses do. Nursing education programs sought courses in the natural sciences (chemistry and physiology) and social sciences (sociology and psychology) to provide a foundation for the nursing courses that were evolving with theories and models. Research became important to confirm nursing's position as a profession, but many of the studies examined the behavior of the nurse or the system of nursing education rather than clinical practice. The endorsement of the scientific approach as a logical, linear, and sequential process concomitantly rejected any indication of intuition or discernment of knowledge in any way other than what could be calculated by quantitative measures. The wisdom that was transferred through generations of nurses almost was lost by the insistence in academic programs of a focus on "hard" science.

By the 1960s, special care areas were surfacing in hospitals. As machines were invented for diagnostic testing and monitoring of patients, as early computers were developed, and as statistics evolved into a special branch of mathematics, physicians and nurses were placing patients into geographic and medically focused units where care could be concentrated. The emergence of coronary care units was quickly followed by the creation of intensive care units that soon became differentiated as surgical, trauma, neonatal, and other narrow domains. Nurses and physicians needed more knowledge and clinical skills to understand the medical, nursing, and technological advances that were occurring, and specialization became formalized into programs.

As nurses came to understand more about what constituted the practice of nursing, the boundaries of nursing expanded. Breaking free of the old-fashioned perspective of the nurse as handmaiden to the physician, nurses in the 1970s and 1980s sought autonomy as independent practitioners of nursing such as clinical nurse specialists. Nurse practitioner programs were created to relieve a shortage of physicians. However, rather than becoming "junior doctors," nurse practitioners pushed out the margins of the discipline of nursing. Physical examinations, formerly limited to the scope of practice of physicians, were incorporated into nursing education programs, and physical examinations became essential to clinical nursing practice. Assertiveness training was taught in schools of nursing, which produced articulate registered nurses who could speak up. The nursing process became the watchword of the profession, and national standards were adopted based on assessment, diagnosis, planning, implementation, and evaluation criteria. Nursing theories were developed and research was conducted to test the theories. Certification in specialty areas acknowledged the clinical competence of nurses in distinct practice areas. Intensive care nurses became certain of and comfortable with their clinical knowledge and used it to provide physicians with indispensable data and to suggest treatment options. The rise in the number of baccalaureate-prepared nurses triggered a move toward graduate education. The number of doctoral programs in nursing was increasing. Although the improving image of nursing still did not command the respect from physicians, nurses gained respect and trust from the public.

By the 1990s, nurses were found in many settings. In addition to staff nurses, hospitals employed nurses as unit managers, educators in staff-development departments, coordinators of outpatient services, senior administrators, and creators of data and information systems. Nurses also served as infection-control officers, materials coordinators, patient-relations officials, and heads of quality improvement. Outside the hospital, nurses provided direct care in hospices and homes, in occupational health departments of business and industry, in prisons and correctional facilities, in schools, in interdisciplinary teams concerned with the health of astronauts, and in a host of military situations. Nonhospital, non-direct care opportunities found nurses directing their own continuing education companies, staffing professional and specialty associations, and combining nursing knowledge and skill with law and business degrees, in marketing and product sales, in pharmaceutical companies (as salespersons, researchers, and lobbyists), and in computer sales. Professional nurses also were contributing their expertise through positions as executive directors or members of boards of directors of social and health-related associations such as Planned Parenthood, Inc. Nurses were appointed to state boards of nursing; a few ran for public office; and some nurses directed or staffed offices of federal and state legislators, legislative committees and commissions, and bureaucratic agencies. The scope of nursing practice had expanded, and most state nurse practice acts reflected the changes in their legal definitions of nursing.

Laws that govern nursing define the practice of nursing and set the scope of practice of professional nurses. Early definitions of practice focused on the provision of direct care; later definitions added functions and roles such as "teaching, counseling, administration, research, consultation, supervision, delegation and evaluation of practice" and "observation, care, and counsel of the ill, injured, infirm, the promotion and maintenance of health" ("Laws governing nursing," 1994, p. 3). Clearly, the role of the nurse had been expanded beyond caring for the sick patient. Laws governing advanced practice have emerged to offer title protection and legal guidance. Because all laws are the result of compromise, nurse practice acts reflect what is acceptable at the time, not the ideal.

The Emerging Political Role of Nurses

As early as the 1960s, social scientists from a broad array of disciplines had investigated the concept of occupational and professional roles. Concepts such as role ambiguity, role congruence, role conflict, and role taking were frequently cited in the literature (Argyris, 1962). Haas's (1964) early study of nurses clarified that their role had four dimensions: task, authority or power, deference or prestige, and affect or feelings. Despite Haas's study, however, the term *role* still is synonymous with task in most of the literature, and readers miss, therefore, a full understanding of the concept.

There has been a major shift in the roles that nurses assume. In addition to clinical experts, nurses have become entrepreneurs, decision makers, and political activists. Many nurses realized that to control practice and move the profession of nursing forward as a major player in the healthcare arena, nursing and nurses had to be involved in the legal decisions about the health and welfare of the public, decisions that often were made in the governmental arena.

For many nurses, political activism meant letting someone else get involved. For some nurses, political activism meant dusting off the page in the high school or college *Problems in Government* textbook that presented an algorithm about how a bill becomes a law. A focus on the legislative process in which bills are drafted and passed by the Senate and the House of Representatives stimulated some grassroots connections between nurses and their legislative members. Nurses began to "tune in" to bills that affected a specific disease entity (e.g., diabetes), a population (e.g., the elderly), an issue (e.g., drunk driving), or a personal passion. Nurses learned to write letters to congresspersons and to visit them in their offices on occasion.

Organized nursing, especially the American Nurses Association (ANA), realized early that decisions that affected nurses and their patients often were made in Washington, DC. ANA moved its national headquarters to that city in 1992 (Kelly & Joel, 1995) to establish visibility and make a statement about the seriousness of purpose of the organization. ANA created political action committees (PACs) that developed processes for endorsing public officials through statements or with financial contributions to their campaigns. ANA also created a department of governmental affairs that employed full-time registered lobbyists who developed ongoing relationships with elected and appointed officials and their staffs. The development of staff relationships was especially critical as nurses learned that the way to access governmental decision makers was through their staff. By developing credibility with those active in the political process and demonstrating integrity and moral purpose as client advocates, nurses slowly became players in the complex process of policymaking.

The ANA and its state and district levels educated nurses about the political process through continuing education programs, legislation committee structures, and the creation of Senate and congressional district coordinators. The latter were nurses who volunteered to create ongoing relationships with their U.S. senators and representatives to serve as liaisons between legislators and organized nursing. The creation of the Nurses Strategic Action Team (N-STAT) and state nurses association Legislative Liaison programs provided a grassroots network of nurses throughout the country who are informed when immediate action is needed and who respond quickly to their legislative representatives.

Political appointments of nurses were sporadic but strong appointments. Kristine Gebbie, RN, served as the "AIDS Czar" in the 1990s. Sheila Burke, RN, was chief of staff to Senate Majority Leader Bob Dole, and Dr. Mary Wakefield, RN, was chief of staff for Senators Quentin Burdick and Kent Conrad. Carolyne Davis, RN, served as head of the Health Care Financing Administration, the agency responsible for the third-largest federal budget and for shaping Medicare and Medicaid policy. Virginia Trotter Betts, RN, a former president of ANA, was appointed senior health policy advisor of the U.S. Department of Health and Human Services during the Clinton administration. Also during that administration, Dr. Beverly Malone, RN, another former ANA president, served as deputy assistant secretary for Health and Human Services. Dr. Malone went on to become the general secretary of the Royal College of Nursing in England, Scotland, and Northern Ireland. These prestigious and powerful appointments came after many years of involvement in politics and with policymakers.

Nurses learned that by using nursing knowledge and skill they could gain the confidence of government actors. Communications skills that were learned in basic skills classes or in psychiatric nursing classes are critical in listening to the discussion of larger health issues and in being able to present nursing's agenda. Personal stories gained from professional nurses' experience anchor altruistic conversations with legislators and their staffs in an important emotional link toward policy design. Nurses' vast network of clinical experts produces nurses in direct care who provide persuasive, articulate arguments with people "on the Hill" during appropriations committee hearings and informal meetings.

Nurses began to participate in formal, short-term internship programs with elected officials and in bureaucratic agencies. Most of the programs were created by nurses' organizations that were convinced of the importance of political involvement. The interns and fellows learned how to handle constituent concerns, how to write legislation, how to argue with opponents and remain colleagues, and how to maneuver through the bureaucracy. They carried the message of the necessity of the political process to the larger profession, although the rank and file still were not active in this role.

As nurses moved into advanced practice and advanced practice demanded master's degree preparation, the role of the nurse in the **policy process** became clearer. Through the influence of nurses with their legislators, clinical nurse specialists, certified nurse midwives, certified registered nurse anesthetists, and nurse practitioners were named in several pieces of federal legislation as duly authorized providers of health care. The process was slow; however, the deliberate way of including more nurse groups over time demonstrated that to "get a foot in the door" is an effective method of allowing change in the seemingly slow processes of government. Some groups of nurses did not understand the political implications of *incrementalism* (the process of making changes gradually) and wanted all nurse groups named as providers at one time. They did not understand that most legislators do not have any idea what registered nurses do. Those nurse lobbyists who worked directly with legislators and their staff bore the brunt of discontent in the profession and worked diligently and purposefully to provide a unified front on the Hill and to expand the definition of provider at every opportunity. The designation of advanced practice nurses as providers was an entree to federal reimbursement for some nursing services, a major move toward improved client and family access and health care. Advanced practice nurses (APNs) became acutely aware of the critical importance of the role of political activist. Not only did APNs need the basic knowledge, they understood the necessity of practicing the role, developing contacts, working with professional organizations, writing fact sheets, testifying at hearings, and maintaining the momentum to move an idea forward.

However, most nurses still focus their political efforts and skills on the legislative process. They do not have an understanding of the comprehensiveness of the policy process, the much broader process that precedes and follows legislation. For APNs to integrate the policy role into the character of expert nurse, they must recognize the many opportunities for action. APNs cannot afford to "do their own thing," that is, just provide direct patient care. They cannot ignore the political aspects of any issue. Nurses who have fought the battles for recognition as professionals, for acknowledgment of autonomy, and for formal acceptance of clinical expertise worthy of payment for services have enabled APNs today to provide reimbursable, quality services to this nation's residents. The American Association of Colleges of Nursing (American Association of Colleges of Nursing, 1996, 1998) underscored the importance of understanding and becoming involved in policy formation, and the organization and financing of health care for the APN with its documents on essential components of baccalaureate and master's education in nursing.

Finding a Foundation in Theory and Research

As nurses in the middle of the 20th century sought more education in institutions of higher learning, they found few nursing programs at the master's and doctoral levels. However, potential nurse scholars were exposed to an array of disciplines from which they could study. Many of those disciplines enjoyed an academic history and were respected for having a body of knowledge. Education, psychology, anthropology, and sociology were the most common academic fields entered by early nurse scholars, and the nurses soon adapted concepts, models, and theories to nursing practice. The process of teaching and learning, principles of adult education, and styles of leadership were drawn from the field of education. Psychology and sociology lent nursing a rational approach to studying behavior, helped nurses ascribe determinants of social and asocial conduct, and provided nursing with a theoretical foundation in interpersonal therapeutic communications. Through the study of anthropology, nurses learned about the customs and values of people different from themselves, the commonalities of human behavior, and the rigors of conducting field research. Aspects of these disciplines became integrated into nursing education, research, and practice.

Nurses became interested in the idea and applicability of theory and within a generation had begun considering the philosophical foundations and theories of nursing. Early nurse theorists, such as Peplau (1952), Orem (1971), and Henderson (1966), concentrated on organizing clinical practice as a deliberate, reasoned response by the nurse to sick people. This move toward intentional activity based on astute observations and thoughtful connections served nursing well. Nursing became "as much an intellectual activity as a physical endeavor" (Halloran, 1983, p. 17). Nursing theories were extrapolated from systems theory as Rogers (1970) and King (1971) developed and refined their thinking about the discipline. Watson (1979) and Benner (1984), building on humanistic concepts and examining the essence of the profession, furthered the theoretical foundation of nursing as they challenged others to conceptualize and redefine commonly held assumptions and relationships. Leininger (1978) confronted nursing's ethnocentricity and provided theoretical groundwork for cultural care from a global perspective. Nurse scholars in other countries, such as

Grijpdonk in Belgium and Van de Brink Tjebbes in the Netherlands, developed theories that were tested for applicability in their own and other cultures (R. Martijn, personal communication, November 12, 1997). These early nurse theorists, among others, changed the direction of nurses from dependent workers to autonomous thinkers.

The link between nursing research and advanced nursing practice became evident as nurses moved into graduate programs. Master's and doctoral education required research courses, practica, theses, and dissertations. The knowledge and skills that nurses developed served as a foundation for study in a wide array of disciplines and in as many areas of nursing as are available. Although much research was completed, not all of it added to the body of knowledge of clinical nursing. Early studies focused on attitudes and behaviors of nurses and nursing students. Inquiry into theories and models of education, instructional methods, and curriculum development and evaluation contributed to improved presentation of nursing in the academic setting and to the teaching/learning processes practiced by nurses in clinical settings.

Clinical nursing research became a focus area in the 1990s when outcome data were needed to defend nurse decisions. Clinical research cited in nursing journals moved from a few published studies to a wave of clinical trials in a variety of patient care areas. Brooten and Naylor (1995) referred to "nurse dose" (the amount and type of nursing needed to produce an effect of nursing care) as critical in determining outcomes. Blank (1997) named nursing case management as the vehicle through which health care will be restructured as the quality of nursing care is measured through clinical outcomes. Clinical pathways were espoused as a successful way to demonstrate the importance of outcomes to healthcare providers and payers (Porter-O'Grady, 1996; Zander, 1990). Hegyvary (1992) expanded the concept and proposed that patient outcomes reflect the economic, organizational, political, and social context within which they are studied. Far beyond local impact, the influence of nurse experts can never be overestimated for their work with the federal Agency for Health Care Policy and Research (AHCPR) in the development of clinical practice guidelines. As AHCPR evolved into the Agency for Healthcare Research and Quality (AHRQ), health services research took on an important role in further defining what nursing is and the value of nurses.

The initial link between nursing and policy can be viewed as beginning in the 1960s when nurses sought federal funding for research. The explosion of social programs and the raising of social consciousness that occurred in the 1960s and 1970s in the United States alerted nurses to the value of political activity. The professional association provided a structure for the voice of nursing and developed a cadre of nurses who contributed to policy formation and were committed to political activism.

Today's nurses have a much clearer understanding of what constitutes nursing and how nurses must integrate political processes into their practices to further the decisions made by policymakers. Nurses continue to focus on the individual, family, community, and special populations in the provision of care to the sick and infirm and on the activities that surround health promotion and the prevention of disease and disability. Advanced practice nurses have a foundation in expert clinical practice and can translate that knowledge into understandable language for elected and appointed officials as the officials respond to problems that are beyond the scale or impact of individual healthcare providers. As nurses continue to refine the art and science of nursing, forces external to the profession compel the nursing community to consider another aspect—the business of nursing—that is paradoxical to the long history of altruism.

A New Organizational Paradigm

The whole economic basis of capitalism, that is, the manufacturing system, had become rapidly outdated by the beginning of the new millennium. Traditional organizational structures that were invented in the late 19th century to accommodate the move from a farm-and-feudal system to an urban-industrial system no longer fit a new age. Hierarchical, bureaucratic institutions had been the norm, and centralized, top-down administration had been the method of control. Information was the new commodity, and communications systems were needed to create and disseminate the plethora of new material. The computer chip had replaced the printing press and forced a move to a new organizational model (Porter-O'Grady & Wilson, 1995). Efficiency and cost containment led to downsizing and rightsizing, which often were euphemisms for "smallsizing" that translated into firings and layoffs. Machine workers had been replaced by technologists, who were being replaced by "knowledge workers" (Drucker, 1959, p. 40). Knowledge workers required new structures and processes for doing their work.

The new paradigm for organizations in the 21st century begins with changes within one's head; that is, a move to a perspective that is outside the usual way of thinking. What work is done, where it is done, and how it is done are mundane questions that demand creative answers. Large manufacturing plants no longer are needed if merchandise can be made elsewhere and retailers can rely on just-in-time inventories. The very question of what product should be produced requires evaluation. The "where" of work has changed. Offices do not have to exist in a skyscraper because a computer can be located at the beach, in a mountain retreat, or in a kitchen. However, the new worker cannot afford the isolation and detachment noted in the title character of Bartleby, the scrivener (Melville, 1853), who simply "preferred not to" be a part of the group. Drucker (1995) insists that knowledge workers have two new requirements: (1) they work in teams, and (2) if they are not employees, they must be affiliated with an organization. He emphasizes that organizations are important because they provide a continuity that enables the worker to convert specialized knowledge into performance. Drucker (1999) also notes that productivity is an organization's greatest challenge. This is especially true in a company in which thinking and making decisions are the major processes. Systems thinking, a metaparadigmatic approach, is crucial to the effectiveness of an organization in the 21st century (Flood & Senge, 1999).

An organization must have a mission that is publicized and in which all workers (both traditional employees and managers) can invest their energies. Structures and processes should be constructed to facilitate the work of the institution (Wheatley, 1992). Part of the new paradigm is based on the assumption that prior worker and manager practices that evolved from the old bureaucratic model are outdated and must be replaced with collaborative communications that can mobilize and empower all people in the organization (Champy, 1995). People do not expect establishments to remain static or stable; organizations learn new lessons continuously or they fail (Senge, 1990). Peters (1988) addresses the chaotic nature of new companies as being patterned and dynamic, two characteristics of organizations in the new paradigm that provide direction for all levels of workers. Complexity science acknowledges patterns in chaos, complex adaptive systems, and principles of self-organization (Zimmerman, Lindberg, & Plsek, 1998). Peters (1997) also notes that innovative organizations are inhabited by innovative people who seek affiliation with others in new, productive coalitions.

Partnerships are valued over competition, and the old rules of business that rewarded power and ownership have given way to accountability and shared risk. Reengineering the old systems to the new systems does not mean merely automating processes or restructuring the organizational chart. Reengineering involves a radical, cross-functional, futuristic change in the way people think (Porter-O'Grady & Malloch, 2002), a reframing or "discontinuous thinking" (Blancett & Flarey, 1995, p. 16). Long-term planning is replaced by strategic planning, and vertical work relationships are replaced with networks and webs of people and knowledge. All workers at all levels share a commitment to the organization and an accountability to define and produce quality work (Covey, 1991). All workers share responsibility for self-governance, from which both the organization and the worker benefit (Porter-O'Grady, Hawkins, & Parker, 1997). Control is replaced by leadership. The new leader does not use policing techniques of supervision but enables and empowers colleagues through vision, trust, and respect (Bennis & Nanus, 1985; Kouzes & Posner, 1987; Porter-O'Grady & Wilson, 1999). Encouragement, appreciation, and personal recognition are celebrated together in an effective organization (Kouzes & Posner, 1999). Exhibit 1–1 presents a framework for organizations in this millennium.

Exhibit 1–1 Framework for Effective Organizations in the 21st Century

■ Mission: Vision, product/outcome

■ Structure: Network, linkages, distribution of power, risk management

■ Processes: Production, challenge, correction

■ Culture: Communication, technology, access, recognition

Kennedy and Charles (1997) assert that, rather than the "authority" or blind obedience of the industrial establishment, the new leader must return to the origin of the word *author* and serve as coach and mentor by helping others learn. Much as Siddhartha learned that knowledge can be transmitted to others but wisdom must be experienced (Hesse, 1951), the worker of the 21st century needs the knowledge that is passed on from those who have learned over time to experience the wisdom necessary to be competent and fulfilled in the new organization.

The Changing Paradigm in Health Care

The impact of the enormous changes occurring in business and industry in the late 20th century was reflected in the healthcare delivery system. Hospitals faced a dinosaur-like future as a result of several changes. The traditional medical model of a complex hospital system of sick care, a profusion of technology, and ethical questions that could not have been anticipated at the beginning of the century were pointing to a serious need for reform in the healthcare system. The United States was spending 13% of its gross national product on health care, a figure that caused great concern to government officials and economists.

Cost containment began with congressional demand for prospective payment for Medicare recipients through diagnosis-related groups (DRGs). Government-funded Medicare, the largest payer in the country of healthcare services for the elderly, replaced the retrospective method of payment for primarily hospital services (i.e., nursing services) with a system that linked medical diagnoses to length of stay (Fuchs, 1993). Private insurance companies followed the government's lead and reinvented their methods of payment, changing to a prospective system.

Hospital administrators, faced with decreasing income, were forced to contain costs. Nursing care long had been considered by financial personnel as an expenditure, and nurses were not usually thought of as income generators. The actual cost of nursing care was unknown, and few nurses knew how to calculate it or even what factors to consider. Financial analysts and business executives who did not understand the value of quality care became focused on costs and profit. Nursing, a profession that had matured over a few short decades into a confident discipline, found itself confronted with assaults from business decisions that affected the type, setting, scope, and quality of nursing care. How nursing services are produced and calculated, how much nursing care is required for each recipient, and how to decide what mix of service providers is needed became very important questions.

A pecking order, which was especially noticeable in hospitals, had been established in which nurses were subservient to physicians. Rules were valued, and compliance with rules was the measure of success. "Doctors orders" were considered inviolate commands, and nurses' clinical knowledge and judgment were discounted. This arrangement generated physician-nurse games in which communication from nurses was couched in passive, circuitous language. Separation of disciplines occurred as health workers focused on distinct parts of the person's illness or problems. Compartmentalization served a pyramidal system but did not contribute to a holistic approach to providing comprehensive health care.

Nurses were confronted with a system that was changing around them and that sometimes produced subtle changes whose impact was not recognized immediately. Nurse managers found themselves dealing with budgets, variances, and other business-related activities for which they had not been educated. Nurses without appropriate education in management and community health were forced to seek referrals for patients who were being discharged after brief hospitalization and to ensure continuity of care in homes and other healthcare agencies.

Corporate mergers and acquisitions and other organizational arrangements resulted in a tumultuous hospital-cum-healthcare system in which layoffs, staff reductions, and elimination of positions and departments affected nurses in many ways. Nurse administrators encountered executive decisions to downsize when new systems and processes were not yet in place. For example, the position of nurse manager was eliminated in many hospitals in the 1990s with the expectation that staff nurses would assume responsibility and accountability for managerial activities, but the requisite education and training were not provided. Licensed nurses were replaced in many institutions with unlicensed assistive personnel who were given inadequate training in a short time and expected to provide comprehensive care with little supervision to ill patients with complex conditions. Staff nurses worried that patient and nurse safety were jeopardized.

The Pew Health Professions Commission (1995) studied the training and practice of healthcare professionals and recommended revolutionary changes in how the professions are regulated and educated.

From interdisciplinary and multidisciplinary courses and programs to single professional licensure, the recommendations focused on preparing nurses, physicians, dentists, pharmacists, and other healthcare professionals for practice within the new healthcare paradigm. The Pew Commission encouraged cross training for multiskilled allied health workers. Nurses understood early that the new definition of *interdisciplinary* means nursing, allied health, medicine, and other health professions. On the other hand, many physicians think *interdisciplinary* means specialists in orthopedics, cardiology, radiology, and pulmonology who work together, and allied health professionals believe the term means collaboration among occupational therapists, physical therapists, and physician's assistants. There still is work to be done to convince all healthcare providers of the value of an interdisciplinary team for the patient and the provider.

Nurses who weathered drastic organizational changes were seldom acknowledged as having to face problems. Noer (1993) was one of the few authors who wrote about the guilt and depression felt by those who did not lose their jobs but were expected to carry on in sometimes deprived circumstances. Nurses took the lead in efforts to redesign nursing systems by proposing systems that replaced the industrial-age concept of responsibility that bred paternalism with accountability, in which empowerment, partnerships, and leadership are fostered (Porter-O'Grady & Wilson, 1995). Reengineering the workplace for nurses demanded a transformation to professional practice (Blancett & Flarey, 1995). Some healthcare systems did not integrate information technology into the new order, resulting in restructured old systems rather than new paradigms of health care, according to nursing informatics expert Roy Simpson (personal communication, June 6, 1998).

Health care in the 20th century was delivered most often through hospitals, although there was a major move to the community in the last decades (Aiken, 1990). In the 1990s, new systems of nurse empowerment were created by visionary nurse leaders such as Blancett and Flarey (1995), Porter-O'Grady and Wilson (1995), and Wolf, Boland, and Aukerman (1994a, 1994b). Nursing responses to external forces of managed care centered on a system of case management in which the nurse, preferably an advanced practice nurse, brokered and coordinated care for clients before, during, and after hospitalization (Ethridge & Lamb, 1989; Genna, 1987; Maurin, 1990; Mundinger, 1984; Zander, Etheredge, & Bower, 1987). Models of case management were created for many organizational structures, acute care facilities, hospices, and community health enterprises (Bower, 1992). As case managers, APNs took the lead in including members of other disciplines in decisions about the health care of clients, families, and communities.

Early in the 21st century, hospitals were investing in corporate partnerships with other health care and business organizations. Many mergers and acquisitions resulted in staff cuts, and nurses and other healthcare professionals (e.g., pharmacists, physicians, physical therapists) were forced to rethink the way in which care was provided. Collaboration became a necessity, and whole departments began to build coalitions with each other to reduce complexity and improve communication. Healthcare report cards provided mixed response as to their utility in making informed choices about hospitals and physicians (Dranove, Kessler, McClellan, & Satterthwaite, 2003). After the 1999 Institute of Medicine report (Koln, Corrigan, & Donaldon, 1999) noted the large number of medical errors in hospitals, more than 90 major industries formed the Leapfrog Group (Milstead, 2003) that recommended urban hospitals adopt computerized physician order entry, evidence-based hospital referrals, and the use of intensivists. Evidence-based nursing practice developed at the same time and provided credibility for nursing interventions.

Venegoni (1996) identifies five significant factors that influenced the changes in healthcare systems for the 21st century: (1) place (site of delivery); (2) people (who receives care); (3) preventive model (reward for health, not sickness); (4) paradigm (quality improvement and customer satisfaction); and (5) process (modern technology). The comparison of the old hospital paradigm and the emerging model, as shown in Exhibit 1–2, illustrates a practical expression of Venegoni's factors.

Nurses were taking on new positions in all types of healthcare systems and had become sophisticated providers of care. Beyond that, nurses were beginning to integrate the roles of educator, researcher, administrator, and political activist. As client advocates, nurses speak out on issues of prevention of illness and disability, safety and environmental hazards, and informed consent. Nurses have come to realize the critical nature of involvement with legislators who make policies such as laws, regulations, and programs that affect nurses, patients, and the healthcare system. A more comprehensive understanding of the societal mandate for nursing services requires that nurses assume an active part of a complex system of sociocultural, economic, and political forces. Nurses, especially those in advanced practice, are expanding the scope of nursing in direct care by addressing healthcare issues that are a matter of public interest. Decisions that affect the public interest are made over time in the policy arena.

What Is Public Policy?

In this chapter, policy is an overarching term used to define both an entity and a process. Although there has not been a clear definition of policy in the nursing literature (Rodgers, 1989), scholars in political science have developed definitions and models from which nursing

Exhibit 1–2 Comparison of Old Healthcare Paradigm with New Paradigm

Old Paradigm	New Healthcare Paradigm
Hospital based, acute care	Short-term hospital: same-day surgery, 23-hour stays; prehospital testing and precertification; tele-health/telemedicine; home health; mobile vans; school and mall clinics
Specialty units	Cross-training (multiskilled workers): LDRP, OR/PACU, CCU/telemetry
Hierarchical management	Decentralization (unit budget, scheduling, variance); shared governance; strategic plan
Physician as captain of ship; others are followers	Inter/multidisciplinary team, collaboration; case management (registered nurse/broker)
Nurse as employee; job focused, "refrigerator nurse"	Nurse as professional: career-focused clinical ladder; continuing credentials; tuition reimbursement, paid certification exam
Medical condition; focus on segment	Holistic person in family/community; pastoral care, parish nurse
"Sick" care; focus on cure	Health care, health promotion, prevention programs; focus on cure, care, and continuity of care; complementary health alternatives
Cost containment; focus on billing	Focus on patient and accountability of caregivers/agency; electronic patient record, patient/continuous quality improvement, care maps
Written medical record	Integrated electronic records: smart card, bedside computers
Fee-for-service	Managed competition (HMO, PPO, IPA)
Physician as employer	Physician as employee; capitation system
One insurance plan	Variety of insurance options ("covered lives"): basic plan, dental, eye, long-term care, cancer, disability
80% to 100%	Greater deductible, lower percentage coverage, or copayment insurance

can benefit. The purpose of **public policy** is to direct problems to government and secure government's response (Jones, 1984). Although there has been much discussion about the boundaries and domain of government and the extent of difference between the public and private sectors, that debate is beyond the scope of this chapter.

The definition of public policy is important because it clarifies common misconceptions about what constitutes policy. In this book, the terms public policy and policy are interchangeable. The process of creating policy can be focused in many arenas and most of these are interwoven. For example, environmental policy deals with health issues such as hazardous material, particulate matter in the air or water, and safety standards in the workplace. Education policy, more than tangentially, is related to health— just ask school nurses. Regulations define who can administer medication to students; state laws dictate what type of sex education can be taught. Defense policy definitely is related to health policy when developing, investigating, or testing biological and chemical warfare. Health policy directly addresses health problems and is the specific focus of this book.

Policy as an Entity

As an entity, policy is seen in many forms as the "standing decisions" of an organization (Eulau & Prewitt, 1973, p. 495). As formal documented directives of an organization, official government policies reflect the beliefs of the administration in power and provide direction for the philosophy and mission of government organizations. Specific policies usually serve as the "shoulds" and "thou shalts" of agencies. Some policies, known as position statements, report the opinions of organizations about issues that members believe are important. For example, state boards of nursing (government agencies created by legislatures to protect the public through the regulation of nursing practice) publish advisory opinions on what constitutes competent and safe nursing practice.

The term policy is used often to refer to goals, programs, and proposals. Although such substitution may be confusing in conceptualizing policy, the term may be seen as a type of verbal shorthand for colleagues who are discussing a specific program or program goal. For example, nurses who talk about the gag-rule policy of the Reagan administration understand that they are discussing programs, such as Title X of the Medicare program related to family planning that forbade health professionals from discussing abortion as an option to clients in agencies that received federal funding. A similar gag rule occurred in the 1990s when many health maintenance organizations forbade physicians to discuss treatment options with patients.

Agency policies can be broad and general, such as those that describe the relationship of an agency to other governmental groups. In the most narrow sense, policies can be specific announcements, such as operational procedures. Procedure manuals in government hospitals that detail steps in performing certain nursing tasks are examples of specific policy activities. Both general and specific policies serve as guidelines for employee behavior within an institution. Although policies and procedures often are used interchangeably, policies usually are considered more broad.

Laws are types of policy entities. As legal directives for public and private behavior, laws serve to define action that reflects the will of society—or at least a segment of society. Laws are made at the international, federal, state, and local levels and have the impact of primary place in guiding conduct. Lawmaking usually is the purview of the legislative branch of government in the United States, although presidential vetoes, executive orders, and judicial interpretations of laws have the force of law.

Judicial interpretation is noted in three ways. First, courts may interpret the meaning of laws that are written broadly or with some vagueness. Laws often are written deliberately with language that addresses broad situations. Agencies that implement the laws then write regulations that are more specific and that guide the implementation. However, courts may be asked to determine questions in which the law is unclear or controversial (Williams & Torrens, 1988). For example, the 1973 Rehabilitation Act prohibited discrimination against the handicapped by any program that received federal assistance. Although this may have seemed fair and reasonable at the outset, courts were asked to adjudicate questions of how much accommodation is "fair" (Wilson, 1989). Second, courts can determine how some laws are applied. Courts are idealized as being above the political activity that surrounds the legislature. Courts also are considered beyond the influence of politically active interest groups. The court system, especially the federal court system, has been called upon to resolve conflicts between levels of government (state and federal) and between laws enacted by the legislature and interpretation by powerful interest groups. For example, courts may determine who is eligible or who is excluded from participation in a program. In this way, special interest groups that sue to be included in a program can receive "durable protection" from favorable court decisions (Feldstein, 1988, p. 32). Third, courts can declare the laws made by Congress or the states unconstitutional, thereby nullifying the statues entirely (Litman & Robins, 1991). Courts also interpret the Constitution, sometimes by restricting what the government (not private enterprise) may do (Wilson).

Regulations are another type of policy initiative. Although they often are included in discussions of laws, regulations are different. Once a law is enacted by the legislative branch, the executive branch of government is charged with administrative responsibility for implementing the law. The executive branch consists of the president and all of the bureaucratic agencies, commissions, and departments that carry out the work for the public benefit. Agencies in the government formulate regulations that achieve the intent of the statute. On the whole, laws are written in general terms, and regulations are written more specifically to guide the interpretation, administration, and enforcement of the law. The Administrative Procedures Act (APA) was created to provide opportunity for citizen review and input throughout the process of developing regulations. The APA ensures a structure and process that is published and open, in the spirit of the founding fathers, so that the average constituent can participate in the process of public decision making.

All of these entities evolve over time and are accomplished through the efforts of a variety of actors or players. Although commonly used, the terms *position statement, resolution, goal, objective, program, procedure, law,* and *regulation* really are not interchangeable with the word *policy.* Rather, they are the formal expressions of policy decisions. For the purposes of understanding just what policy is, nurses must grasp policy as a process.

Policy as a Process

In viewing policy as a guide to government action, nurses can study the process of policymaking over time. Milio (1989) presents four major stages in which decisions are made that translate to government policies: (1) agenda setting, (2) legislation and regulation, (3) implementation, and (4) evaluation. Agenda setting is concerned with identifying a societal problem and bringing it to the attention of government. Legislation and regulation are formal responses to a problem. Implementation is the execution of policies or programs toward the achievement of goals. Evaluation is the appraisal of policy performance or program outcomes.

In each stage, formal and informal relationships are developed among actors both within and outside of government. Actors can be individuals, such as a legislator, a bureaucrat, or a citizen. Actors also can be institutions, such as the presidency, the courts, political parties, or special-interest groups. A series of activities occurs that brings a problem to government, which results in direct action by the government to address the problem. Governmental responses are political; that is, the decisions about who gets what, when, and how are made within a framework of power and influence, negotiation, and bargaining (Lasswell, 1958).

Even as this book explains each of the stages of the policy process and explores them for areas in which nurses can provide influence, one must recognize that the policy process is not necessarily sequential or logical. The definition of a problem, which usually occurs in the agenda-setting phase, may change during legislation. Program design may be altered significantly during implementation. Evaluation of a policy or program (often considered the last phase of the process) may propel onto the national agenda (often considered the first phase of the process) a problem that differs from the original. However, for the purpose of organizing one's thoughts and conceptualizing the policy process, the policy process is examined from the linear perspective of stages.

Even before the process itself can be studied, nurses must understand why it is so important to be knowledgeable about the components and the functions of the process and how this public arena has become an integral part of the practice of advanced nursing.

Why Nurses and Public Policy?

Registered professional nurses have studied the basics of how a bill becomes a law in their baccalaureate programs. An extension of the focus on legislation usually is provided in graduate schools. However, most nurses (and most nurse educators) do not have a clear understanding of the total policy process. To focus on legislation misses a whole range of governmental and political activities—activities in which professional nurses should have a central place.

In the 1990s, the healthcare delivery system was the subject of a major thrust of reform. Reform is a political process in which priorities are determined and public policy decisions are made. Nurses, as the largest group of healthcare professionals in the country and as the providers of the most direct and continuous care to individuals and groups, were "at the table." That is, nursing was included in the short list of groups convened by a presidential mandate that were instrumental in assisting the government in the mid-1990s to make changes that would directly affect the health of citizens and the legal purview of the healthcare professions. The nursing presence was a direct result of the many years of leadership exerted by a few nurses (mostly through the professional association) who have understood the importance and have worked tirelessly to develop relationships, to suggest problems and alternative solutions, and to demonstrate willingness to compromise in the present to secure greater gain in the future. Although the federally directed process of reform did not result in substantial change, all of the issues that nursing brought to the discussion were still being addressed after legislation failed. These issues, such as universal access to health care, a basic services package, an emphasis on health promotion and disease prevention, catastrophic coverage for long-term care, and an initial emphasis on at-risk populations such as women and children (ANA, 1994), fell to the states for discussion.

Nurses and nursing are at the center of issues of tremendous and long-lasting impact, such as access to providers, quality of care, and reasonable cost. In addition, issues crucial to the profession are being decided, such as who is eligible for government reimbursement for services and what is the appropriate scope of practice of registered nurses in advanced practice. If nurses wait until legislation is being voted on before they become involved, it is too late to affect decisions.

Nurses have learned the legislative process. Nurses have written letters and made visits to their legislators. Now nurses must move forward and apply the knowledge of the whole policy process by speaking out to a variety of appropriate governmental actors and institutions so that nursing can move issues onto the national agenda, lobby Congress with alternatives, and provide nursing expertise as policies and programs are being designed. In addition, nurses must be the watchdogs as programs are implemented so that target groups are served and services are appropriate. Nurses should be experts at program evaluation and continuing feedback to ensure that old problems are being addressed, new problems are being identified, and appropriate solutions are being considered.

The opportunities for nursing input throughout the policy process are unlimited and certainly not confined narrowly to the legislative process. Nurses are articulate experts who can address both the rational shaping of policy and the emotional aspects of the process. Nurses cannot afford to limit their actions to monitoring bills; they must seize the initiative and use their considerable collective and individual influence to ensure the health, welfare, and protection of the public and healthcare professionals.

An Overview of the Policy Process

Most of the chapters in this book address specific components of the policy process in depth and from a theoretical perspective. However, at the outset, advanced practice nurses should have an overview of the total process so that they do not get stuck on legislation. Many useful articles and books have been written about policy in general and even about specific policies, but few have addressed the scope of the policy process or defined the components. The elements of agenda setting (including problem definition), government response (legislation, regulation, or programs), and policy and program implementation and evaluation are distinct entities but are connected as parts of a whole tapestry in the process of public decision making.

Agenda Setting

Getting a healthcare problem to the attention of government can be a tremendous first step in getting relief. The actual mechanism of defining a healthcare problem is a major political issue in which APNs can participate, especially in a collective manner as an interest group. Problem definition often is influenced by special-interest groups. When acquired immune deficiency syndrome (AIDS) was first diagnosed in the 1980s, the disease was perceived as a problem of homosexuals and intravenous drug users. Within this definition, assumptions were made by government officials that the disease might be confined to a small population. Federal health agencies were not likely to obtain a large budget for a disease that affected small groups, especially those considered outside the mainstream of American values. Gay rights activist organizations such as the Gay Men's Health Crisis (GMHC) and AIDS Coalition to Unleash Power (ACTUP) were special-interest groups that were instrumental in persuading the government to alter the definition of the AIDS problem by broadening it to include persons other than homosexuals. As AIDS became known in hemophiliacs, infants, and heterosexual men, the problem became redefined as a community health problem. From this perspective, AIDS was perceived as having an impact on a larger segment of the population, including mainstream Americans. Government officials in the administrative and legislative branches were pressured to assume responsibility for addressing an epidemic. Officials were able to identify a variety of departments and agencies beyond the traditional health and human services, such as the Department of Defense and the Bureau of Indian Affairs, that could seek funding for programs of research and treatment. Defining the problem differently increased access to the national agenda.

APNs must come to understand the concepts of windows of opportunity, policy entrepreneurs, and political elites. "Sound bites" and "word bites" are tools that were introduced by people who were invested in getting the AIDS crisis onto the national agenda (Milstead, 1993). Gay rights groups used radical political action tactics borrowed from the civil rights movement of the 1960s and 1970s to get their message heard by those in Washington, DC. Activists conducted sit-ins and marches, testified at hearings, ridiculed weak efforts to provide research and treatment, and held press conferences. During the press conferences, self-taught activists learned that although a person may be recorded by microphone or video camera during a speech, only a few seconds would be broadcast on the news. Activists prepared written scripts of selected material from their interviews in advance of the interviews and presented the scripts to the media people. This allowed the speakers to talk at length about their issues and yet focus the media replay to ensure that a specific message was promoted.

Government Response

The government response to public problems often emanates from the legislative branch and comes in three forms: (1) laws, (2) rules and regulations, and (3) programs. Because only senators and representatives can introduce legislation (not even the president can bring a bill to the floor of either house), these elected officials command respect and attention. The work of legislation is not clear cut or linear. Informal communication and influence are the coin of the realm when trying to construct a program or law from the often vague wishes of disparate groups. The committee structure of both houses is a powerful method of accomplishing the work of government. Conference committees are known as the "Third House of Congress" (*How our laws*, 1990) because of their power to force compromise and bring about new legislation. APNs must appreciate the difference between the authorization and appropriations processes and seek influence in both arenas. Becoming involved directly with legislators and their staffs has been a training ground for many APNs. Supporting or opposing passage of a bill often has served as the first contact with the political process for many nurses. However, this place often has been the stopping point for many nurses because they were unaware of other avenues of involvement, such as the follow-up process of regulations and rulemaking.

Lowi (1969) notes that administrative rulemaking often takes place as an effort to bring about order in environments that are unstable and full of conflict. Some regulations codify precedent; others break new ground and address issues not previously explicated. An example of the latter is the Federal Trade Commission's (FTC) Trade Regulation Rules. In 1964, the FTC, whose mission is to protect the consumer and enforce antitrust legislation, wrote regulations requiring health warnings on cigarette packages. The tobacco industry reacted so fiercely that Congress quickly passed a law that nullified the regulations and replaced them with less stringent ones (West, 1982). Other ways to sanction agencies whose rules are viewed as too restrictive are to reduce budget allocations and increase the number of adjudications or trial-like reviews. Advanced practice nurses must become knowledgeable about the regulatory process so that they can spot opportunities to contribute or intervene prior to final rulemaking (The regulatory process, 1992).

Programs are concrete manifestations of solutions to problems. Program design often is a joint effort of legislative intent, budgetary expediency, and political feasibility [the latter meaning "an interest group arrangement hammered out in Congress" (Skocpol, 1995, p. 283)]. There are many opportunities for nurses in advanced practice to become involved in the design phase of a program. Selecting an agency to administer the program, choosing the goals, and selecting the tools that will ensure eligibility and participation are all decisions in which the APN should collaborate.

Policy and Program Implementation

It is important that APNs keep reminding their colleagues that the phases of the policy process are not linear and that policy activities are fluid and move within and among the phases in dynamic processes. The implementation phase includes those activities in which legislative mandates are carried out, most often through programmatic means. The implementation stage also includes a planning ingredient. Problems occur in program planning if technological expertise is not available. This is particularly important to nurses, who are experts in the delivery of health care in the broadest sense.

If government officials do not know qualified, appropriate experts, decisions about program planning and design often are determined by legislators, bureaucrats, or staff who know little or nothing about the problem or the solutions. As excellent problem solvers, APNs have many opportunities to offer ideas and solutions. One strategy is to employ second-order change to reframe situations and recommend pragmatic alternatives to implementers (de Chesnay, 1983; Watzlawick, Weakland, & Fisch, 1974). Bowen (1982) uses probability theory to demonstrate how program success could be improved. She suggests putting several clearance points (instances where major decisions are made) together so that they could be negotiated as a package deal. She also advocates beginning the bargaining process with alternatives that have the greatest chance for success and using that success as a foundation for building more successes, a strategy she refers to as a "bandwagon approach" (p. 10). In the past, nurses have done the opposite: focused on failure and perceived lack of nursing power. APNs have begun to note successes in the political arena and are building a new level of success and esteem. The nurse in advanced practice today uses the strategies of packaging, success begets success, and persistence in a deliberate way so that nurses can increase their effective impact in the implementation of social programs.

Although nurses most often work toward positive impact, they have found that opposition to an unsound program can have a paradoxical positive effect. Although not in the public arena, an example of phenomenal success in the judicious use of opposition occurred when the professional body of nursing rose up as one against the American Medical Association's 1986 proposal to create a new type of low-level healthcare worker called a registered care technician. The power emerged as more than 40 nursing organizations stood together in opposition to an ill-conceived proposal that would have placed patients in jeopardy and created dead-end jobs.

Policy and Program Evaluation

For nurses who have worked in the nursing process of clinical reasoning (Pesut & Herman, 1999), the process of evaluation seems to be a logical component of the policy process. Evaluation is the systematic application of methods of social research to public policies and programs. Evaluation is conducted "to benefit the human condition to improve profit, to amass influence and power, or to achieve other goals" (Rossi & Freeman, 1995, p. 6). Evaluation research is a powerful tool for defending viable programs, for altering structures and processes to strengthen programs, and for providing rationale for program failure. Goggin, Bowman, Lester, & O'Toole (1990) propose that researchers investigate program implementation within an analytical framework rather than a descriptive one. They argue that a "third generation" of research established within a sound theory would strengthen the body of knowledge of the policy process. APNs can contribute to both the theory and the method of evaluation.

Evaluation must be started early and continued throughout a program. An unconscionable example of a program that should have been stopped even before it was begun is the Tuskegee "experiment." From 1932 to 1972, a group of African Americans was used as a control group and denied antibiotic treatment for syphilis even after treatment was known to be successful (Thomas & Quinn, 1991). Beyond evaluation research, this study clearly points out the moral and ethical concerns that are mandated when researchers work with human beings. Should a study or program be started at all? At what point should it be stopped? What is involved in "informed consent"? If a program involves experimental therapy, what are the methods for presenting subjects with relevant data so that participation preferences are clear (Bell, Raiffa, & Tversky, 1988)? These kinds of questions should be considered automatically by today's researchers, but it is the responsibility of APNs as consumer agents to ask the questions if they have not been asked or if there is any doubt about the answers.

A Bright Future

The multiple roles of the APN—provider of direct care, researcher, consultant, educator, administrator, consumer advocate, and political activist—reflect the changing and expanding character of the professional nurse. Today is the future; nursing action today sets the direction for what health care becomes for projected generations. As true professionals with a societal mandate and a comprehensive body of knowledge, nurses function as visionaries who are grounded in education, research, and experience. APNs serve as the link between human responses to actual and potential health problems and the solutions that may be addressed in the government arena.

Full integration of the policy process becomes evident when professional nurses discern early the social implications of health problems, seize the opportunity to inform public officials with whom the nurses have credible relationships, provide objective data and subjective personal stories that help translate big problems down to a level of understanding, propose alternative solutions that acknowledge reality, and participate in the evaluation process to determine the effectiveness and efficiency of the outcomes.

Educating Our Political Selves

Nurses in advanced practice should be expert in the knowledge and skills of political activity. Basic content in undergraduate nursing programs must be reexamined in light of the needs of the profession. Educators must do more than plant the seeds of interest and excitement in baccalaureate students. Educators must model activism by talking about the bills they are supporting or opposing, by organizing students to assist in election campaigns, and by demanding not only that students write letters to officials but that they mail them and provide follow-up.

Educators can develop games in which students maneuver through a virtual bureaucracy to move a health problem onto the agenda. Brainstorming techniques can lead students to discover innovative alternative solutions. Baccalaureate students can analyze policy tools to discover how and when to use them. Teachers of research methods and processes can use political scenarios to point out how to phrase clinical questions so that legislators will pay attention. Program effectiveness can be studied in research and clinical courses. The theoretical components taught in class and followed by practical application through participation in political and legislative committees in professional organizations must serve as "basic training" for the registered nurse.

Graduate education must demand demonstrated knowledge and application of more extensive and sophisticated political processes. Nursing must increase the total of those with master's degrees and doctoral degrees beyond 9.6% and 0.6%, respectively, of nearly 2.9 million registered nurses (ANA, 2007; Spratley, Johnson, Sochalski, Fritz, & Spencer, 2000). All graduate program faculty should serve as models for political activism. The atmosphere in master's and doctoral programs should heighten the awareness of students who are potential leaders.

Faculty can motivate students by displaying posters that announce political events and by including students in discussions of nursing issues framed in a policy context. Students who spot educators at rallies and other political and policy occasions are learning by example. Faculty should advertise their experiences as delegates to political and professional conventions. A few faculty can serve as mentors for students who need to move from informal to sustained, formal contact with policymakers and who have a policy track in their career trajectories. Both faculty and students should consider actual experience in government offices as a means of learning the nitty-gritty of how government functions and of demonstrating their own leadership capabilities. The Nurses' Directory of Capitol Connections (Bull, Sharp, & Wakefield, 2000) is an excellent resource for identifying a wide range of opportunities for participation of nurses who work in the policy arena.

If students hesitate and seem passive about involvement, educators must help these nurses determine where their passions are. This may help students focus on where they might start. Often the novice can be enticed by centering on a clinical problem.

Identifying Problems

Advanced practice nurses, by definition, are "professional nurses who have successfully completed a graduate program in nursing or a related area that provides specialized knowledge and skills that form the foundation for expanded roles in health care" (American Nurses Association [ANA] House of Delegates, 1993, p. 5). According to this denotation, APNs function in the provision of direct clinical care; as educators, administrators, and researchers; in consultative and counseling roles; and with a variety of titles. Within this broad interpretation, APNs have the capacity and opportunity to identify and frame problems from multiple sources.

Clinical Problems

The choice of a clinical problem on which to focus one's energy is a major decision. A nurse may be working in a specialized area and may see a need for more research or alternatives to treatment. For example, those who work with patients and families with breast cancer already may have a passion for issues critical to this area. Other current topics receiving attention include diabetes, obesity, AIDS, early detection and treatment of prostate cancer, child and parent abuse, cardiac problems in women, and empowering caregivers (Hash & Cramer, 2003; Pierce & Steiner, 2003).

Professional problems that are especially critical to nurses in advanced practice include reducing barriers that prevent practice autonomy and reimbursement for nursing services. Workplace issues include advocacy for workplace safety and management strategies for training and redeploying nurses as work sites change. Related social problems that affect nurses include the increase of street violence and bioterrorism.

A plethora of problems and "irritations" can arouse the passion of a nurse in advanced practice.

Funding for Education

Preparing nurses at the graduate level, either with master's or doctoral degrees, has been a problem on several levels. The first concern was with a cyclical shortage of nurses, especially during wartime when nurses left hospital employment and entered the armed forces. The Social Security Act of 1935 and, a decade later, the National Mental Health Act of 1946 provided some federal funding for graduate education and research (Lash, 1986).

By the 1950s, nurses were seeking graduate degrees, but there were not enough programs in nursing. Part of the problem was that not enough nurses held doctoral degrees and could teach in graduate programs (Aiken, 1986). Organized nursing knew that federal legislators had initiated a GI bill that provided money to attend college for those who served in World War II. Nursing advocates convinced legislators that nurses were a scarce national resource, and funds were appropriated for nursing education through the Nurse Training Acts (NTAs) that began in 1943. Funding encouraged the initiation of new graduate nursing education programs, such as nurse-practitioner and clinical nurse specialist programs. By 1966, an amendment created grants for students, and the 1972 bill awarded capitation grants to nursing education programs to expand enrollment and increase graduations. With the infusion of federal dollars, the quantity and quality of educators and education improved (Kelly & Joel, 1995, p. 399).

Nursing education as a functional area lost ground with the expansion of technology, the explosion of knowledge, and the increase in clinical master's degrees that began in the 1990s. Nursing's heritage of experienced teachers (education majors were acceptable routes for women/nurses who pursued higher education in the first half of the 20th century) was supplanted with clinically competent APNs who often were not schooled in principles of teaching and learning. Funding for nurses who sought baccalaureate and master's degrees focused on clinical nursing. Although this was appropriate to accommodate new knowledge about genetics, immunology, pharmacology, ethics, and other important content, teaching was slowly squeezed out.

In the first decade of the 21st century, academic institutions face not only a shortage of faculty, but a shortage of faculty who have backgrounds in the principles of education. A few colleges and universities have begun doctoral programs with a focus on teaching, and many master's programs offer an education track. Funding for scholarships and loans in the early 2000s reflects a beginning recognition of the need for adequately prepared nurse-teachers.

Support for Nursing Administration

The only area in which federal funding was not provided directly was in nursing administration. Even though NTA criteria for student qualifications clearly eliminated those studying nursing administration by denying their eligibility, potential leaders in that specialty became very important as managed care schemes replaced traditional fee-for-service arrangements. Nurses' need for knowledge about budgets, organizations, change theory, human resource strategies, and other formerly tangential material became critical in the 1990s. Federal money for education in that area had not been a priority, and nurse administrators have had to shoulder the burden of their education alone with the hope of executive and entrepreneurial opportunities through which they could recoup some of their financial investment. Federal nurse traineeships did change the eligibility in the late 1990s to include nurses with administration majors, but the funding competed with that for clinical scholarships.

Investment in Nursing Research

From early nurse scientist programs that encouraged research training in physical and behavioral science programs to later grants that allowed nursing education programs to develop researchers in nursing, federal funds have provided the impetus for scientific inquiry into nursing concerns. Pre- and postdoctoral fellowships for nurse scientists and new investigator awards fostered research activity and the education of future researchers. Faculty development grants and research conferences made it possible to study and disseminate findings. The creation of the National Center for Nursing Research and its later elevation to the National Institute of Nursing Research (NINR) were outgrowths of struggles in the profession and between nursing and federal officials in efforts to secure funding for nursing research, especially clinical research (Brown, 1986). Although funding increased slowly over the years, NINR remains the lowest-funded institute of National Institutes of Health (NIH).

Government responds to social problems that either are too big for the private sector or are particular to the mission of government. The leadership role of government has been pictured by Osborne (1992) as "steering" rather than "rowing" in the 1800s with the provision of land grants for colleges and in the 1990s with funding for advanced practice nurses. Nurses must steer the course as healthcare experts by staying involved in the political process and influencing health policy. All registered nurses, especially those in advanced practice, have an extraordinary investment in the new structures and processes that will continue to be negotiated to provide health care to the citizens and residents of the United States.

Expanding the Framework

Nurses were central players in early discussions of a new healthcare delivery system (Backer, Costello-Nikitas, & Mason, 1993). The 1990s **nursing agenda for healthcare reform** was a timely and fresh approach that rejected the traditional medical model and instead focused on the consumer as well as the provider. Nurse practitioners, clinical nurse specialists, and those in the new paradigm of the blended role in advanced practice spoke out as agents of patients and families to ensure that critical elements that affect healthcare cost, quality, and access are incorporated into current and future organizational arrangements for the delivery of care. Nurses and nursing were a strong political force in discussions of what healthcare delivery should be.

Practice the Rules of Debate

Nurses absolutely must "get their act together" and work toward a unified voice on issues that affect the public health and the nursing profession. Whatever their differences in the past—anger from entry-into-practice arguments that have dragged on for over half a century; disparagement and animosity among those with varied levels of education; cerebral and pragmatic concerns about gaps between education and practice, practice and administration, or administration and education—nurses must put these kinds of divisive, emotional issues behind them if they expect to be taken seriously as professionals by elected and appointed public officials and policymakers.

Nurses cannot afford to stop arguing critical issues internally, but they must learn how to argue heatedly among themselves—and then go to lunch together. Nurses can learn lessons from television shows such as The O'Reilly Factor and The McLaughlin Group about how to challenge, contest, dispute, contend, and debate issues passionately and then shake hands and respect the opponent's position. Passionate issues must not polarize the profession any longer and, more important, must not stand in the way of a unified voice to the public.

Strengthen Organized Nursing

The most productive and efficient way to act together is through a strong professional organization. As organizations in general have restructured and reengineered for more efficient operation, so will the professional associations. APNs have a knowledge base that includes an understanding of how organizations develop and change. This theoretical knowledge must serve as a foundation for leadership in directing new organizational structures that are responsive to members and other important bodies. National leaders must talk with state and local leaders as new configurations are conceived. States must confer among themselves to share innovations and knowledge about what works and what does not.

The Nursing Organizations Alliance (Saver, 2003), composed of the presidents and executive directors of more than 50 major nursing organizations, held an inaugural meeting in 2003. The alliance is a loose collection of groups that provides a forum to discuss and debate issues important to a wide range of perspectives. Time will tell how effective this organization will be in serving as an internal medium for airing differences and coming to consensus.

Issues such as the role of collective bargaining units within the total organizational structure, the position of individual membership vis-à-vis state membership, the political role of a specialized interest group (nurses) in creating public policy, and the issue of international influence in nursing and health care require wisdom and leadership that APNs must exert as the American Nurses Association addresses its place as a major voice of this country's nurses. One united voice is necessary to carry nursing's messages to the public. For example, the ANA, American Association of Colleges of Nursing, and the American Organization of Nurse Executives took a single message to Congress to increase funding for NINR and to authorize and appropriate funding for the Nurse Reinvestment Act (to create scholarships for students and faculty).

Issues inherent in multistate licensure are being debated today, and the outcome will reflect the extent to which nurses will use concepts of telehealth in their practices. Because APNs already are eligible for Medicare reimbursement for telehealth services that are provided in specified rural areas (Burtt, 1997), these nurses are rich resources and must be included in reasoned discussions on this issue. State boards of nursing in every state and jurisdiction face issues of appropriate methods of recognizing advanced nursing practice, the role of the government agency in regulating nursing and other professions, and the analysis of educationally sound and legally defensible examinations for candidates.

Nurses who have been reluctant to become "political" cannot afford to ignore their obligations any longer. Each nurse counts, and, collectively, nursing is a major actor in the effort to ensure the country's healthy future. Nurses have expanded their conception of what nursing is and how it is practiced to include active political participation. A nurse must choose the governmental level on which to focus: federal, regional, state, or local. The process is similar at each level: Identify the problem and become part of the solution.

Advanced practice nurses understand the scope of service delivery, continuity of care, appropriate mix of caregivers, and the expertise that can be provided by multidisciplinary teams. By being at the forefront of understanding, nurses have a moral and ethical mandate to lead the public-policy process. Dynamic political action is as much a part of the advanced practice of nursing as is expert direct care.

Work with the Political System

By now, many APNs have developed contacts with legislators and have appointed officials and their staffs. A new group that holds great potential for nurse interaction is the Congressional Nursing Caucus in the U.S. House of Representatives, begun in 2003 by Representatives Lois Capps (D-CA) and Ed Whitfield (R-KY). This bipartisan group assembles to educate Congress on all aspects of nursing—education, practice, research, leadership. Members hold briefings on the nurse shortage, patient and nurse safety issues, preparedness for bioterrorism, and other relevant and pertinent issues and concerns. The caucus will serve as a "clearinghouse for information and a sounding board for ideas brought forth by the nursing community" (American Nurses Association, 2003, p. 1).

APNs must stay alert to issues and be assertive in bringing problems to the attention of policymakers. It is important to bring success stories to legislators and officials—they need to hear what good nurses do and how well they practice. Sharing positive information will keep the image of nurses in an affirmative and constructive picture. Legislators must run for office (and U.S. Representatives do this every 2 years), so media coverage with an APN who is pursuing noteworthy accomplishments is usually welcomed eagerly.

Conclusion

Nurses in advanced practice must have expert knowledge and skill in change, conflict resolution, assertiveness, communication, negotiation, and group process to function appropriately in the policy arena. Professional autonomy and collaborative interdependence are possible within a political system in which consumers can choose access to quality health care that is provided by competent practitioners at a reasonable cost. Nurses in advanced practice have a strong, persistent voice in designing such a healthcare system for today and for the future.

The policy process is much broader and more comprehensive than the legislative process. Although individual components can be identified for analytical study, the policy process is fluid, nonlinear, and dynamic. There are many opportunities for nurses in advanced practice to participate throughout the policy process. The question is not whether nurses should become involved in the political system, but to what extent. In the whole policy arena, nurses must be involved with every aspect. Knowing all of the components and issues that must be addressed in each phase, the nurse in advanced practice finds many opportunities for providing expert advice. APNs can use the policy process, individual components, and models as a framework to analyze issues and participate in alternative solutions.

Nursing has a rich history. The professional nurse's values of altruism, respect, integrity, and accountability to consumers remain strong. In some ways, the evolution of nursing roles has come full circle, from the political influence recognized and exercised by Nightingale to the influence of current nurse leaders with elected and appointed public officials. The APN of the 21st century practices with a solid political heritage and a mandate for consistent and powerful involvement in the entire policy process.

Discussion Points and Activities

1. Read Nightingale's *Notes on Nursing* and other historical sources of the mid-1800s and discuss how Nightingale used personal and family influence to move her agenda for the Crimea and for nursing education.
2. Read articles about Mildred Montag's proposal for associate degree nursing education and discuss the implications of moving nursing out of hospitals and into institutions of higher learning.
3. Read the 1965 ANA Position Paper on Educational Preparation for Professional Nursing and articles in response to the position paper before discussing the impact among nurse educators and among types of nursing programs.
4. Compare the definition of nursing according to Nightingale, Henderson, the ANA, and your own state nurse practice act. What is the difference in a legal definition and a professional definition? What are the similarities? What did definitions include or not include that reflected the state of nursing at the time? Construct a definition of nursing for today and for 10 years from now.
5. Discuss the role of research in nursing. What has been the focus over the past century? What is the pattern of nursing research vis-à-vis topic, methodology, relevance? To what extent do you think nursing research has had an impact on nursing care? Cite examples.
6. Trace the amount of federal funding for nursing research. Do not limit your search to federal health-related agencies; that is, investigate departments (commerce, environment, transportation, etc.), military services, and the Veterans Administration. What opportunities does this present for nurse scientists?
7. Read books (e.g., Blancett and Flarey, Covey, Noer, Porter-O'Grady and Wilson) and articles (e.g., Curtin, Milstead, O'Malley, Wolf) about the changing paradigm in healthcare delivery systems. Discuss the change in nursing as an occupation and nursing as a profession. What does this mean in today's transformational paradigm?

8. Consider a thesis, graduate project, or dissertation on a specific topic (e.g., clinical problems, healthcare issues) using the policy process as a framework.

9. Identify policies within public agencies and discuss how they were developed. Interview members of an agency policy committee to discover how policies are changed.

10. Have faculty and students bring to class official governmental policies. What governmental agency is responsible for developing the policy? For enforcing the policy? How has the policy changed over time? What are the consequences of not complying with the policy?

11. Identify nurses who are elected officials at the local, state, or national level. Interview these officials to determine how the nurses were elected, what their objectives are, and to what extent they use their nursing knowledge in their official capacities. Ask the officials if they tapped into nursing groups during their campaigns. If so, what did the nurses contribute? If not, why not?

12. Discuss the major components of the policy process and discuss the fluidity of the process. Point out how players move among the components in a nonlinear way.

13. Using Exhibit 1–1 as a framework, construct a healthcare organization in which access is provided and quality care is assured.

14. Develop an assessment tool by which students can determine their own level of knowledge and involvement in the policy process. Reminder: Stretch your thinking beyond legislative activity.

15. Watch *The O'Reilly Factor* and *The McLaughlin Group* or a similar television program and analyze the verbal and nonverbal communication patterns, pro-and-con arguments, and other methods of discussion. Discuss your analysis within the framework of gender differences in communication and utility in the political arena.

16. Construct a list of ways in which nurses can become more knowledgeable about the policy process. Choose at least three activities in which you will participate. Develop a tool for evaluating the activity and your knowledge and involvement.

17. Select at least one problem or irritation in a clinical area and brainstorm with other APNs or graduate students on how to approach a solution. Discuss funding sources; be creative.

18. Attend a meeting of the state board of nursing, the district or state nurses association, or a professional convention. Identify issues discussed, resources used, communication techniques, and rules observed. Evaluate the usefulness of the session to your practice.

19. Using Exhibit 1–2 as a guide, write in activities and practices that you see or in which you are involved within the new paradigm.

20. Discuss what skills (task, interpersonal, etc.) and attitudes are required for the nurse in the new paradigm. Who is best prepared to teach these skills,

and what teaching techniques should be used? How will they be evaluated? Develop a worksheet to facilitate planning (see Exhibit 1–3).

21. Discuss at least five strategies for helping nurses integrate these skills into their practices.

Exhibit 1–3 Requirements for the New Paradigm of Healthcare Delivery for the 21st Century		
Skill	Teaching Technique	Evaluation Measure

References

Aiken, L. H. (1986). Nursing education: The public policy debate. In J. C. McCloskey and H. K. Grace (Eds.), Current issues in nursing (2nd ed., pp. 680–696). Boston: Blackwell Scientific.

Aiken, L. H. (1990). Charting the future of hospital nursing. Image: Journal of Nursing Scholarship, 22(2), 72–78.

American Association of Colleges of Nursing. (1996). The essentials of master's education for advanced practice nursing. New York: Author.

American Association of Colleges of Nursing. (1998). The essentials of baccalaureate education for professional nursing practice. New York: Author.

American Nurses Association. (1994). Nursing's agenda for health care reform. Washington, DC: American Nurses Publishing, Inc.

American Nurses Association. (2003, March 19). American Nurses Association commends Reps. Capps, Whitfield for forming congressional nursing caucus. Retrieved July 20, 2007, from: www.nursingworld.org/pressrel/2003/pr0319.htm

American Nurses Association. (2007). About ANA. Retrieved July 11, 2007, from: www.nursingworld.org/about

American Nurses Association (ANA) House of Delegates. (1993). Regulation of advanced nursing practice (action report). Washington, DC: American Nurses Publishing Co.

Argyris, C. (1962). Interpersonal competence and organizational effectiveness. Homewood, IL: Dorsey Press.

Backer, B. A., Costello-Nikitas, D., & Mason, D. J. (1993). Power at the policy table—when women and nurses are involved. Revolution, 3(2), 68–71, 74–76.

Bell, D. E., Raiffa, H., & Tversky, A. (1988). *Decision making.* Cambridge, MA: Cambridge University Press.

Benner, P. G. (1984). *From novice to expert: Excellence and power in clinical nursing practice.* Menlo Park, CA: Addison-Wesley.

Bennis, W., & Nanus, B. (1985). *Leaders.* New York: Harper and Row.

Blancett, S. S., & Flarey, D. L. (1995). *Reengineering nursing and health care: The handbook for organizational transformation.* Gaithersburg, MD: Aspen.

Blank, A. E. (1997). Linking the restructuring of nursing care with outcomes. In E. L. Cohen & T. G. Cesta (Eds.), *Nursing case management* (2nd ed., pp. 261–273). St. Louis, MO: Mosby.

Bowen, E. (1982). The Pressman-Wildavsky paradox: Four addenda on why models based on probability theory can predict implementation success and suggest useful tactical advice for implementers. *Journal of Public Policy, 2*(1), 1–22.

Bower, K. A. (1992). *Case management by nurses.* Washington, DC: American Nurses Publishing.

Brooten, D., & Naylor, M. D. (1995). Nurses' effect on changing patient outcomes. *Image: Journal of Nursing Scholarship, 27*(2), 95–99.

Brown, B. J. (1986). Past and current status of nursing's role in influencing governmental policy for research and training in nursing. In J. C. McCloskey & H. K. Grace (Eds.), *Current issues in nursing* (2nd ed., pp. 697–712). Boston: Blackwell Scientific.

Bull, J., Sharp, N., & Wakefield, M. (2000). *Nurses' directory of Capitol connections* (5th ed.). Fairfax, VA: George Mason University Center for Health Policy, Research and Ethics.

Burtt, K. (1997, November/December). Nurses use telehealth to address rural health care needs, prevent hospitalizations. *The American Nurse, 29*(6), 21.

Champy, J. (1995). *Reengineering management.* New York: Harper Business.

Covey, S. R. (1991). *Principle-centered leadership.* New York: Summit Books.

de Chesnay, M. (1983). The creation and dissolution of paradoxes in nursing practice. *Topics in Clinical Nursing, 5*(3), 71–80.

Dranove, D., Kessler, D., McClellan, M., & Satterthwaite, M. (2003). Is more information better? The effects of "report cards" on health care providers. *Journal of Political Economy, 3*(11), 555–585.

Drucker, P. F. (1959). *Landmarks of tomorrow.* New York: Harper.

Drucker, P. F. (1995, February). The age of social transformation. *Quality Digest,* 36–39.

Drucker, P. F. (1999). Knowledge worker productivity: The biggest challenge. *California Management Review, 4*(21), 79–94.

Ethridge, P., & Lamb, G. (1989). Professional nursing case management improves quality, access, and cost. *Nursing Management, 20*(3), 30–35.

Eulau, H., & Prewitt, K. (1973). *Labyrinths of democracy.* Indianapolis, IN: Bobbs-Merrill.

Feldstein, P. J. (1988). *The politics of health legislation.* Ann Arbor, MI: Health Administration Press.

Flood, R. L., & Senge, P. M. (1999). *Rethinking the fifth discipline: Learning within the unknowable.* London: Routledge.

Fuchs, V. R. (1993). *The future of health policy.* Cambridge, MA: Harvard University Press.

Genna, J. (1987, November/December). AIDS management. *Healthcare Forum Journal,* 18–48.

Goggin, M. L., Bowman, A. O'M., Lester, J. P., & O'Toole, L. J., Jr. (1990). *Implementation theory and practice: Toward a third generation.* New York: HarperCollins.

Haas, J. E. (1964). *Role conception and group consensus* (Research Monograph No. 17). Columbus, OH: The Ohio State University, Bureau of Business Research.

Halloran, E. J. (1983). Staffing assignment: By task or by patient. *Nursing Management,* 14(8), 17.

Hash, K. M., & Cramer, E. P. (2003). Empowering gay and lesbian caregivers and uncovering their unique experiences through the use of qualitative methods. *Journal of Gay and Lesbian Social Services. Issues in Practice, Policy and Research,* 15(1/2), 47–64.

Hegyvary, S. (1992). *Outcomes research: Integrating nursing practice into the world view: National Institutes of Health, Patient Outcomes Research: Examining the Effectiveness of Nursing Practice* (pp. 17–24). (DHHS Publication No. 93-3411). Bethesda, MD: Department of Health and Human Services.

Henderson, V. (1966). *The nature of nursing: A definition and its implications for practice, research, and education.* New York: Macmillan.

Hesse, H. (1951). *Siddhartha.* New York: Bantam Books.

How our laws are made. (1990). (House Document 101–139). Washington, DC: U.S. Government Printing Office.

Jones, C. O. (1984). *An introduction to the study of public policy* (2nd ed.). Monterey, CA: Brooks/Cole.

Kelly, L. Y., & Joel, L. A. (1995). *Dimensions of professional nursing* (7th ed.). New York: McGraw-Hill.

Kennedy, E., & Charles, S. C. (1997). *Authority.* New York: Simon & Schuster.

King, I. M. (1971). *Toward a theory for nursing.* New York: John Wiley and Sons.

Koln, L. T., Corrigan, J. M., & Donaldon, M. S. (Eds.). (1999). *To err is human: Building a safer health system. A report from the Committee on Quality of Healthcare in America,* Institute of Medicine, National Academy of Sciences. Washington, DC: National Academy Press.

Kouzes, J., & Posner, B. (1987). *The leadership challenge.* San Francisco: Jossey-Bass.

Kouzes, J., & Posner, B. (1999). *Encouraging the heart: A leader's guide to rewarding and recognizing others.* San Francisco: Jossey-Bass.

Lash, A. A. (1986). Federal financing and its effect on higher nursing education. In J. C. McCloskey & H. K. Grace (Eds.), *Current issues in nursing* (2nd ed., pp. 663–679). Boston: Blackwell Scientific.

Lasswell, H. D. (1958). *Politics: Who gets what, when, how.* New York: Meridian Books.

Laws governing nursing in South Carolina. (1994). Columbia: South Carolina Department of Labor, Licensing, and Regulation.

Leininger, M. (Ed.). (1978). *Transcultural nursing: Concepts, theories and practices.* New York: John Wiley & Sons.

Litman, T. J., & Robins, L. S. (1991). *Health politics and policy* (2nd ed.). Albany, NY: Delmar.

Lowi, T. (1969). *The end of liberalism.* New York: Norton.

Manier, J. (2002, July 7). U.S. quietly OKs fetal stem cell work. *Chicago Tribune Online.*

Maurin, J. (1990). Case management: Caring for psychiatric clients. *Journal of Psychosocial Nursing,* 28(7), 8–12.

Melville, H. (1853). Bartleby, the scrivener: A story of Wall Street. *Putnam's Monthly Magazine,* 2(911), 546–577.

Milio, N. (1989). Developing nursing leadership in health policy. *Journal of Professional Nursing,* 5(6), 315.

Milstead, J. A. (1993). *The advancement of policy implementation theory: An analysis of three needle exchange programs.* Doctoral dissertation. University of Georgia, Athens.

Milstead, J. A. (2003). Leapfrog group: A prince in disguise or just another frog? *Nursing Administration Quarterly,* 26(4), 16–25.

Mundinger, M. (1984). Community-based care: Who will be the case managers? *Nursing Outlook,* 32(6), 294–295.

Noer, D. M. (1993). *Healing the wounds.* San Francisco: Jossey-Bass.

Orem, D. E. (1971). Nursing: Concepts of practice. Scarborough, Ontario: McGraw-Hill.

Osborne, D. E. (Ed.). (1992). Reinventing government: How the entrepreneurial spirit is transforming the public sector. Reading, MA: Addison-Wesley.

Peplau, H. (1952). Interpersonal relations in nursing. New York: Springer.

Pesut, D., & Herman, J. (1999). Clinical reasoning: The art and science of critical and creative thinking (2nd ed.). Albany, NY: Delmar Learning.

Peters, T. J. (1988). Thriving on chaos. New York: Knopf.

Peters, T. J. (1997). The circle of innovation: You can't shrink your way to greatness. New York: Knopf.

Pew Health Professions Commission. (1995, November). Critical challenges: Revitalizing the health professions for the twenty-first century (3rd report). San Francisco: UCSF Center for the Health Professions.

Pierce, L., & Steiner, V. (2003). The male caregiving experience: Three case studies. Stroke, 34(1), 315.

Porter-O'Grady, T. (1996). Accountability and the role of advanced practice. In C. E. Loveridge & S. H. Cummings (Eds.), Case management in the new paradigm (pp. 477–480). Gaithersburg, MD: Aspen.

Porter-O'Grady, T., Hawkins, M. A., & Parker, M. L. (1997). Whole-systems shared governance: Architecture for integration. Gaithersburg, MD: Aspen.

Porter-O'Grady, T., & Malloch, K. (2002). Quantum leadership: A textbook of new leadership. Gaithersburg, MD: Aspen.

Porter-O'Grady, T., & Wilson, C. K. (1995). The leadership revolution in health care: Altering systems, changing behaviors. Gaithersburg, MD: Aspen.

Porter-O'Grady, T., & Wilson, C. K. (1999). Leading the revolution in health care: Advancing systems, igniting performance (2nd ed.). Gaithersburg, MD: Aspen.

The regulatory process. (1992, December 4). Capitol Update, 10(23), 1.

Rodgers, B. L. (1989). Exploring health policy as a concept. Western Journal of Nursing Research, 11(6), 694–702.

Rogers, M. E. (1970). An introduction to the theoretical basis for nursing. Philadelphia: F. A. Davis.

Rossi, P. H., & Freeman, H. E. (1995). Evaluation: A systematic approach (5th ed.). Beverly Hills, CA: Sage.

Saver, C. (2003). Alliance takes another step. Nursing Spectrum Midwestern Edition, 4(1), 12.

Senge, P. (1990). The fifth discipline: The art and practice of the learning organization. New York: Doubleday.

Skocpol, T. (1995). Social policy in the United States. Princeton, NJ: Princeton University Press.

Spratley, E., Johnson, A., Sochalski, J., Fritz, M., & Spencer, W. (2000). The registered nurse population: Findings from the 2004 National Sample Survey of Registered Nurses. Retrieved June 19, 2007, from: http://bhpr.hrsa.gov/healthworkforce

Thomas, S. B., & Quinn, S. C. (1991). The Tuskegee syphilis study, 1932 to 1972: Implications for HIV education and AIDS risk reduction education programs in the black community. American Journal of Public Health, 8(11), 1498–1505.

Venegoni, S. L. (1996). Changing environment of healthcare. In J. V. Hickey, R. M. Ouimette, & S. L. Venegoni (Eds.), Advanced practice nursing: Changing roles and clinical applications (pp. 77–90). Philadelphia: Lippincott.

Watson, J. (1979). Nursing: The philosophy and science of caring. Boston: Little, Brown.

Watzlawick, R., Weakland, C. E., & Fisch, R. (1974). Change. New York: W. W. Norton.

West, W. F. (1982, September/October). The politics of administrative rulemaking. Public Administration Review, 420–426.

Wheatley, M. (1992). *Leadership and the new science*. San Francisco: Berrett-Koehler.

Williams, S. J., & Torrens, P. R. (Eds.). (1988). *Introduction to health services* (3rd ed.). Albany, NY: Delmar.

Wilson, J. Q. (1989). *American government institutions and policies* (4th ed.). Lexington, MA: D. C. Heath.

Wolf, G., Boland, S., & Aukerman, M. (1994a). A transformational model for the practice of professional nursing—Part I: The model. *Journal of Nursing Administration*, 24(4), 51–57.

Wolf, G., Boland, S., & Aukerman, M. (1994b). A transformational model for the practice of professional nursing—Part II: Implementation of the model. *Journal of Nursing Administration*, 24(5), 38–46.

Zander, K. (1990). The 1990s: Core values, core change. *Frontiers in Health Service Management*, 2(1), 39–43.

Zander, K., Etheredge, M., & Bower, K. (Eds.). (1987). *Nursing case management: Blueprints for transformation*. Boston: New England Medical Center.

Zimmerman, B., Lindberg, C., & Plsek, P. (1998). *Edgeware: Lessons from complexity science for health care leaders*. Dallas: VHA, Inc.

Agenda Setting

Elizabeth Ann Furlong, JD, PhD, RN

Key Terms

- ➤ **Contextual dimensions** Studying issues in the real world, in the circumstances or settings of what is happening at the time.
- ➤ **Iron triangle** Legislators or their committees, interest groups, and administrative agencies that work together on a policy issue that will benefit all parties.
- ➤ **Stakeholders** Policy actors, policy communities, and policy networks; people and groups that have a say in what goes on.
- ➤ **Streams** Kingdon's concept of the interaction of public problems, policies, and politics that couple and uncouple throughout the process of agenda setting.
- ➤ **Window of opportunity** Limited time frame for action.

Introduction

"And, we must persist to eliminate the words collaboration and supervision from every statute and regulation in the country. Though frustrating and time-consuming, each time legislators open the Nurse Practice Act for revision, they become better informed of our issues" (Pearson, 2003b, p. 8). This advanced nurse practice concern is one of many political and legislative concerns faced by nurse practitioners. This chapter emphasizes the agenda-setting aspect of policy by using exemplar case studies at both the state and national levels. *Agenda setting* is the process of moving a problem to the attention of government so that solutions can be considered. Advance practice nurses (APNs) can apply the knowledge from these case studies to the many current concerns they face, such as the just-listed scope of practice issues.

"At the end of my pilgrimage, I have come to the conclusion that among the sins of modern political science, the greatest of all has been the omission of passion" (Lowi, 1992, p. 6). This criticism does not apply to public policy researchers' current scholarly interest in agenda setting, policy design, and alternative formulation, nor does it apply to certain policy communities who push for selected public policies. The passion of the former group, the researchers, is seen in their search and inquiry for a better understanding of public policy. The passion of the latter, policy communities, is reflected in their tenacity on policy design, in pushing to make sure that a policy is put into practice as was intended.

Advanced practice nurses, as well as policymakers and citizens, are interested in the best public policy to address society's concerns. In the past, political science researchers have mostly studied the latter steps of policymaking—implementation and evaluation—to gain an understanding of public policy and knowledge that could be used by policymakers to create better public policy. Although all stages of the policy process have been studied, the need for more research on the earlier parts of policymaking—agenda setting, policy formulation, and policy design—has drawn more discussion in recent years (Bosso, 1992; Ingraham, 1987; May, 1991). Thus, research interest in these latter areas grew during the 1980s and 1990s and it continues into the 21st century.

In this chapter, examples are given of agenda setting at both the state and the federal levels. First, the state example is discussed. This exemplar case study can inform the APN of an issue that attempted to get on the Nebraska state agenda by a petition amendment to change the state constitution. Although this endeavor failed to be on the November 2006 General Election ballot, the controversy it raised resulted in a parallel issue being put on the state legislative issue in January 2007. Further, many interest groups expect this again, to be a petition amendment for the November 2008 General Election ballot. By discussing this case study, APNs can learn two ways that issues can get on state agendas (constitutional amendment petition initiatives and introduction of a law), how interest groups both propose and block such agenda issues, how such interest groups persist over years to accomplish their goals, and/or how opponents plan strategies to prevent such agenda items. Following the state agenda-setting example, a classic national legislative example is given.

The Nebraska Humane Care Amendment

Issues get on political agendas because of what Kingdon (1995) describes as problem **streams** and Longest (2006) discusses as the saliency of an issue. The attempt to pass a state constitutional amendment, called the Nebraska Humane Care Amendment, can be understood in the context of the famous Terri Schiavo case that occurred in 2005. "A Florida court judge ruled that a feeding tube keeping her alive in a persistent vegetative state could be removed" (Longest, p. 103). This court case received much national lay, health professional, and ethical media attention (Mason, Leavitt, & Chaffee, 2007). There was unprecedented action by Congress on her behalf. A federal judge refused to order the reinsertion of the feeding tube.

The history and context of the outcome of the court case led to the petition amendment initiative for a state constitutional change in Nebraska during the summer of 2006. An interest group external to Nebraska created the amendment initiative ("Outsiders fueled", 2006). The group organized and financially funded this initiative during the summer of 2006. The knowledge implication for APNs is that once a state constitution has been changed, it is very difficult to undo the change. If the amendment proponents accomplished their goal, it would result in more permanent policy change than passage of a state law by the legislative branch of state government, which, in Nebraska, is the only unicameral legislative body of the 50 states.

A state constitution is the highest law of the state—no other state law can be in conflict with it. If a law is in conflict, the state constitution trumps the other law. Thus, from the proponents' interest group perspective, attempting to change the state constitution is a smart political strategy. As noted earlier, a group external to Nebraska, called America at Its Best, with a postal address in Kalispell, Montana, totally funded the expenses for the Nebraska Humane Care Amendment petition endeavor at a cost of $835,000. The only Nebraskans involved were those who were minimally and perfunctorily involved with legal documents. America at Its Best lists the following organizations as some of its supporters: Americans for a Limited Government, Club for Growth, Funds for Democracy, and the National Taxpayers Union.

In Nebraska, 10% of registered voters are needed on a petition ballot for the issue to be voted on at an election ("Humane care", 2006; "Outsiders fueled", 2006). This means 113,721 valid signatures must be obtained. Although the petition signature gatherers obtained 137,200 signatures, the final decision by the Nebraska Secretary of State was that there were not enough valid signatures, and thus, this issue did not get on the agenda for Nebraska voters to vote on in the General Election in November 2006.

There were many reasons why 20% of the signatures were invalid ("Humane care", 2006). One reason for concern was that Nebraskans were given incorrect and/or fraudulent information when asked to sign the petition by the petition seeker. Some Nebraskans noted a dissonance between the title of the amendment and its substantive content. The goal of the Humane Care Amendment was to prohibit medical interventions, food, or water from being withheld or withdrawn in terminal conditions (Nebraskans for Humane Care Committee, 2006). In addition, it proposed to eliminate parental decision making about a child's condition. If the petition had become a state constitutional amendment, it would have the highest legal authority mandate of the state. Although it did include a statement of respecting advance directives of those who had fully expressed language about the withholding of food and water in terminal conditions, this proposed constitutional amendment raised many clinical, professional, best practice, and ethical issues for APNs.

Why was the state of Nebraska chosen for this agenda-setting issue? First, Nebraska is known and recognized for its more conservative and traditional political ideology compared to other states. Second, the out-of-state organizers had conducted polling in Nebraska in March 2006 to seek Nebraskans' views on this topic. Push polling had been conducted to see if Nebraska was a ripe state for such an amendment (P. Zieg, personal communication, October 23, 2006). The survey data results were positive that such a petition drive could be successful in Nebraska. Third, funding of the petition amendment was in concert with another petition amendment being funded by the same external group. The group spent $861,998 for a petition titled "Stop Over Spending" that would limit state spending. Although $1,998 was donated by others besides America at Its Best, the majority of the funding came from the external group ("Outsiders fueled", 2006). An attorney opponent noted that both initiatives were strategies to increase partisan voter turnout for the Republican party (P. Zieg, personal communication, October 23, 2006). Fourth, when comparing state constitutional procedures for change, Nebraska's procedures are relatively easy to create constitutional change (P. Zieg, personal communication, October 23, 2006). Not all states provide for such changes; that is, Nebraska is one of 18 states that permit this (Weissert & Weissert, 2006).

Finally, Nebraskans, like most individuals in other states, do not all have advance directives and would be subject to the mandated constitutional amendment had it passed. A range of statistical data can be found in the literature about the use of advance directives. For example, Tilden (1999) reports 80% of nursing home residents nationwide do not have an advance directive, whereas 90% of nursing home residents in Oregon do have an advance directive. A recent survey conducted by the Nebraska Hospice and Palliative Care Organization notes that 33% of Nebraskans have an advance directive, 96% said, "it's important to be off machines that extend life," and 74% wouldn't want medical interventions to keep them alive as long as possible if they were dying ("Survey probes", 2007, pp. E 1). In addition, 75% said they felt total physical dependency on others was worse than death. The APN can note the discrepancy between these data and the data obtained from the push polling efforts, which reflected that Nebraskans were "ripe" for such a state constitutional amendment. In summary, the result of a court case (the Terri Schiavo case) that drew national attention became the impetus for getting an issue on one state's agenda. The preceding five reasons are why one state was chosen as the place to pursue a certain policy. It is thought that if the proponent group is successful in one state, such policy could be pursued in other states.

Several **stakeholder** interest groups were either proponents or opponents of this amendment proceeding on the government agenda. In addition to the external group (America at Its Best), proponents also included the citizens who correctly understood the amendment and signed the petition initiative. It is also possible that some citizens were neutral or opposed to the issue, but wanted the opportunity for Nebraskans to vote on the issue. A resource helpful to the proponents was faculty at Ave Maria Law School, who drafted the amendment language (Dr. L. A. Sojka, personal communication, October 23, 2006).

Opponents included a variety of individuals and interest groups. Many of these were patients, family members, health providers (including many nurses), state legislators, and community leaders (nurses, ethicists, attorneys, physicians) who formed a coalition during the summer of 2006 to plan strategies to block this item from getting on the agenda. The coalition continued to fight the issue in the spring of 2007 as a bill was introduced into the Nebraska Unicameral to make such petition initiatives more difficult in the future. The coalition is preparing for potential educational and lobby work in the summer and fall of 2008 to prevent such an amendment on the November 2008 ballot.

The failed November 2006 state constitutional petition amendment continues to have agenda-setting repercussions. In January 2007, some Nebraska state senators introduced legislation to change petition signature verification. Legislative Bill 311 has been unanimously voted out of committee and proceeds to floor debate ("Bills would", 2007).

Other senators introduced another legislative bill that would modify the signature thresholds for both constitutional amendments and statutory initiatives. The intent of this state legislative bill is to make it more difficult to change the state constitution. This bill has also been voted out of committee. Senator Avery, who introduced the bill, says, "I also have deep respect for our state constitution. It deserves to be protected from the desires and whims of out-of-state organizations. It's not written in pencil so that whoever has the biggest eraser can come in and erase it all willy-nilly" ("Bills would", 2007, p. 7). Finally, a third bill has been introduced that also relates to petition signatures. Senator Harms argued the following during Unicameral debate: "That's what got people fired off, it was people putting money into telling Nebraskans what to do. That's wrong" ("Petition restrictions", 2007, p. B2).

This section has discussed examples of issues getting on the public agenda at the state level of government, whether by petition initiative or by law. The next section includes an example of a national issue of interest to nurses and APNs getting on the Congressional agenda.

The National Center for Nursing Research Amendment

Victor Hugo wrote, "Greater that the tread of mighty armies is an idea whose time has come" (Kingdon, 1995, p. 1). For nurses, one example of this was the initiation of legislation in 1983 that increased the funding base for nursing research. An amendment to the 1985 Health Research Extension Act, which created the National Center for Nursing Research (NCNR) on the campus of the National Institutes of Health, is the focus of this chapter's national example of agenda setting.

Creation of the NCNR came about because of a goal of a group of nurse leaders during 1983 and 1984 to create a national institute of nursing. To pass the legislation in 1985, a political compromise was made with legislators to create a center instead of an institute. However, in 1993, the NCNR was changed to an institute. Today the agency continues as the National Institute of Nursing Research (NINR). Discussion in this chapter of the NCNR amendment focuses on agenda setting and policy formulation that occurred from 1983 to 1985.

The Influence of National Nursing Groups

The creation of the National Center for Nursing Research (NCNR) on the campus of the National Institutes of Health (NIH) was a policy victory for national nursing organizations. Despite the victory, those nursing organizations still need a better understanding of agenda setting, policy formulation, and policy design as they work for other policy changes in the future. Although nurses' groups traditionally have not been considered strong political actors, these groups recognize the importance of political activity to bring about public policies that enhance patient care (Warner, 2003).

In the last decade of the 20th century, nurses' groups were just emerging as actors in policy networks. "Yet a full cadre of nurse leaders who are knowledgeable and experienced in the public arena, who fully understand the design of public policy, and who are conversant with consumer, business and provider groups does not yet exist" (DeBack, 1990, p. 69).

In a study of significant national health organizations that play a key role in the health policymaking area (Laumann, Heinz, Nelson, & Salisbury, 1991), no nursing organizations were cited. The scope and nature of nursing care and certain restrictions to providing that care are closely related to public policy. APNs are well aware of this because state legislative activity daily affects their professional practice. Raudonis and Griffith (1991) and Warner (2003) are three of many nurse leaders who challenged nurses to be more knowledgeable about health policy. These leaders also urged nurses to become more empowered on health policy issues. If that were to happen, public policy could better reflect the contributions of nursing to patient care, to the health of citizens, and to cost-effective quality solutions for the financial crisis of the health care system. Nagelkerk and Henry (1991) echo this concern: "To date, few studies in nursing can be classified as policy research. Leaders in our field, therefore, have identified this type of undertaking as a priority" (p. 20).

Research on the NCNR amendment is important because it studies political actors who are not generally studied, that is, nurses' interest groups. This research contributes to public policy scholars' knowledge of all actors in policy networks. Laumann et al. (1991) acknowledges that "we may even run a risk of misrepresenting the sorts of actors who come to be influential in policy deliberation" (p. 67). The significance of this research becomes obvious when the Schneider and Ingram (1993a) model of "social construction of target populations" in policy design is applied to the nurse interest groups. For example, how nurses were viewed by policymakers—the social construction of nurses as a target population—influenced not only the policy that nurses were interested in, but also passage of the total NIH reauthorization bill.

Dohler (1991) compared health policy actors in the United States, Great Britain, and Germany and found that it is much easier to have new political actors in the United States because there are multiple ways to become involved. He has written of the great increase in new actors since 1970. Baumgartner and Jones (1993) also describe multiple paths of access to becoming involved.

Overview of Models

Several researchers have developed models of agenda setting and policy formulation (Baumgartner & Jones, 1993; Cobb & Elder, 1983; Kingdon, 1995). Several political scientists are developing theoretical modeling of policy design (Hedge & Mok, 1987). Ingraham (1987) is one of several authors who has noted the lack of one design, one theory, or one model in policy design. Meanwhile, public policy scholars are pushing for more empirical study of agenda setting, alternative formulation, and policy design (Schneider & Ingram, 1993a).

Data analysis reveals the importance of the Schneider and Ingram model (1993a) of the social construction of target populations and of the Kingdon model (1995) for an understanding of the agenda-setting process of this amendment to the NIH reauthorizing legislative bill. Analysis of this legislation over a period of a decade also underscores the importance of the Dryzek (1983) definition of policy design. An analysis of the legislation supported the importance of studying the contextual dimension that has been advocated by Bobrow and Dryzek (1987), Bosso (1992), deLeon (1988–1989), Ingraham and White (1988–1989), May (1991), and Schneider and Ingram (1993b). The value of other models—institutional, representational communities and institutional approach, and the congressional motivational model—is addressed because these models contribute to an understanding of this example. Finally, during the study of interest groups opposed to this legislation, the researcher noted two occurrences of **iron triangles** in the early 1980s. These findings are discussed in more detail.

Kingdon Model

Kingdon (1995) addresses two public policy questions: How do issues get on the political agenda? And after the issues are there, how are alternative solutions devised? In describing his model, Kingdon identifies both participants and processes that explain the emergence of the agenda and the alternatives. The participants can be actors inside or outside of government. The processes are conceived as three streams that he labels policy streams, problem streams, and political streams. These processes are affected by a **window of opportunity** that allows for the merger of the streams and the setting of an agenda. He distinguishes between items on the nongovernmental-systemic agenda and the governmental-formal agenda. The formal agenda consists of those issues that governmental officials are actively discussing and trying to resolve. Kingdon's research reports that the two types of agendas are affected differently by the three streams.

Of the actors in the federal government who are participants, the ones most influential in agenda setting are the administration (the president and his or her advisors), members of Congress, and, to a lesser extent, congressional staff. In the overall ranking, members of Congress ranked second to the administration in importance in agenda setting. This was true despite all the barriers that Congress members face. The ability of a member of Congress to set agendas is furthered if he or she is a committee chairperson, a ranking minority member on a committee, or viewed as a powerful representative.

Kingdon notes that members of Congress become involved in agenda setting to initiate policy to meet constituent needs, to enhance members' reputation in Washington regarding their ability and power, and to put sound public policy into effect. Although congressional staff members are not viewed as having as important a role as the administration and congressional members, the interdependence of the staff and the member is noted. Staff frequently act as conduits of ideas and issues to the representative or senator. Staff are in a position, by virtue of their ready access to important members of Congress, their ability to concentrate all their energies on given subjects, and their straddling of political and technical worlds, to have considerable impact on the alternatives considered by important people and even on the agendas of those people. It is important to remember, however, that staffers do all of these things within the limits that are set by the senators and representatives who hire and can fire them (Kingdon, 1995).

Kingdon suggests that elected officials are more important to agenda setting whereas staffers are more important to alternative formulation. In comparing governmental versus nongovernmental actors, he finds that the former are more instrumental in agenda setting. He finds that the latter (especially interest groups) sometimes play more of a key role in blocking agendas than in promoting agendas. An application of this concept can be seen in the state agenda-setting example given earlier in this chapter, that is, a coalition interest group is attempting to block the goal of the Nebraska Humane Care Amendment. Further, nongovernmental actors are more important in formulating alternative solutions to problems than they are in agenda setting.

An interest group is most influential if it can "convince governmental officials that it speaks with one voice and truly represents the preferences of its members. If the group is plagued by internal dissension, its effectiveness is seriously impaired" (Kingdon, 1995, p. 55). In discussing this idea, Kingdon alludes to different groups being treated differently by elected officials depending on the group's organizational unity, income, and education. Although the language is different, this is similar to what Schneider and Ingram (1991) investigate in more detail with their model of the social construction of target populations and the importance of such models when analyzing policy. APNs can be more effective when they are united and speak with one voice. One example is how all four groups of APNs in Nebraska organized in a unified manner to change state legislation in 2004 relative to scope of practice.

Although Kingdon studied the various participants who are responsible for agenda setting, he also emphasizes the fact that an idea can come from anywhere and that in some ways its source of origin does not matter. He emphasizes that it is essential for an idea to land on fertile soil and be nurtured. "Thus the key to understanding policy change is not where the idea came from but what made it take hold and grow" (Kingdon, 1995, p. 76). His research focuses on an idea that suddenly takes off, "an idea whose time has come" (p. 1). His model is adapted from the Cohen-March-Olsen model of organizational decisions. Both models see decision making as a dynamic, fluid process rather than a linear, sequential process. "A problem is recognized, a solution is available, the political climate makes the time right for change, and the constraints do not prohibit action" (p. 93).

A problem stream can be marked by systematic indicators of a problem, by a sudden crisis, or by feedback that a program is not working as intended. In Kingdon's research, 50% of the interviewees reported on the importance of systematic indicators (such as studies and reports) in getting an issue on the agenda. He differentiates between a *condition* and a *problem*: conditions become problems when people believe that something ought to be done about them. Thus, APNs can convert conditions of concern into problems.

The second stream, policy, is characterized by the policy community, the presence of ideas, the softening-up phase, criteria for the survival of ideas, and the presence of available alternatives. Policy communities are those groups of specialists who have a concern and expertise in certain areas, such as health. This fluid group of both governmental and nongovernmental actors is known to each other by their writings, their professional organizations, and their networking.

In some policy areas, there are specific policy entrepreneurs who are willing to invest "their resources—time, energy, reputation, and sometimes money—in the hope of a future return" (Kingdon, 1995, p. 129). For example, Gray (1992) categorizes John Wennberg as an entrepreneur in the setting of a health services research agenda. Although such entrepreneurs sometimes solve problems, Kingdon suggests that many times such individuals are looking for problems to which they can attach their pet solution. APN policy entrepreneurs can identify problems to which they can apply their health policy solutions.

To be placed on an agenda, an idea must have been softened up. The principle here is that people have to get used to new ideas, and then someone must build support and acceptance for new proposals. This can be done by policy entrepreneurs, policy communities, or agenda-setting participants through education or by freeing trial balloons and making speeches. This phase is known as "getting your ducks in a row," "greasing the skids," and "get[ting] people to talking" (Kingdon, 1995, pp. 135–136).

The third stream of Kingdon's model is the political stream, which consists of the public mood, pressure group campaigns, election results, partisan or ideological distributions in Congress, and changes of administration. Factors that can be influential in this stream include committee jurisdictional boundaries and turf concerns among agencies and government branches. APNs must understand that in the political stream, it is necessary to study coalition building by government officials. Negotiation and persuasion are effective techniques. In wanting a winning coalition, elected officials may more likely say, "You give me my provision, and I'll give you yours" rather than, "Let me convince you of the virtue of my provision" (Kingdon, 1995, p. 167).

Finally, agenda setting occurs as a coupling of streams during a critical time when a window of opportunity appears. "Policy windows open infrequently, and do not stay open long" (Kingdon, 1995, p. 166). It is important for policy entrepreneurs or policy communities to be alert to opportunities. Agendas are affected more by the problem and political streams, whereas alternatives are affected more by the policy stream. Windows of opportunity open because of changes in the political stream or because new problems capture officials' attention.

Interview data and a review of the literature show many ways in which the Kingdon model can explain the agenda setting for the NCNR amendment. For example, these were variables for the problem stream: (1) the need for nursing research was recognized by many, that is, Representative Madigan (R-IL), legislative staffers, and national nurse leaders; (2) the data about financial disparity in funding for nurses; and (3) the timing of an Institute of Medicine (IOM) report on this problem. These were the variables for the political stream: (1) this policy would be valuable for Rep. Madigan's reelection; and (2) this was an important policy proposal for the Republican party to secure increased voting by women voters. For the policy stream, it was sound public policy.

A window of opportunity opened as the timing of the release of the IOM report in conjunction with the election cycle, the presence of many national nurse leaders who were policy and politically knowledgeable, and a representative who initiated the idea for this bill all came together quickly and at an opportune time. In summarizing these findings in relation to the Kingdon model, this example validates the importance of the political and problem streams. However, the NCNR amendment was passed without meeting the policy stream processes described by Kingdon, that is, that it goes through a softening-up phase.

Advanced practice nurses can apply the Kingdon model to ongoing priority practice issues with which they are concerned. For example, APNs can be attentive to the three streams (policy, problem, and political) and a window of opportunity in which to move their agenda. Every year a legislative update is printed in *The Nurse Practitioner*. This is one way to recognize the advances made in state policies in the areas of scope of practice, prescriptive authority, reimbursement practices, title protection, and emerging issues (Pearson, 2003a).

APNs also need to be aware of taking political action in regulatory agencies when that is the best way to problem solve. For example, nurse practitioners find it increasingly difficult to have mail-order pharmacies recognize and fill their prescriptions (Edmunds, 2003). Two nurse practitioners from New York and South Carolina addressed this problem stream by working with the Food and Drug Administration and the Federal Trade Commission because they recognized that the venue of working through regulatory agencies was the best initial solution for this problem (Edmunds).

Importance of Contextual Dimensions

Some authors, notably Bobrow and Dryzek (1987), Bosso (1992), DeLeon (1988–1989), Ingraham and White (1988–1989), May (1991), and Schneider and Ingram (1993b), have emphasized the need to analyze the political context in which policies get on the agenda, alternatives are formulated, and policies are put into effect. Although this is neither a definitive nor an exhaustive list, five **contextual dimensions** are suggested by Bobrow and Dryzek (1987) for studying the success or failure of any designed policy: (1) complexity and uncertainty of the decision-system environment; (2) feedback potential; (3) control of design by an actor or group of actors; (4) stability of policy actors over time; and (5) the audience must be stirred into action.

DeLeon (1988–1989) writes that sometimes researchers, because of their unstructured environment, have chosen to study approaches and methodologies that may meet scientific rigor better, but in doing so come "dangerously close to rendering the policy sciences all-but-useless in the real-life political arenas" (p. 300). DeLeon notes that it is difficult to impossible for researchers to "structure analytically the contextual environment in which their recommended analyses must operate" (p. 300).

Researchers work in a world of great social complexity, extreme political competition, and limited resources. Of the previously mentioned writers, Bosso and May are especially strong in their advocacy of this contextual approach to the study of public policy. Bosso (1992) echoes DeLeon's concern: "In many ways, the healthiest trend is the admission, albeit a grudging one for many, that policymaking is not engineering and the study of policy formation cannot be a laboratory science. In policy making contexts do matter, people don't always act according to narrow self-interest, and decisions are made on the basis of incomplete or biased information" (p. 23).

Data from congressional documents, archival sources, and personal and telephone interviews show the importance of the political context to all aspects of policy design—how the policy arrived on the agenda, how policy alternatives were formulated, the legislative process, implementation, and redesign of the legislation 8 years later resulting in new legislation within 2 years to accomplish the original goal (Bobrow & Dryzek, 1987; Bosso, 1992; deLeon, 1988–1989; Ingraham & White, 1988–1989; May, 1991; Schneider & Ingram, 1993b).

Examples of Political Contextual Influence

First, partisan political party conflict in Congress influenced the initial agenda setting of the amendment and the legislative process throughout the 2 years. Opposition to Rep. Waxman's (D-CA) NIH bill in the spring and summer of 1983 resulted in Rep. Madigan's initiating a substitute policy. As noted by two congressional staffers, this was an example of partisan conflict. Another example of partisanship, noted by an interviewee, was that the appointment of Dr. Ada Sue Hinshaw as the first director of the NCNR was made easier because she was Republican. (The administration at the time was Republican.)

Second, a U.S. Representative's concern with his reelection chances influenced the initial agenda setting because of the congressional perception that nurses were a target population that could help his reelection chances. Several respondents noted that this was an important factor in the initial decision for this type of public policy.

A third contextual dimension was the bipartisan negotiation to enact policy. Such negotiations by Rep. Waxman and Rep. Madigan in early fall 1983 resulted in a firm resolve during the 97th and 98th Congresses to stay with the proposed NIN policy and during the 99th Congress to accept a compromise of an NCNR. Another example of bipartisan negotiation was the early committee work by Rep. Madigan, Rep. Broyhill (R-NC), and Rep. Shelby (D-AL) to forge a simple bipartisan amendment that was four lines long. The bipartisan effort of these three representatives smoothed the way for passage of this amendment by the subcommittee. Bipartisan support for issues increases the chances the legislation will pass. Thus, legislators use this strategy early in the legislative process.

Fourth, interest group unity on a policy was a factor. Such unity by nurse groups was considered by many interviewees to be a crucial factor in the bill's passage. This factor also was important in explaining why no other policy alternatives were pursued. Because the decision to support Rep. Madigan was officially made by the Tri-Council in the summer of 1983, and although other policy alternatives were considered after that, the priority of presenting unity with Rep. Madigan was maintained. Dohler (1991) reports on the importance of the unity of policy communities. He concludes that the deregulation of two organizations, the Professional Standards Review Organization and the Health Systems Agencies, occurred because of the "weakened stability of the network segment" (p. 267). Dohler determined that if there is not a stable united policy community, programs falter. If there is such stability (as with the nursing community in this research), there is an increased chance of success.

Fifth, lack of interest group unity with a congressperson was seen as a negative factor. Such behavior by the American Association of Medical Colleges disillusioned Rep. Madigan and increased his interest in initiating the NIN policy.

Sixth, partisan conflict between the White House and an interest group (nursing) that supported Democratic presidential and vice presidential candidates had an influence on this legislation's history. This campaign support by the American Nurses Association (ANA) for the Democratic candidates was evaluated as the reason for the 1984 Republican presidential veto of the NIN amendment and the NIH bill that had passed Congress. Interviewee data reported one congressperson's concern with how the ANA political action committee (PAC) distributed its money—mainly to Democratic candidates. Research by Makinson (1992) a decade later on the 1990 election reflects that the ANA PAC gave 85% of its money to Democratic candidates.

Seventh, ideological and partisan conflicts over other issues within the larger NIH bill affected the bill's legislative history. Concerns about fetal tissue research and animal rights research caused much difficulty in the early 1980s. Concerns about immigration laws and immigrants with HIV infection raised concerns in the 1990s and affected compromises and passage of the bills. Other such issues, although not about the NINR amendment, had a major effect on the bill's legislative history. APNs need to understand bills in their holistic content and the many pressures on a particular bill.

Eighth, concerns with the federal deficit influenced discussion of the bill and decision making. The creation of new federal entities was opposed because of the deficit concern. President Reagan consistently used this argument as a reason not to create a NINR.

Ninth, legislation passed during a lame-duck presidential term was a factor. The NIH bill with the NCNR amendment was passed in 1985 when President Reagan was beginning his second term. Republican congresspeople did not feel as constrained to vote along party lines, and that was reflected in the 1985 legislative vote and the override vote. Thus, the timing of this vote in President Reagan's lame-duck term helped the bill's passage. When the president vetoes legislation, another option for passage is for Congress to secure the necessary number of votes and override the president's decision. As is explained later in discussion of the 13th contextual variable, this was a significant political event for this nursing issue.

Tenth, the history of Congress with selected administrative agencies influenced the political context. Rep. Waxman's attempted control of NIH was a factor in Rep. Madigan's initiation of NIH legislation during the summer of 1983. Data support the analysis that of all administrative agencies, the NIH consistently was regarded positively by Congress members. This was reflected in ample funding levels on a consistent basis. Contrary to this usual positive regard was the negative situation between Rep. Dingell (D-MI) and the NIH. He had "captured" letters sent by NIH officials to research scientists asking them to lobby their Congress members for increased funding. Rep. Dingell reminded NIH officials that this activity violated law. Further, this situation led Rep. Dingell and other Congress people to ask who was and who should be in charge of the NIH.

Eleventh, the interaction of Congress, administrative agencies, and the Office of Management and Budget (OMB) also influenced the political context. The congressional funding pattern identified in the 10th factor changed somewhat in the early 1980s. NIH officials became anxious when OMB dictated that NIH make a last-minute revised budget to honor a 1980 promise to fund 5,000 new grants yearly. This mandated division of NIH's economic pie contributed to NIH officials' not wanting new research entities on their campus that would further erode current programs and projects. A second similar budgetary crisis occurred at NIH in spring 1985 that again caused much consternation for NIH officials and research scientists.

Twelfth, the internal political dynamics of Congress also influenced this legislation. Rep. Waxman was a member of the congressional class of 1974, when the dynamic in Congress was a decentralization of power and increased congressional staff. A *congressional class* refers to that cohort of elected officials in a certain election. The data revealed that Rep. Waxman was interested in gaining more power and control over NIH. Although his committee had authorizing power over NIH, it did not have the greater power of the appropriations committee that was responsible for funding. However, with his ability to authorize legislation, Rep. Waxman had leverage to gain more power. His attempt to micromanage NIH resulted in Rep. Madigan's initiating substitute policy.

Thirteenth, interaction between the White House and Congress affected the legislation. For example, President Reagan publicly vetoed the legislation in 1984, although he could have done it quietly by not signing the bill. This was done to alert Congress to expected conflict the following year if the bill's provisions were kept the same. The override vote in 1985 is an example of the negative relationship between the White House and Congress. Data showed that members of Congress (and many of the president's party) felt betrayed over their work on this legislation and over what they thought their communication had been with the president about passing this policy and putting it into effect. This sense of betrayal spurred their work in securing the veto override vote. Another example of the relationship between the White House and Congress was the number of presidential vetoes by President Reagan of congressional legislation and the few veto-override votes. Since his inauguration, President Reagan had vetoed 41 legislative bills; this override of the NIH bill veto was the fifth successful override vote since 1981 ("Senate approves", 1985).

Fourteenth, even international political relations were a consideration. During the fall of 1985, the Senate waited until the Geneva Summit was finished before beginning the veto-override vote. This was done to keep President Reagan from losing any credibility during the summit meeting because the Soviet leader would be aware of the veto-override vote.

Fifteenth, the skills and abilities of an interest group in furthering its intended policy had an influence on the context of legislation. Data revealed that in the early 1980s many factors influenced the ability of the nursing interest group to promote this policy after it was on the agenda. These influences were (1) the formation of the Tri-Council; (2) a special interest in public policy of the executive director of the National League of Nursing; (3) the coming need to reauthorize the Nurse Education Act; (4) many deans of nursing education programs who were policy oriented; (5) a combination of people who saw the need; (6) much networking by nurses; (7) the presence of highly motivated people who were interested in furthering the nursing profession; (8) nurses appointed to positions in the White House; (9) more nurses working on the Hill; and (10) the study conducted by Dr. Joanne Stevenson (personal communication, 1990) on nurse researchers' inability to obtain NIH grants. These 10 factors were obtained from interview data. Many of these influences demonstrate the increased numbers of nurses who were active in policy and politics in many dimensions and in many places—at state and national governmental levels, in professional associations, in executive and legislative branches of the government, in schools of nursing, and in networking circles. Further, the research by Dr. Stevenson showed that nurses had an increased opportunity of receiving NIH grants when they omitted their RN credential on their grant and only listed their PhD.

Sixteenth, the adage that all politics is personal influenced the legislation at various points. Data revealed the importance of personal relationships in getting the idea on the agenda, in gaining strategic information, in sharing needed information, and in asking for requests. For example, strategic networking at certain cocktail parties helped, as did carpooling with selected political actors. Savvy nurse leaders facilitated other nurses meeting legislators and legislative aides in these settings so that nurses could lobby effectively.

Finally, the importance of congressional staffers to the initiation and passage of legislation must be noted. Several interviewees spoke of the importance of certain staffers in their tenacity to ensure that the NCNR amendment was passed. Other staffers noted the importance of the professional education background and socialization of staffers in influencing the types of policy options that are initiated and worked on with vigor. Interview data attested to the tenacity of one Capitol Hill staffer during the conference committee.

Two of Bobrow and Dryzek's (1987) five contextual dimensions were in evidence and contributed to the success of this policy, both because the NCNR was passed as legislation in 1985 and because the NCNR became a national institute of nursing research in 1993. The two criteria are related in this instance: the control of design by an actor or group of actors and the stability of policy actors over time. Once this policy was on the agenda and once nurses were united, the nursing interest group was committed to it. The nursing interest group showed unity in working with Rep. Madigan and staying the course. Thus, although there were other policy alternatives discussed, they were never vigorously pursued by the nurse interest group. Once the compromise for NCNR was made in 1985, the nurse interest group found that acceptable because they knew they had a foot in the door and because they planned to accomplish their original design (a NINR) at a later date.

The second dimension, stability of policy actors, also relates to the nurse interest group. This group of nurse leaders was stable over a decade and kept tenaciously to its goal. Although the policy arrived on the formal agenda because of Rep. Madigan, once the policy was there, a very stable group of nurse actors worked more than a decade to see that the original policy design eventually was enacted (change from a NCNR to a NINR).

May (1991) writes that regardless of how one defines policy design there is the "emphasis on matching content of a given policy to the political context in which the policy is formulated and implemented" (p. 188). This statement describes the contextual dimension of how this public policy arrived on the formal agenda. Rep. Madigan was going to introduce substitute legislation for Rep. Waxman's NIH bill. Rep. Madigan's NIN amendment was based on an appraisal of what policy content would best work in that political context.

Ingraham and White (1988–1989) write: "Politics can influence both design process and design outcome in a number of ways. It can constrain problem definition and the range of alternative solutions available for consideration. . . . It can, in fact, eliminate the process of design altogether" (p. 316). Data indicate that this happened. Partisan politics and reelection politics influenced the design process—the policy option that was chosen (the NINR proposal). That policy option moved quickly to the formal agenda, where it then moved forward in the legislative process. The politics of that option kept other alternative solutions from being considered seriously. Thus, the politics of this situation influenced the design process and the selection of the policy option and constrained the availability of other policy alternatives.

Schneider and Ingram Model

In addition to the political context emphasis, Schneider and Ingram (1991, 1993a, 1993b) specifically push for empirical research that studies the social construction of target populations (those groups affected by the policy). They propose that one can best understand agenda setting, alternative formulation, and implementation by knowing how elected officials perceive different target populations; in other words, by knowing the "social construction"—images, symbols, and traits— of such populations.

In their beginning work in this area, Schneider and Ingram proposed a theory in which there is a continuum of target populations categorized as the advantaged, contenders, dependents, and deviants. Their model suggests that there are pressures to initiate beneficial policy that help those groups that are seen positively, while groups that are seen negatively will receive punitive policy. They argue that groups that are viewed positively are the "advantaged" and the "dependents" whereas the negatively perceived groups are the "contenders" and the "deviants." This is a beginning categorization, and they call for empirical research in this area. They admit that their theory needs three items:

1. A definition of target populations and of social constructions
2. An explanation of how social constructions influence public officials in choosing agendas and designs of policy
3. An explanation of how policy agendas and designs influence the political orientations and participation patterns of target populations

To better understand the idea of social construction of target populations, examples are given from the model proposed by Schneider and Ingram. Positively viewed target populations could be on a continuum of being viewed as those with and without power. For example, the elderly, business people, military veterans, and scientists are examples of target populations that are viewed positively and as having power. Target populations who are considered more dependent, such as children, mothers, and the disabled (the dependent), are viewed positively but as having less power.

There is a category of negatively viewed target populations. These groups can be viewed as with and without power as well. Examples that Schneider and Ingram (1991) provide of negatively perceived target populations that have power include the rich, big unions, minorities, cultural elites, and the moral majority (the contenders). Target populations viewed negatively and as not having political power include criminals, drug addicts, communists, flag burners, and gangs (the deviants).

The authors describe how this model could be applied to understand agenda setting. Social constructions of target populations help provide better answers to Lasswell's (1936) enduring question: Who gets what, when, and how? Conventional political science hypotheses about the characteristics that determine groups' influence in setting policy agendas and influencing policy content become significantly more robust when augmented by assessments of social constructions. Further, understanding social construction of target populations helps to explain how elected officials behave, and why—in some circumstances— officials support policy provisions that distribute benefits at odds with their apparent self-interest, as determined by their assessment of interest group and constituency opinion (Schneider & Ingram, 1993b).

Because research (Hall, 1987; Kaji, 1993) shows that important motivations for congressional members are their interests in winning reelection and in initiating sound policy that addresses social problems, Schneider and Ingram's model of congressional members' perception of groups is relevant to the agenda setting, alternative formulation, and legislative action in which they participate. This model predicts that certain types of policy tools are used more frequently with certain types of target populations.

The need for empirical research in this approach to public policy study is a ripe area for APNs. For example, a 1997 study by Declercq and Simmes examined how "drive-through deliveries" got on the state legislative agendas and were passed as legislation by several states quite quickly. This clinical issue has implications especially for nurse practitioners and nurse midwives. Some of the findings correlate with similar findings in this NINR case study examination—use of Kingdon's model, importance of contextual dimensions, and importance of symbols.

The Schneider and Ingram theory, together with Kingdon's research, provides the best explanation for understanding the process of the NCNR legislation. Schneider and Ingram (1991, 1993a, 1993b) say that one can best understand agenda setting, alternative formulation, and implementation by knowing how elected officials see different target populations and by knowing the social construction, or images, symbols, and traits of such populations. The data consistently revealed that this NCNR policy was initiated by Rep. Madigan because of the social construction of this target population. Proposing public policy for this target population would help him pass his substitute NIH legislation. Nurses, as a target population, would be on the continuum of positively viewed groups. Although Schneider and Ingram acknowledge that theirs is an emerging model that needs empirical testing to refine and define several of its phenomena, this author found it to be of explanatory value and extreme importance.

Mueller (1988) wrote: "Politicians must be convinced that they will gain from new policies—either through political success or through program effectiveness" (p. 443). The selection of nurses as a target population when Congress members, especially Republicans, needed the female vote contributed to a convincing argument for potential political success for them.

Conclusion

"No data are ever in themselves decisive. Factors beyond only the data help decide which policy is formulated or adopted by the people empowered to make the decision to form policy" (James, 1991, p. 14). James is referring to data in a problem stream as described by Kingdon. The accuracy of this quote was demonstrated in this research because the Schneider and Ingram theory of the "social construction of target populations," together with the Kingdon model and the contextual dimension, explained the policy process.

The contextual dimension influenced all aspects of the policy, from agenda setting in 1983 through policy redesign in 1991, with passage of the amended legislation in 1993 that accomplished the original 1983 goal. The importance of studying the political context was demonstrated by the 17 contextual dimensions that influenced this legislative policy process.

Of particular explanatory value in the early agenda-setting and policy-alternative formulation of this legislation were the Schneider and Ingram model and the Kingdon model. The particular amendment was pursued because of application of the "social construction of target populations." That is, the target population of nurses was chosen because they would help Rep. Madigan's and other Congress members' chances for reelection. The Kingdon theory adds to the further understanding of this legislation. Within Kingdon's model, neither the problem stream nor the policy stream was decisive for the process of this legislation; rather, the political stream was. The factors of the political stream (reelection chances for Rep. Madigan and other congresspeople, partisan ideology in Congress, the public mood about gender issues, and turf concerns between government agencies) all strongly influenced the setting of this issue on the agenda. The following hypotheses supported by this empirical research include the fact that policy is more likely to be initiated for those target populations who are positively viewed by Congress members, issues are more likely to reach the formal agenda when the political stream factors are related to positively viewed target populations, and policy process is best understood in a contextual perspective.

For APN scholars these case studies contribute to an understanding of agenda setting and policy design by evaluating the importance of the Schneider and Ingram model, the Kingdon model, policy design, and the contextual dimension to policy initiation, development, implementation, and policy redesign in the creation of the National Institute for Nursing Research and in a state issue relating to end-of-life care.

Discussion Points and Activities

1. How did the Kingdon model explain how the NCNR amendment got on the political agenda?
2. How can APNs become aware of factors in the problem stream to which Kingdon alludes?
3. What are examples of policy streams that APNs could be advancing relative to their practice?
4. How can APNs be involved in the political stream?
5. How can APNs anticipate windows of opportunity?
6. According to Schneider and Ingram, to which of the four target populations do nurses belong? Discuss the relevance to agenda setting.
7. What are ways that APNs can network with congressional members and their staffers?
8. How can APNs promote unity among themselves and with other nurses?
9. What current contextual dimensions can promote APN practice?
10. How can APNs use the Kingdon model and the Schneider and Ingram model?

References

Baumgartner, F. R., & Jones, B. D. (1993). *Agendas and instability in American politics.* Chicago: University of Chicago Press.

Bills would change petition requirements. (2007, January 26). *Unicameral Update, XXX*(4), 1, 7.

Bobrow, D. B., & Dryzek, J. S. (1987). *Policy analysis by design.* Pittsburgh, PA: University of Pittsburgh Press.

Bosso, C. J. (1992). Designing environmental policy. *Policy Currents,* 2(4), 1, 4–6.

Cobb, R. W., & Elder, C. D. (1983). *Participation in America:The dynamics of agenda-building* (2nd ed.). Baltimore: Johns Hopkins University Press.

DeBack, V. (1990). Public policy—nursing needs health policy leaders. *Journal of Professional Nursing, 6*(2), 69.

Declercq, E., & Simmes, D. (1997). The politics of "drive-through deliveries": Putting early postpartum discharge on the legislative agenda. *Milbank Quarterly, 75*(2), 175–202.

DeLeon, P. (1988–1989). The contextual burdens of policy design. *Policy Studies Journal, 17*(2), 297–309.

Dohler, M. (1991). Policy networks, opportunity structures, and neo-conservative reform strategies in health policy. In B. Main & R. Mayntz (Eds.), *Policy networks: Empirical evidence and theoretical considerations* (pp. 235–296). Frankfurt am Main: Campus Verlag.

Dryzek, J. S. (1983). Don't toss coins in garbage cans: A prologue to policy design. *Journal of Public Policy, 3*(4), 345–368.

Edmunds, M. (2003). Advocating for NPs: Go and do likewise. *Nurse Practitioner, 28*(2), 56.

Gray, B. H. (1992). The legislative battle over health services research. *Health Affairs, 11*(4), 38–66.

Hall, R. L. (1987). Participation and purpose in committee decision making. *American Political Science Review, 81*(1), 105–127.

Hedge, D. M., & Mok, J. W. (1987). The nature of policy studies: A content analysis of policy journal articles. *Policy Studies Journal, 16*(1), 49–62.

Humane care voted could be in '08. (2006, September 19). *Omaha World Herald,* 1-A.

Ingraham, P. W. (1987). Toward more systematic consideration of policy design. *Policy Studies Journal, 15*(4), 611–628.

Ingraham, P. W., & White, J. (1988–1989). The design of civil service reform: Lessons in politics and rationality. *Policy Studies Journal, 17*(2), 315–330.

James, P. (1991). Bravo to the nursing emphasis on policy research. *Reflections, 17*(1), 14–15.

Kaji, J. T. (1993). *A simple theory of legislative advocacy.* Paper presented at the annual meeting of the Midwest Political Science Association, Chicago.

Kingdon, J. W. (1995). *Agendas, alternatives, and public policies.* New York: HarperCollins College Publishers.

Lasswell, H. (1936). *Who gets what, when and how?* New York: McGraw-Hill.

Laumann, E. O., Heinz, J. P., Nelson, R., & Salisbury, R. (1991). Organizations in political action: Representing interests in national policy making. In B. Marin & R. Mayntz (Eds.), *Policy networks: Empirical evidence and theoretical considerations* (pp. 63–96). Frankfurt am Main: Campus Verlag.

Longest, B. B. (2006). *Health policymaking in the United States.* Washington, DC: AUPHA Press.

Lowi, T. J. (1992). The state in political science: How we become what we study. *American Political Science Review, 86*(1), 1.

Makinson, L. (1992). Political contributions from the health and insurance industries. *Health Affairs, 11*(4), 120–134.

Mason, D. J., Leavitt, J. K., & Chaffee, M. W. (2007). *Policy and politics in nursing and health care.* St. Louis: Saunders Elsevier.

May, P. J. (1991). Reconsidering policy design: Policies and publics. *Journal of Public Policy, 11*(2), 187–206.

Mueller, K. J. (1988). Federal programs to expire: The case of health planning. *Public Administration Review, 48*(3), 719–725.

Nagelkerk, J. M., & Henry, B. (1991). Leadership through policy research. *Journal of Nursing Administration, 21*(5), 20–24.

Nebraskans for Humane Care Committee. (2006). *Nebraskans for humane care*. Retrieved June 19, 2007, from: www.nehumanecare.com

Outsiders fueled two petition drives. (2006, August 10). *Omaha World Herald*, pp. B1–B2.

Pearson, L. (2003a). Fifteenth annual legislative update. *Nurse Practitioner, 28*(1), 26–58.

Pearson, L. (2003b). NPs stand ready for 2003. *Nurse Practitioner, 28*(1), 8.

Petition restrictions advance. (2007, February 2). *Omaha World Herald*, pp. B1–B2.

Raudonis, B. M., & Griffith, H. (1991). A model for integrating health services, research, and health care policy formation. *Nursing and Health Care, 12*(1), 32–36.

Schneider, A., & Ingram, H. (1991). *The social construction of target populations: Implications for citizenship and democracy*. Paper presented at the annual meeting of the American Political Science Association, Washington, DC.

Schneider, A. L., & Ingram, H. (1993a). How the social construction of target populations contributes to problems in policy design. *Policy Currents, 3*(1), 1–4.

Schneider, A. L., & Ingram, H. (1993b). Social construction of target populations: Implications for politics and policy. *American Political Science Review, 87*(2), 334–347.

Senate approves NIH authorization. (1985, July 27). *Congressional Quarterly*, p. 1493.

Survey probes attitudes on death, dying. (2007, February 5). *Omaha World Herald*, pp. E, 1.

Tilden, V. (1999). Ethics perspective on end-of-life care. *Nursing Outlook, 47*, 162–167.

Warner, J. R. (2003). A phenomenological approach to political competence: Stories of nurse activists. *Policy, Politics, and Nursing Practice, 4*(2), 135–143.

Weissert, C. S., & Weissert, W. G. (2006). *Governing health*. Baltimore: Johns Hopkins University Press.

Government Response: Legislation

Mary Wakefield, PhD, RN, FAAN

Key Terms

➤ **Caucus** An association of members of Congress, a political party, or other group created to advocate a political ideology or a regional or economic interest.

➤ **Constituents** Residents of a geographic area who can vote for a candidate and whom a member of Congress represents.

➤ **Interest group** An organized group with a common cause that works to influence the outcome of laws, regulations, or programs.

➤ **Issue specialists/Policy analysts** A loose network of researchers, academics, and government staff who are knowledgeable about a particular topic and who often discuss ideas and critique or suggest policy solutions.

➤ **Legislative assistant (LA)** An employee of a Senator or Representative who is responsible for keeping the member apprised of legislative proposals, negotiations, and hearings. LAs often draft reports and serve as liaisons among elected and appointed officials. LAs may be politically neutral or partisan advocates of an issue.

➤ **Member** An elected participant of a lawmaking body.

➤ **Staff** Personnel hired to work in an agency, committee, or other organization. These employees carry out the day-to-day business of the office.

Introduction

The purpose of this chapter is to provide advanced practice nurses (APNs) and others with an understanding of the multiple factors that influence the development of public policy through the legislative branch of government. Many of the factors considered in this chapter are operationalized in both state and federal legislative arenas. Consequently, this discussion is relevant to nurses interested in affecting policy in state capitals or the nation's capital.

In today's environment, an understanding and the ability to influence policy development are critically important. The health policy work undertaken in the legislative arena directly or indirectly affects virtually every facet of the APN's work—whether it is the medication one prescribes, the license one holds, the telehealth technology used to access a specialist, or the level of reimbursement received for providing care. Given the pervasive effect of policy on nursing practice, it is imperative that those in advanced practice know how to influence the policy that ultimately affects their practice and their patients.

The policymaking process, in general, and the development of legislation, specifically, can be likened to a murky river that runs its course through many twists and turns. On the surface, the river may appear almost placid, inviting, hardly moving. However, beneath the surface, subtle, then strong currents push and pull, doing much of the work of moving the water and sweeping whatever is within it downstream. This chapter explores some of the currents that are often unseen, yet pivotal, in moving policy initiatives through the legislative process.

The Players

Six general categories of players exert notable influence in the legislative process. Although other categories can be named, individuals in the categories discussed here commonly engage in public health policy development and exert considerable influence throughout the process. The six categories include the following:

1. Member of Congress
2. Congressional staff
3. Special-interest groups and their lobbyists
4. Executive branch
5. Constituents
6. Media

These categories are not listed in order of importance or ability to influence legislation. For example, a powerful lobbyist often can exert far more influence than a freshman member of the House of Representatives, especially if the latter is a member of the minority party. Rather, the influence of individuals from each of these categories ebbs and flows, varying with the policy issue at hand.

Members of Congress

Currently, there are 535 **members** of Congress: 100 senators and 435 representatives. The political party with control of the majority of seats wields considerable influence in significant ways, ranging from setting the legislative agenda to chairing all congressional committees. The identification of problems and possible solutions largely emanates from the political ideology of the party in control. Because of this, statements of belief and priorities expressed by the majority party serve as an important framework for subsequent legislation.

With few exceptions, tradition dictates that members of Congress with the greatest seniority move into positions of influence and are more likely than their junior counterparts to be given the committee assignments they desire. For example, a senior senator from an agricultural state who wishes to obtain a committee assignment on the Agricultural Appropriations Subcommittee is more likely to be given that assignment than is a newly elected senator interested in the same position. Seniority is an important factor in determining who is at the table when key decisions are made by legislative bodies. It comes as no surprise, then, that discussion of the power incumbents wield by virtue of seniority or a committee assignment important to **constituents** back home frequently constitutes a major theme in incumbents' political advertising and campaigning during reelection.

Though there is often a direct relationship between seniority and ability to wield power, personal characteristics tend to influence the degree of attention that members choose to give legislative issues. Some of these personal characteristics include the member's occupation prior to election, the home state or district the member represents, personal experience with the healthcare system, and even the gender and ethnic background of the legislator. Personal factors are important enough that effective lobbyists, such as APNs interested in obtaining the support of a legislator, will have reviewed the legislator's biography before the first meeting occurs.

The significance of these characteristics is readily exemplified. For example, some members of Congress with backgrounds in health care, one a social worker and the other a nurse, are extremely active in a range of health policy initiatives. They frequently draw on their personal experiences in the healthcare field when, in committee meetings or on the floor of the Senate or House, members make a case for the importance of proposed legislation. Clearly, health legislation is not the sole prerogative of legislators who are former healthcare professionals. However, drawing on personal experience, their explanations speak volumes to their less knowledgeable colleagues when critical decisions about complex health legislation are being made. In cases where members have specific healthcare backgrounds, lobbyists will often seek out the guidance or assistance of members whose professional backgrounds are similar to the organizations they represent.

Beyond the professional background of the member, it is not uncommon for lobbyists to know of any ties to health care that the legislator's family may have. For example, knowing that the spouse of a member is a nurse is often useful information to nurse lobbyists, while knowing that an influential senator has a son-in-law who is a chiropractor may be useful information to chiropractic lobbyists. One can assume that, at the very least, such members would be more knowledgeable about these healthcare providers than many of their congressional counterparts. From the perspective of special-interest groups, in the best of all worlds, members with family who have ties to the healthcare field may be favorably predisposed toward policy supportive of similar provider groups.

It is also generally the case that members of Congress reflect the interests of their home district or state. One commonly used strategy is referred to as "earmarking" legislation with descriptions of funding for projects that route resources back to specific projects and places in home districts. This practice is increasing. This priority spending circumvents established federal programs and formulas that determine the allocation of federal funds (Utt, 1999). In addition to routing federal resources explicitly back home, members of Congress also can be found supporting issues seemingly relevant to their home state to negotiate support for their initiatives. For example, a senator from a tobacco-producing state is much more likely to oppose strict regulation of the tobacco industry than is a senator from a non-tobacco-producing state. However, personal phone calls from a senate colleague or a promise to provide support for an initiative important to the non-tobacco-state senator at some future date can often result in support from members who, on the surface, might appear to have no particular interest or stake in tobacco legislation.

Because passage of legislation requires a majority vote, it is quite common for members to "buttonhole" their colleagues on the floor of the Senate or House, at a reception, or by phone at home in the evenings to enlist support or opposition. Likewise, it is not uncommon for members working with lobbyists to target uncommitted members, bringing pressure to bear on them from both inside and outside Congress. Working in tandem with congressional offices, nursing organizations frequently use grassroots efforts, meetings, and other strategies to sway uncommitted policymakers to obtain sufficient support or opposition for proposed legislation.

Even personal experience with the healthcare system can affect a member's views. For example, both Senator Inouye (D-HI) and former Senator Dole (R-KS) underwent lengthy rehabilitation following life-threatening wounds received in battle while serving in the military. Both men often publicly credited the nurses who cared for them with being instrumental in their successful recoveries. Senators with immediate family members with mental illnesses have been staunch advocates of parity in health insurance coverage for this category.

Finally, although the vast majority of members of Congress are white males, there is an increase in ethnically diverse and female legislators elected to office. Although members of Congress are sent to Washington, DC, to represent all of their constituents as well as the interests of the country at large, race and gender are factors that can unify members around policy activities. For example, the Congressional Black **Caucus** is an informal group of black members of the House of Representatives who meet to discuss shared interests. Likewise, female members of Congress have banded together to push for increased federal funding for breast cancer, and male members of Congress have cosigned and circulated letters urging support for prostate cancer research.

Knowledge of these fundamental characteristics and how they may be brought to bear on legislation helps to guide nurse lobbyists who solicit support for policy positions. Although it is important to be familiar with the positions policymakers take on various issues, it is equally important to look for cues as to why they have taken or whether they are likely to take certain positions. Identifying these personal characteristics that extend beyond political party affiliation can help APNs determine how malleable an individual's position may be in the future.

Congressional and Personal Office Staff

Members of Congress employ a number of professional **staff** in their Washington, DC, offices. Over the past 30 years, Congress has greatly expanded the number of staff in response to increasing workloads brought about by the complexity and breadth of policy issues about which members are expected to be knowledgeable. In congressional offices, there is usually a chief of staff or administrative assistant responsible for overseeing the press, political, and public relations activity; directing office and personnel management; and maintaining oversight of the legislative operations. It is not uncommon for this individual to have political ties to the member, perhaps even having served as the campaign manager for the member's election to office.

Congressional offices also have legislative directors who are responsible for day-to-day legislative activities. These individuals tend to have more policy expertise and less political involvement than does the administrative assistant/chief of staff. Offices also have a press operation with at least one press secretary responsible for interacting with the media and disseminating information regarding the member's policy-related activities. The press secretary writes and distributes press releases about the member's work, organizes press conferences, and arranges interviews with media representatives.

Specific legislative work is done by **legislative assistants (LAs)**. Also worth noting is the fact that many offices welcome interns (often college students), fellows (often professionals with expertise in particular fields such as medicine or psychology) who may be participating in policy fellowship programs, or volunteers interested in learning about the legislative process or acquiring policy-related experience. The latter two categories may consist of university faculty, corporate executives, or any number of professionals, including advanced practice nurses.

On the staff of every member of Congress is an LA responsible for health policy. Legislative assistants generally assume responsibility for a number of issues. For example, in one congressional office, an LA may handle health, transportation, and banking while an LA in another congressional office may be responsible for health, welfare, education, and social security. Because of smaller office budgets, there tend to be fewer LAs in the offices of members of the House of Representatives than in the Senate offices. Also, Senate staff tend to receive higher salaries than their House counterparts receive. Senate positions are generally more sought after and are filled with more experienced individuals. The average tenure for legislative assistants is 2 to 3 years, after which many staff capitalize on their Hill experience by moving to higher paying lobbying positions for special-interest groups.

The majority of health LAs are in their mid- to late 20s and, increasingly, are women. Even though legislative assistants are usually extremely influential in terms of crafting legislation, few have an educational background in health care. Nevertheless, because these positions are highly competitive, individuals who fill them are motivated, intelligent, and learn quickly. Given this description, clearly APNs, as their first task, must ascertain the knowledge level of the LA on policy issues of importance to the nursing community. Nurses in advanced practice cannot assume that legislative assistants have even a rudimentary knowledge of the education and practice of the APN. Quite unintentionally, LAs unfamiliar with the scope of practice of these nurses can exclude advanced practice nurses from health-policy initiatives.

As the key health advisor to members of Congress, these staff are influential in a number of ways. Health LAs are responsible for "staffing" members at committee hearings that focus on health policy, often writing the members' statements for them as well as crafting questions to ask witnesses who testify at hearings. Health LAs generally accompany members to meetings with lobbyists or constituents and are responsible for briefing the member prior to the meeting as well as completing any staff work necessary to implement decisions or commitments the member may make during the meeting.

Health LAs may be responsible for writing speeches or drafting letters to the editor of a local newspaper to be submitted under the member's name. LAs (or their assistants, referred to as legislative correspondents) draft responses to constituent letters that will go out under the member's signature. Perhaps most important, the health legislative assistant advises the member on health policy issues. These issues can range from a request for federal support for a health-related research project conducted at a clinic in the member's home state to a request for co-sponsorship of a bill that would increase the utilization of telehealth technology.

The LA's advice may be provided in a briefing memo or verbally to the member. In terms of legislation alone, hundreds of health-related bills are introduced in each session of Congress. It is the LA's responsibility to track those that might be of greatest interest to the member or viable during the session. Because of the tremendous demands on the member's schedule, it is not uncommon to see an LA providing "last-minute" information and advice while accompanying the member to the floor of the Senate for a vote on the health-related bill. It is the LA's responsibility to work with the office referred to as Legislative Council to draft bill language incorporating policy ideas that the member wishes to pursue.

Almost without exception, legislative assistants are pivotal to informing and influencing policymakers. An astute LA provides guidance based on knowledge of how a member's position will likely be greeted by constituents (e.g., nurses in the home state or district may oppose a particular stance while hospital administrators may support it and consumers may not have a strong opinion). This kind of legwork by the health LA is critically important in helping to keep the member informed of positions his or her constituents have and the related risks of antagonizing certain constituencies. Silence on an issue may be interpreted as indifference. Consequently, APNs must make their views known if they are to exert influence on policy initiatives under consideration.

Legislative assistants generally craft initiatives or advise their members based on information the LAs receive, not on personal experience with health care. Consequently, LAs welcome information and recommendations from nurses who are constituents of the member for whom they work. Initiating and maintaining communication with the health LAs of one's congressional delegation enhances the likelihood that an APN will be sought out for policy advice on proposed legislation. The goal of individual APNs and their associations should be to have the LA view them as a content expert and as an available resource for a range of reasons, from eliciting ideas for legislation to critiquing provisions of health-related bills.

Although the health LA in Washington, DC, is a pivotal link, members maintain offices in major cities in their districts or states that are staffed by assistants who serve as conduits of information between the district or state office and the Washington, DC, office. Despite the fact that these offices are readily accessible, they are often underutilized. Staff in local offices have a number of responsibilities, and nurses in advanced practice can access staff for a host of reasons. Requests for a meeting with the member or health LA, information about bills, the member's position on a specific piece of legislation, or an invitation to address a nurses' conference can generally be routed through the local office. Local staff are aware of the member's schedule when back in the district or state and often accompany the member on tours, meetings, and other events. Consequently, staff in local offices can be an excellent resource, are accessible, and are often less harried than their Washington, DC, counterparts.

Committee Staff

In addition to personal staff, Congress employs hundreds of experienced professional staff responsible for supporting the work of congressional committees. Committees generally have separate staff responsible to the majority and the minority committee members, with a smaller number allocated to the minority. Although personal staff are responsible for a wide range of issues (e.g., in addition to nonhealth legislative issues, even within the health portfolio, personal staff may advise on Medicare, Medicaid, NIH appropriations, the Public Health Service, and numerous other federal health programs), committee staff tend to have a narrow focus. For example, on the Senate Finance Committee with jurisdiction over Medicare and Medicaid, one staff member working for the chairperson and majority members may be responsible only for Medicaid.

Generally, committee staff are older than the personal office staff and have significant expertise from either advanced educational degrees or professional experience in the content area for which they are responsible. Previously, committee staff may have worked in personal offices of members of Congress or as lobbyists. Committee staff may also come from or move to federal agencies over which the committee has responsibility. Committee staff that are seasoned in the work of the committee become highly valuable to the committee chair and members and often exert influence directly related to their expertise. Although members of Congress tend to be generalists, responsible for an array of issues, committee staff function as specialists. Because of the depth of knowledge in specific areas, committee staff can usually command high salaries after they leave Capitol Hill.

Committee staff are usually responsible for planning the committee agendas, coordinating hearing schedules and witnesses, and preparing legislation for committee and floor action. They gather and analyze information upon which policy is based and they draft committee reports. They staff the committee chair and ranking member in meetings and when the committee's legislation is considered in the full House or Senate chamber.

Personal office staff interact closely with committee staff, communicating their member's requests related to legislation before the committee. Committee staff tend to be most responsive to requests from their committee members. Consequently, lobbyists will always seek support for legislative provisions from committee members first and only if necessary will seek out the help of other members of Congress to intercede with the committee.

To facilitate moving legislation, the committee staff in one chamber are in frequent contact with their counterparts in the other chamber, working out details and compromises. In fact, "Committee staff are expected to maintain continuous contact with their counterparts on other House and Senate committees, with executive agency officials responsible for programs, and with private sector organizations and groups and knowledgeable staff in the congressional support agencies" (Rundquist, Schneider, & Pauls, 1992, p. 13). Because committees almost always serve as the gateway through which legislation must pass, committee staff are in pivotal positions to influence legislative products.

Special-Interest Groups and Their Lobbyists

Interest groups are defined as "individuals who have organized themselves around some common interest and who seek to influence public policy. . . . They clarify and articulate citizens' preferences, warn policy makers of problems with their proposals, and suggest ways to make them more palatable" (Weissert & Weissert, 1996, p. 102). Lobbyists represent interests ranging from academic institutions to the balloon industry to flight attendants.

With approximately 20,000 lobbyists in Washington, DC (DeVries & Vanderbilt, 1992), it is likely that an APN walking through the halls of a Senate or House office building is passing by individuals who are neither constituents nor members of Congress but, rather, are lobbyists. Furthermore, though congressional offices may be inundated with correspondence from constituents, much of the mail and e-mail delivered to offices is produced by special-interest groups. The mail takes many forms, ranging from study-and-opinion poll results to analysis of a bill to magazines or videotapes presenting policy information. "Lobbying is the art of persuasion—attempting to convince a legislator, a government official, the head of an agency, or a state official to comply with a request" (DeVries & Vanderbilt, p. 1). In addition to sending unsolicited information, it is not uncommon for lobbyists to produce specific data at the request of a congressional office or even to write statements that can be incorporated into speeches given by the member.

In addition to meetings, mailings, conversations with LAs, and other strategies applied locally, lobbyists augment their efforts as necessary with grassroots campaigns; that is, to bring additional pressure to bear on a member, special-interest groups often orchestrate phone and letter campaigns that involve voters from the member's home district or state. When statements, postcards, e-mail messages, or telephone calls convey identical verbatim messages, it quickly becomes clear that the contacts are organized. However, volume often matters, regardless of whether the message appears organized or not. It is common for members to inquire about the number of letters and phone calls coming in that support or oppose a particular piece of legislation.

Regarding congressional and presidential elections, it is important to note that many special-interest groups exert influence through political action committees (PACs). For example, in 1974 the American Nurses Association established a PAC "to support candidates who share ANA's views on health care quality and access issues and to advance nursing's political agenda." The American Nurses Association Political Action Committee (ANA-PAC) is the campaign funding arm of the ANA. "The purpose of ANA-PAC is to assist candidates who are friends of nursing win elections for federal office, thus increasing the number of federally elected officials who understand and support the ANA's policy agenda" (Malone, Chaffee, & Wachter, 2002, p. 632). The ANA-PAC amasses contributions from ANA members and converts them into financial support for political candidates.

Special-interest groups with shared views often combine resources through temporary coalitions to wield greater influence. For example, in 1997 more than 10 nurse organizations worked together to track legislative proposals related to graduate medical education. Within the profession, the nursing community must speak with a unified voice. To induce policymakers to act, not only must the message be communicated to them, it must be consistent. Strategies employed by coalitions include meeting with members and/or LAs with a few representatives of the coalition and sending letters that are signed by multiple associations. These strategies convey broad support and not infrequently represent hundreds of thousands of members of associations.

It is not uncommon to find organizations coalescing around one policy issue and assuming opposing positions on another policy issue. It is vital that APNs learn to focus on issues and not take it personally if a person or group is supportive on one issue and not on another. The APN must recognize that an opponent in one circumstance may be an essential ally in another.

The Executive Branch

Even though regulatory agencies are dealt with elsewhere, it is important for APNs to note that considerable interaction occurs formally and informally between the legislative and executive branches of government and, consequently, the latter merits mention in the development of legislation. A few examples readily highlight this relationship. During the appropriations process, heads of federal agencies appear at appropriations committee and subcommittee hearings to present the administration's funding proposals for the coming fiscal year. For example, the head of the National Institute for Nursing Research appears before both the House and Senate Appropriations Subcommittees for Labor, Health and Human Services, and Education and related agencies. The testimony presented generally highlights major initiatives under way as well as activities that are being planned.

Frequently, the agency head is knowledgeable of particular issues of concern to committee members, in particular the chairperson. For example, if the chair is known to have a special interest in mental health, references will be made to planning, implementation, evaluation, or research of any programs in that area. Although these hearings are often poorly attended by committee members, and the development of proposed funding levels may be well under way prior to the hearing, it is nevertheless an important opportunity for federal agency representatives to use this forum to bring their cases to both the Congress as well as the public because the work of federal agencies is not automatically embraced (Gray, Gusmano, & Collins, 2003).

Informally, there is significant contact between members, congressional staff, and agency officials. This contact is frequent in cases where the executive branch and members are of the same political party affiliation and between the executive branch and House and Senate leadership offices and chairs of congressional committees. Requests for information and negotiation on legislative proposals are common interactions. Likewise, although relatively few invitations can be filled, federal agency heads often will be invited by the member to the home state or district for tours, conferences, and other events. Appointed officials generally are accompanied by members of the congressional delegation, and their visits are often related to federal policy that has local implications. For example, the head of the Centers for Medicare and Medicaid Services (CMS) has attended public meetings in the home districts of the cochairs of the House Rural Healthcare Coalition to hear concerns about perceived Medicare payment inadequacy in those rural regions.

Constituents

Opinions may be held that Washington politicians are "bought and paid for" by special interests and, in truth, special interests can wield tremendous influence. Ultimately, voters send individuals to Washington, DC, and voters can replace them. Much of the legislation considered in the nation's capital is debated without stirring considerable interest by most constituents. However, in circumstances where it appears that a proposal may negatively affect constituents, informed consumers may be quick to respond. The Medicare Modernization Act (MMA), legislation that enacted sweeping healthcare reform, is one illustration. Typically the purview of healthcare providers and other special-interest groups, this legislation prompted a widespread reaction. Senior citizen groups, family advocacy organizations, and others all had opinions about the proposal and freely expressed their views to elected representatives.

Most members of Congress go to great efforts to stay informed regarding the views of their constituents. Even members who represent states at great distances from Washington, DC, make frequent trips home to meet with individuals and participate in local activities. Likewise, major newspapers from the area a policymaker represents serve as an extremely important source of information about views back home. Even letters to the editor that reflect policy concerns are usually scanned by appropriate staff. Talk radio shows may be monitored on occasion by district or state staff to learn the views of individuals who call in as well as the program guests.

Although the average voter's view is important, a professional with expertise and knowledge of a particular issue often brings added value to the message. Consequently, advanced practice nurses who serve as resources, highlight health problems affecting constituent groups, and propose policy solutions can be very effective with their own congressional delegation. In communicating with members or their staff, providing national data that describe the problem is helpful (e.g., projected shortages of registered nurses). However, members are most interested in descriptive information about the impact of a problem on the constituents they represent. Presented in conjunction with data, an anecdote about the effect of a particular problem helps to illustrate its significance.

Generally, there is no better source of information on health policy concerns than healthcare professionals who reside in a member's home district or state. Although health issues deliberated by Congress are national in scope, members of Congress place a high priority on protecting and promoting the health and welfare of their constituents. Consequently, an APN's opinion matters.

Nurses are most powerful when their elected representatives serve on committees with jurisdiction over health programs. That is, on any particular legislative proposal, nurses may be much more influential in one state than in another, depending on their representatives' committee assignments.

The Media

An APN may be surprised by the activity under way early in the morning in most congressional offices. Walking past staff desks, many individuals can be found taking a few moments to review articles online from morning newspapers published in the home state or district. Legislative assistants commonly review articles relevant to their issue portfolio at the same time that constituents are reading their local newspapers over breakfast.

One of the first tasks of the day in the member's local office is to review and fax all newsworthy articles to the Washington, DC office. These articles are then packaged by the press staff and distributed to legislative assistants. Likewise, the member is frequently provided with a packet of articles drawn from home state newspapers to review. It is not uncommon to find staff in local offices responsible for videotaping local evening news shows and reviewing them for information that may be useful to the congressional office.

Using these mechanisms, staff stay well informed about which issues are highlighted in the press and how they are reported. The media, then, serve as an important conduit of information and opinion. Furthermore, news stories often serve as the catalyst for policy-related initiatives. Stories that focus on negative outcomes of medical errors have prompted significant legislation designed to address the identified problems. In addition to influencing policy, congressional members invest significant time in communicating directly or through their press secretaries with the media back home. Press releases are faxed to media outlets, and videotape of the member is fed back to television stations in the hope that a position taken or a vote cast will become a positive story on the local evening news or in the next morning paper.

Therefore, the media can serve as both a catalyst for legislative initiatives and also as a means of communicating to constituents about legislative activity. The information presented by the press influences not just the public but policymakers and their staffs as well. This important function is one that can be capitalized on by knowledgeable nurses who use the media to express their views about particular health issues. It is important to note that when health-related stories run in the press and the stories do not reference nurses, the profession is invisible to both the public and policymakers. Often, views expressed by large numbers of individuals will have greater impact on policymakers than those that are expressed by a few. This simple principle underscores the importance of widespread engagement by nurses in advanced practice in the policy development process. Although many voices, using various channels and strategies, are heard by policymakers and their staff, strength in communicating a message comes from a chorus of voices clearly articulating the problem and proposing policy solutions.

The Process

Although expert nurses need to know who the major stakeholders are in policy development, they also must know how the policymaking process works and what strategies can be used to influence the product of this process. Just as healthcare providers have a common lexicon, individuals interested in public policy must understand terms and processes commonly used. Although entire textbooks are written describing in detail facets of the policymaking process, the purpose of this section is to facilitate an understanding of a few selected aspects of it.

Legislation may be introduced at any time that the House or Senate is in session. Proposed legislation is termed a bill until it is passed in identical form by both the House and the Senate and is either signed by the president or becomes law without the president's signature. Hundreds of bills are often introduced in the first few days of a legislative session and may be offered through the final hours prior to adjournment, resulting in about 5000 bills introduced annually (DeVries & Vanderbilt, 1992). Bills are assigned numbers in the order in which they are introduced during the congressional session. Once introduced in the House or Senate chamber, the bill is then referred to the committee with jurisdiction over the substance of the bill.

Complicating consideration of a bill are referrals that are made to multiple committees. This occurs when different provisions of the bill are the purview of different committees. For example, a bill that includes public health service programs as well as malpractice provisions may be considered by both the Senate Judiciary Committee and the Committee on Health, Education, Labor, and Pensions. APNs must note that significant health policy is often developed in committees not thought of as having jurisdiction over health programs. For example, the Agriculture Appropriations Committee funds the Food and Drug Administration of the Department of Health and Human Services. Knowing the committee of jurisdiction is important to target members with the most influence over the bill.

There are three general types of committees in Congress: oversight, appropriations, and authorization committees. Each merits a brief description. Oversight committees do not act on legislation. Instead, they hold hearings to illuminate issues related to the committee focus. For example, the Senate Special Committee on Aging does not act on legislation related to the aged. However, it does play an active role in examining issues related to the elderly that can help inform members. For example, this committee may hold a hearing on the use of multiple prescription medications by nursing home residents or compromised quality in long-term care. Recommendations by individuals testifying before the committee could eventually be incorporated into bills considered by other health committees.

Authorizing committees are responsible for establishing or making changes in federal programs as well as setting a limit on the amount of federal funding that can be spent to implement the particular program. Most federal programs are evaluated by the committee of jurisdiction through a reauthorization process that usually occurs every 3 to 5 years. The time frame for evaluation is set in the authorizing legislation. Generally, bills authorizing the establishment or continuation of a federal program are enacted before money is appropriated to support the particular program. For example, the Nurse Education Act is authorizing legislation that established the Division of Nursing. At established time intervals, this law is reevaluated by the committees of jurisdiction. If agreement cannot be reached on provisions in reauthorizing legislation, a federal program such as the Division of Nursing may be allowed to continue without the benefit of current authorization. When this situation occurs, it is often viewed as problematic. For example, an unauthorized program can be more susceptible to decreased funding or even elimination.

Appropriations committees are responsible for allocating federal funding on a fiscal year basis to support programs. Membership on these "purse-string" committees is often highly sought because the committee can serve as a conduit of funds to support programs important to constituents back home. For example, a legislator from a farm state will often seek membership on the Agriculture Appropriations Committee, an assignment of significant importance to constituents back home. Appropriations bills originate in the House, and funding levels may not exceed the ceilings established by the authorizing legislation. Likewise, the appropriations committee may choose to fund a particular program at a level significantly below that set by the authorizing committee. Although appropriations bills should only address funding levels, it is not uncommon for members of Congress to insert provisions that "authorize on an appropriations bill." This means that members may make significant programmatic changes by including related legislative language in appropriations bill that should be reserved for authorizing bills.

The appropriations process is an annual event, and fiscal year (FY) funding begins on October 1 and ends on September 30 of every year. A fiscal year is identified by the prefix "FY" followed by the last two digits of the ending year. For example, U.S. government FY08 means that the funding year began October 1, 2007, and ended September 30, 2008. Determining funding levels can be especially arduous when the executive branch and the legislative branch are controlled by members of different political parties with differing views about the importance of various programs, for example, funding for defense versus funding for health care. As a result, it is not uncommon for Congress to fund federal programs after the start of the fiscal year through bills called "continuing resolutions" until such a time as the appropriations bills are finalized.

Of hundreds of bills that may be referred to an authorizing committee in any given legislative session, committee chairs determine which will be considered by the committee. For those bills that are considered, hearings usually are held to obtain information from individuals or organizations with interest in the legislation. This information is referred to as testimony and may be presented verbally during the hearing or in written form. Individuals wishing to comment on a particular bill may forward their views directly to the committee. However, communication can be most effective when a member of one's congressional delegation serves on the committee and constituents share their views with that elected representative.

Following committee consideration, bills may be "reported out," which means sent to the floor of the Senate or House for a vote. Both chambers must act on proposed legislation for a bill ultimately to be enacted into law. After a vote by each chamber, successful bills are forwarded to a conference committee composed of members from both the Senate and the House. This committee is responsible for negotiating any differences in the bills as they were passed by the two chambers. Although the conference committee is not allowed to introduce new provisions for consideration at this point in the process, such action does occur on occasion.

Finally, successful bills are reported out of the conference committee and final votes are cast by both the full Senate and the full House. With congressional work completed, the bill is forwarded to the president for signature and, thereby, is enacted into law. This brief description highlights some of the main events in the process of enacting legislation. Although there are nuances and considerable complexity not reflected in this description, understanding the basic processes is integral to nurses who wish to influence the policymaking process.

With the legislative process in mind, specific strategies that may be effective in influencing the process merit consideration. Nurse involvement in political and policymaking activity can consist of a range of activities along a continuum from paid membership in a nursing organization that has an active government relations department to running for elective office. The question for APNs today is not whether to become involved in influencing policy, but rather, how and to what extent each nurse expert will operationalize his or her involvement. A menu of activities is described in the remainder of this chapter, most of which can be conducted without ever traveling to Washington, DC.

Research

Concrete efforts should be made by individual nurses and professional associations to link health policy with the activities in which nurses are involved. For example, when relevant, the policy implications of nursing research should be delineated, whether the research is a master's thesis or a study conducted by a seasoned nurse researcher.

Too frequently, health policy is developed without the benefit of research-based knowledge. Nurses producing or even just reviewing research can help inform public health policy by linking findings to policy initiatives. Even though APNs find it important to share research findings with colleagues through professional journals, other equally important audiences for much of nursing research are consumers and policymakers. APNs may themselves be researchers, but equally important is the role of translating research findings to meaningfully inform public health policy. The role of **issue specialist** or **policy analyst** may be new for the APN, but is critical as nurse researchers scrutinize problems and dissect solutions with government staff and academics.

For example, research findings described in a Centers for Disease Control and Prevention report may be useful to help illustrate a concern of a public health nurse. Furthermore, citing such findings in correspondence to a policymaker and in a letter to the editor of a local newspaper are useful strategies for informing both the public and policymakers. As data accumulate, policymakers become increasingly aware of problems and their potential solutions, whether these data are numbers of uninsured persons or increasing costs associated with home health care. Based on data, policy may be revised to more effectively address particular problems.

Using every available opportunity, advanced practice nurses need to conduct and present research so that it serves the public and influences the development of sound public policy. Beyond individual nurses, nurse organizations also give voice to the work of nurse researchers and disseminate relevant findings to policymakers.

Putting Issues in Context

Most health policy initiatives are designed to address a triad of concerns that includes cost, access, and quality. For example, concerns regarding increasing costs of prescription drugs and decreasing access to drug therapy for Medicare beneficiaries put this provision in the centerpiece of Medicare reform legislation introduced in 2003. APNs interested in getting an issue on the policy agenda need to consider and package their issue in the context of cost, access, and/or quality.

Ideally, the proposed policy can be depicted as part of a solution to one or more of these major catalysts for healthcare policy. This is especially true when the policy sought appears to primarily benefit APNs. For example, the expansion of Medicare reimbursement for all nurse practitioners included in the Balanced Budget Act of 1997 lent itself to being described as a mechanism for increasing access of the elderly to healthcare providers in underserved urban, as well as rural, areas. Health legislative assistants considering legislative proposals almost always view requests in two ways. First, what is the impact of the proposal on the interest group or individual requesting legislative change? Second, and more important, what is the impact of the proposal on the public's health? The policy recommendation may well meet the needs of both groups. For example, when flight attendants lobbied for a ban on smoking on all domestic flights, their actions were designed to benefit the members of their profession. However, the ban also limited exposure to smoke by nonsmoking passengers. When interacting with policymakers, the benefits that may be derived from a legislative proposal by constituents back home or the broader public need to be thoroughly described.

APNs can be most effective when they take positions on issues that are priority concerns for segments of the public. For example, if domestic violence and teenage smoking are community concerns, nurses should engage in discussing elements of the problem as well as proposing solutions. Being in touch with and responding to the health concerns of the community is no different from responding to the needs of a patient. Applying the APN's expertise to community concerns, whether the health concerns emanate from the local chapter of the American Association of Retired Persons (AARP) or the business community, results in two important benefits. Nurses' expertise contributes to the health of the community as well as to increasing the visibility of the profession.

Visibility

To increase the likelihood that policymakers will incorporate nurses' views into health policy initiatives, APNs need to ensure that their views are visible. For example, at health-related events where the media, policymakers, and the public meet, APNs also need to be represented. Nurses can bring informed opinions to most discussions regarding health care, whether the topic is health professions workforce trends in a state or the health problems of school-age children. Using public forums, whether it is a city council meeting or a town meeting held by a member of one's congressional delegation, nurses in advanced practice should use these important opportunities to educate the public and policymakers about both the topic discussed as well as the role of the APN. Only by capitalizing on and creating new opportunities that enhance the visibility of the profession will nurses increasingly be viewed as content experts, better represented in news stories, and more readily incorporated into policy initiatives.

Effective Communication

To be effective in their work, nurses need to be adept at tailoring their communications in ways that will be readily understood. Nurses are very effective at conveying information, whether the audience is a 15-year-old or an 85-year-old, a high school dropout or a nuclear physicist. Communication with policymakers, whether oral or written, also needs to be targeted and free of terminology unique to medicine and nursing. With multiple competing requests and demands, messages conveyed in the jargon of the discipline frequently are lost on policymakers too busy to seek clarification or not sufficiently clear on the merits of the issue.

Because scores of problems are competing for the attention of members and staff at any point in time, how nurses present an issue is critically important. Identifying one's expertise with the issue is the first place to start. In both written and oral communications, nurse experts first must briefly describe their education and experience. This is an opportunity to educate the policymaker about the work and expertise of APNs and also convey the fact that the information being shared is grounded in professional experience.

In addition, the relevance of the issue to individuals beyond nursing should be identified. Providing information regarding the impact of the issue on the member's constituents enhances the likelihood that the policymaker will act. All information that is presented must be accurate. Credibility and interest are quickly lost when lobbyists or constituents oversell or inaccurately depict a particular problem. Advanced practice nurses need to convey information in an organized, thorough, and concise form that reflects data when available and uses anecdotes that clearly illustrate the concern.

Written Communication

Individuals write letters to policymakers to express opinions, acknowledge the member's work either positively or negatively, follow up on meetings or phone calls, or share knowledge about a particular problem and recommend policy solutions. A few rules should guide the development of correspondence. First, e-mail is the common communication vehicle. Because of screening procedures in place to prevent substances such as anthrax from reaching congressional offices, mail can take weeks to be delivered.

Whether mail or e-mail is used, correspondence should be no longer than two pages and focused on one or two issues at most. The purpose of the correspondence should be stated at the beginning. Compelling rationale for the writer's concern or position on an issue must be clearly presented. If the purpose of the letter is to express disappointment regarding a stance on an issue or a vote that has been cast, the letter should be as positive as possible. Conversely, writing letters thanking a member for taking a particular position on an issue and public acknowledgment of the policymaker's work is very important. A letter to the editor of the local newspaper or a nursing newsletter lauding a member's position (with a copy forwarded to the member) is welcome publicity, especially during an election year.

Letters should always be sent following meetings or even conversations that occurred in passing at large events. Correspondence should include a reiteration of the major points covered in person as well as answers to questions that were raised during the course of the conversation. Business cards should be included and the member and staff encouraged to contact the APN or the professional association for further information.

Oral Communication

Regardless of whether a meeting is held in the member's Washington, DC, office or at a healthcare facility, the first question to raise is to determine the amount of time the staff or member is able to allocate. Too frequently, constituents engage in small talk at the beginning of the conversation only to find out that additional appointments have been added to the schedule or a vote on the floor is imminent. Also, the time available needs to be structured so that the issue can be succinctly presented followed by an opportunity for the staff or member to seek clarification or raise questions.

The APN must not assume that the staff or member is as well informed on the issue as the nurse. Given the scores of policy concerns ranging from foreign affairs to transportation, members cannot keep abreast of every policy concern. If the meeting concludes and confusion exists regarding important aspects of the issue, the chance of a policymaker acting on the information is markedly diminished. To help ensure understanding, a one-page summary that underscores key points should be provided at the conclusion of every meeting.

Finally, in letters and in meetings, numbers count. Noting that the views expressed are shared by a local nurses' organization, nurses employed at a healthcare facility, or even better, the numbers represent concerns of a coalition of groups brings added clout to an issue.

Advanced practice nurses should not hesitate to invite members and their staff to conferences, meetings of nurses' organizations, or tours of nursing education or clinical facilities. The likelihood that the member will incorporate the request into a scheduled trip back home increases markedly when the policymakers are told that they will have the opportunity to meet with large numbers of nurses, patients, and/or other constituents. Also, if appropriate, invite the media and let the member know. If a member or his or her staff are unable to accept one invitation, do not hesitate to send future invitations. The likelihood of acceptance can increase with the size of the audience and proximity to an upcoming election.

Eleven Lessons Learned from Nine Years on Capitol Hill

After serving as a legislative assistant to one U.S. Senator and as chief of staff to three Senators, this author left "The Hill" in 1996. Since then, she has served on multiple health committees that are advisory to either the U.S. Congress, executive branch agencies, or both. The following are prescriptions for other nurses in advanced practice who choose to engage actively in the exciting, rewarding, and frequently stressful world of public health policy.

1. You can gain a lot by giving a little. Within a few years of graduating from my baccalaureate nursing program, I became very involved in my state nurses' association. The opportunities available through membership in a professional association allowed me to build communication and leadership skills, increase my knowledge about a range of professional issues, and expand and strengthen my professional network. Serving on committees and in elected positions provided an opportunity for real-world application for much of what I learned in my formal education.

2. A lot of what you can accomplish does depend on who you know. In my view, although financial support for campaigns in Washington, DC, does enhance access to policymakers, the real currency in the nation's capital is relationships. Furthermore, nurses need to build relationships, not just within the profession, but also with representatives of public and private sector organizations with an interest in health care.

3. Politicians pay attention to numbers. Even though I witnessed the difference one well-connected voice could make in terms of influencing a policy decision, in general, the more broad based the pressure that is brought to bear, the more likely a policymaker will respond. Twenty letters or phone calls supporting a particular

position can be much more effective than two at capturing the attention of a legislator.

4. You have to get off the porch to run with the big dogs. This phrase was often repeated by one of my employers during my tenure on Capitol Hill. It is highly unlikely that a health legislative assistant or policymaker will call an advanced practice nurse and ask whether he or she can meet to discuss issues in which APNs have an interest. It is equally unlikely to find a legislative assistant on Capitol Hill poring through a nursing journal to get new ideas about health problems and solutions from nursing's perspective. If APNs want to be sought out as resources and have their views reflected in health policy debates and decisions, they must deliberately set out to build the foundation for involvement in public policy.

5. Occasionally other people really do know what's better for you than you know yourself. Early on in my work on Capitol Hill, I was encouraged to participate in political activities outside of the office. Initially, I resisted the offer, believing that I could accomplish what I needed to and expand my knowledge base by focusing just on health legislation—a policy purist, if you will. Very quickly I recognized that broader experiences would enhance the quality of work in which I was engaged and have application in other arenas. For example, after involvement with two congressional campaigns, I amassed significant knowledge about polling, the media, working with different national organizations, communicating messages, and even marketing a product—in these cases, U.S. Senators. Virtually everything learned has been transferable and useful in other facets of my professional career.

6. Knowledge helps to build bridges. We need to continue to expand both our depth and breadth. In the world of health care and health policy, I learned that one cannot just engage in "nurse speak." Parochial concerns often appear self-serving. To help others view a nursing issue as important, I needed to be able to articulate how nursing was part of a solution to an important health policy problem. It became clear that nurses need to be aware of what is going on in health care, well beyond the environment and the practice in which they work. Being well-informed across a range of health-related issues allowed me to converse more readily with policymakers, business leaders, and consumer advocates; that is, others did not have to engage me on nursing's turf regarding nursing issues. Rather, I had a knowledge base from which I could reach out and find common concerns and interests as points of departure for discussion.

7. Wear your profession like a badge of honor. Of the hundreds of individuals with whom I interacted while I was on Capitol Hill, very

few were unaware that I was a nurse. In fact, when introducing me as his chief of staff, the last senator for whom I worked always pointed out that I had a doctorate in nursing. I firmly believe that it was important to the profession that my nurse identity—and the associated education and expertise—was recognized as part and parcel of my policy work. At the same time, most of my peers were lawyers or political science majors. Being different helped me establish a separate identity that, because of its uniqueness in the policy arena, helped people to remember me and the profession from which I hailed. It is important that people know that nurses are capable of functioning in many different roles and making substantial contributions. Ultimately, my nursing experience turned out to be a strength, not a handicap. Though I had to learn the policymaking process, confidence came from knowing the health issues for which policy was being developed.

8. Blow up a bridge only if you're sure you'll never need to cross there again. Partisan politics have fueled highly publicized gridlock and hostility. However, this approach to conducting "the people's business" has been roundly criticized. Ideally, at the end of the day policymakers typically sit down and negotiate compromises. Congress is a prime example of a group of people with very different views who must work together to accomplish agreed-upon objectives. Initial inflexibility generally gives way to negotiate agreements on issues. Throughout the process of working on contentious issues, it became clear that if an organization or another member of Congress would not join in on one issue of importance, he or she may be the critical player on another. Consequently, the bridge burned behind you may have provided, on another occasion, the only route to getting you where you want to go.

9. There is no advantage to being a wallflower. Initially, I often had to resist the primordial "flight" response at receptions, meetings with international dignitaries, and experts across a range of fields. I eventually convinced myself that most individuals were friendly and all of them were interesting. What was most helpful was finding a standard "icebreaker" to use. Mine was simply "Hello, I don't believe that we've met. My name is . . . and I work for. . . ." The worst that could come of this opener is a response such as "Well, in fact, we have met."

10. If you have expertise—share it. As a neophyte in the policy arena, I cast a wide net in search of nurses and others who were willing to take a few minutes to answer my questions and provide counsel. Lending a hand to nurses coming up after us benefits all of us—and, although these willing mentors may never have thought that I could someday provide assistance in return, they were nevertheless generous with both their time and assistance.

11. If you need expertise—seek it out. For nurses new to the policy arena in local communities, state capitols, or the nation's capital, guidance and support can come from many people of diverse backgrounds. Accomplished people, nurses and non-nurses alike, are often the same individuals who value mentoring others. In the process of seeking or providing support, using strategies to nurture relationships leaves lasting impressions. A quick note of congratulations or a well-timed phone call were efforts made by some of the busiest people with whom I came in contact.

Conclusion

Public concern typically puts health care in the top set of domestic problems facing the nation. With this level of attention, public policy in the health arena is an important vehicle for influencing professional nursing practice as well as the health of individuals, families, and communities.

With an understanding of the players and factors that can influence the policymaking process, APNs can play a pivotal role in shaping the future of health care. Advance practice nurses can capitalize on the favorable attitudes of the U.S. public toward the profession not the least of which are survey findings that indicate that a significant majority of adults (63%) believe that one important factor in improving quality of care is to expand the role for nurses and have doctors and nurses work as a team (Schoen, How, Weinbaum, Craig, & Davis, 2006).

At the start of the 21st century, competition for resources is serious and the need to find new solutions to complex problems is great. When policymakers acknowledge problems, potential solutions are identifiable, and when favorable political circumstances exist, a window of opportunity opens, although often only briefly (Longest, 1998). In this dynamic, when nurses in advanced practice communicate their contributions (i.e., solutions) to increased quality, enhanced access, and decreased cost of health services (i.e., problems), health policymakers should be responsive. Knowledge coupled with action can help to ensure that responsiveness.

Discussion Points and Activities

1. Describe the role of legislative assistants for health. Discuss how relationships between APNs and LAs can be developed and why such relationships are important.
2. Explain the significance of media to public health policy and the nursing profession.

3. Contrast appropriations committees with authorizing committees and describe their roles in the formulation of health policy.
4. Explain the following statement: APNs can enhance the likelihood of influencing health legislation when they advocate a specific concern couched within a broad health policy context.

References

DeVries, C., & Vanderbilt, M. (1992). *The grassroots lobbying handbook.* Washington, DC: American Nurses Association.

Gray, B. H., Gusmano, M. K., & Collins, S. R. (2003). AHCPR and the changing politics of health services research: Lessons from the falling and rising political fortunes of the nation's leading health services. *Health Affairs—Web Exclusive.* Retrieved June 19, 2007, from: http://content.healthaffairs.org/cgi/reprint/hlthaff.w3.283v1 .pdf

Longest, B. B., Jr. (1998). *Health policymaking in the United States* (2nd ed.). Chicago: Health Administration Press.

Malone, P. S., Chaffee, M. W., & Wachter, M. B. (2002). *Policy and politics in nursing and health care: The power and influence of special interest groups in health care* (4th ed.). St. Louis, MO: Saunders.

Rundquist, P., Schneider, J., & Pauls, F. (1992, January 24). *Congressional staff: An analysis of their roles, functions, and impacts.* Congressional Research Service Report for Congress. Washington, DC: Congressional Research Service, Library of Congress.

Schoen, C., How, S., Weinbaum, I., Craig, J., & Davis, K. (2006). *Public views on shaping the future of the U.S. health system.* New York: Commonwealth Fund. Available online at: www.cmwf.org/usr_doc/schoen_publicviewsfuturehltsystem_948.pdf

Utt, R. (1999, April). *How congressional earmarks and porkbarrel spending undermine state and local decision-making.* Washington, DC: Heritage Foundation.

Weissert, C., & Weissert, W. (1996). *Governing health.* Baltimore: Johns Hopkins University Press.

Government Regulation: Parallel and Powerful

Jacqueline M. Loversidge, MS, RN, C

Key Terms

- ➤ **Board of nursing** A state government administrative agency charged with the power and duty to enforce the laws and regulations governing the practice of nursing in the interest of public protection.
- ➤ **Certification** A form of voluntary credentialing that denotes validation of competency in a specialty area with permission to use a title.
- ➤ *Federal Register* A daily publication of the federal government that contains current executive orders, presidential proclamations, rules and regulations, proposed rules, notices, and sunshine act meetings.
- ➤ **Interstate compact** The legal agreement between states to recognize the license of another state to allow for practice between states. The compact must be passed by the state legislature and implemented by the board of nursing.
- ➤ **Licensure** A form of credentialing whereby permission is granted by a legal authority to do an act that would without such permission be illegal, a trespass, a tort, or otherwise not allowable.
- ➤ **Lobbying** The act of influencing a governmental entity to achieve a specific legislative or regulatory outcome.
- ➤ **Multistate regulation** The provision that allows a profession to be practiced in more than one state based on a single license.

➤ **Mutual recognition** A method of multistate regulation in which boards of nursing voluntarily agree to enter into an interstate compact allowing the state to recognize and honor the license issued by the other state.

➤ **Prescriptive authority** Legal authority to prescribe drugs and therapeutic devices, usually within a practice-specific formulary.

➤ **Professional self-regulation** Voluntary process of compliance to a set of moral, ethical, and professional standards agreed to by a profession.

➤ **Public hearings** Meetings held by state or federal administrative agencies for the purpose of receiving testimony from witnesses who support or oppose regulations or to receive expert testimony.

➤ **Recognition (official recognition)** A form of credentialing that denotes a government authority has ratified or confirmed credentials of an individual.

➤ **Registration** A form of credentialing that denotes enrolling or recording the name of a qualified individual on an official roster by an agency of government.

➤ **Regulation** Governing or directing according to a rule, or bringing under the control of a constituted authority, such as the state or federal government.

➤ **Rules/Regulations** Orders that outline methods of procedure issued by government to operationalize a law.

Introduction

Regulation of the U.S. healthcare delivery system and the healthcare providers who practice within the system is complex. Much of the complexity is attributable to the vastness of the industry, the manner of financing health care, and the proliferation of laws and regulations that govern practice and reimbursement in the interest of public welfare.

This chapter focuses on the major concepts of the regulation of health professionals with emphasis on advanced practice nurses (APNs). Understanding the process of **licensure** and credentialing and its impact on the practice of advanced practice nursing is fundamental to practicing as a competent practitioner. Understanding the regulation of the healthcare system empowers the APN to advocate on behalf of the profession and consumers of health care.

Regulation versus Legislation

The legislative process is one approach to governance. A parallel, yet equally powerful approach is the regulatory process. Together, laws and regulations shape the way public policy is implemented. It is important for the APN to understand both processes and know how to influence each process. Major differences between the two processes are described here.

Laws are promulgated and passed by the legislative branch of government (Congress at the federal level or the state legislature for state laws) and establish the framework and authority base for the regulatory process. Once passed, laws must be implemented by administrative agencies (the executive branch) of government. Laws are written using broad language to provide for flexibility and adaptability in application of the law over time. The administrative agency charged with implementing the law promulgates *regulations* and/or *rules* (terms used interchangeably with the same meaning) that amplify the law describing how the administrative agency will implement the law.

> EXAMPLE: One provision in the nurse practice act provides that a duty of the **board of nursing** is to examine, license, and renew the license of duly qualified individuals. The regulations amplifying that provision of law specify the criteria for eligibility, application procedures, and how and when examinations are conducted.

It is important to note that regulations may never exceed the parameters of the statute they intend to amplify; however, both statute and regulation have the force and effect of law.

The first step in establishing a new law or revising an existing law begins with the introduction of a bill by a legislator or group of legislators (sponsor) during a legislative session. The sponsor may introduce legislation to address an issue or concern of his or her constituents. Also, an administrative agency may seek a legislative sponsor to modify its practice act for a variety of reasons. The bill must be passed during the legislative session in which it is introduced or it "dies" and must then be reintroduced in a subsequent session.

Legislators may amend bills at any time during the legislative process. Amendments may be made to a bill during several points of review: during a subcommittee hearing, a full committee hearing, on the floor of the House or Senate, or in a conference committee. Amendments may be favorable to the sponsor and constituency, or they may be unfavorable as a result of political maneuvering. Some amendments may change the intent of the original bill. There is always risk involved when bills are up for discussion and debate. For example, provisions in nurse practice acts may be changed through passage of a bill that affects another healthcare law or a statewide budget bill. It is important for the APN to monitor a bill throughout the legislative process and exert influence for positive outcomes. It is equally important for the APN to be aware of any legislation that may influence practice and the interests of healthcare consumers.

Regulations, on the other hand, can be promulgated at any time during the year by an administrative agency. The time frame for implementation of the regulation varies according to the administrative procedures act (APA) of the state, but generally the regulation becomes effective within 30 to 90 days of publication of the final regulation. Regulations may be amended by the issuing agency based on public input prior to the publication of the final regulation. The administrative agency promulgating the regulation has discretion in determining what amendments, if any, are made; however, public comment may be very influential in determining the final outcome.

Health Professions Regulation and Licensing

Definitions and Purpose of Regulation

Regulation, as defined in *Black's Law Dictionary*, means "the act or process of controlling by rule or restriction" (Garner, 2004, p. 1311). Health professions regulation provides for an ongoing monitoring and maintenance of an acceptable standard of practice for the professions in the interest of public welfare.

Regulation is needed to protect the public because of the technical complexity of the healthcare system. Diversity in educational credentialing, proliferation of types of providers, lack of public information about competency of healthcare providers, and the bundling of healthcare services make it difficult for the public to understand and evaluate options. The public trusts that every healthcare provider is competent to perform the duties assigned, particularly those who are licensed or registered by a state authority. Because the secondary harm that can come to an individual by an incompetent provider may be life threatening, a major role of the regulatory agency is to ensure the public safety. In addition, the regulatory process provides the public a forum to resolve complaints against healthcare providers (Sheets, 1996).

The laws (statutes) that credential and govern a profession are called *practice acts*. The practice act generally includes sections governing practice, education and credentialing, licensure and **certification**, disciplinary action, and continuing education, the composition and scope of authority of its governing board, and its rule-making authority. Accompanying regulations (rules) specify the details related to initial licensing requirements, standards for acceptable practice, disciplinary procedures, and standards for continuing education. Some states regulate both continuing education and competence; because continuing competence is difficult to measure, however, many states focus on the more measurable outcome of continuing education.

The regulatory process clarifies and amplifies enabling statutes and defines the methods that the governing authority will use to enforce an existing law. Regulations cannot be promulgated by an administrative agency without the expressed intent of a law. Silence of the law on an issue cannot be presumed to be the will of the legislature. When there is no prior statutory authority or legislative precedent to address an issue, the legislative process must be initiated.

> EXAMPLE: An APN petitions the board of nursing to clarify whether **prescriptive authority** is within the scope of practice for the APN. The board staff refer the APN to a provision in the statute that allows the APN to "diagnose and treat" common, well-defined health problems under approved written protocols. The staff conclude that "treatment" may include prescriptive authority as an "additional act" if permitted in the approved written protocols of the nurse and physician preceptor. No specific language is found in the statute that authorizes writing prescriptions by the APN. When the medical board receives the board of nursing opinion, an attorney general's opinion is requested. The attorney general concludes that the board of nursing may not extend the scope of practice of the APN through regulation. The expressed will of the legislature in regard to the scope of practice for the APN must be sought using the legislative process. Note that not all state boards of nursing are granted statutory authority to express formal opinions and must rely on the express language in the practice act and regulations, the attorney general's office, or the courts.

History of Health Professions Regulation

At the end of the 19th century, physicians were the first healthcare providers to gain legislative **recognition** for their practice. The definitions of the practice of medicine are all-encompassing and include any act to diagnose or treat, or attempt to diagnose or treat, any individual with a physical injury or deformity. Herein lies the problem faced by APNs and other healthcare providers who are not physicians: to define a scope of practice that does not overlap with this broad definition. The history of nursing regulation is characterized by efforts to accommodate this medical preemption (Safriet, 1992).

The early regulation of nurses was permissive (voluntary) providing for nurses to register with the governing board, hence the title "registered nurse." In some states, nurses were registered by the medical board prior to the establishment of a separate board of nursing. During this period, there was no competency assessment. Nurses seeking registration provided evidence of graduation from an approved nursing-education program, and "good moral character" was evaluated by requiring references or endorsements from nurses registered by the board.

The first board of nursing and nurse practice acts were passed in 1903 by North Carolina, followed by New York, New Jersey, and Virginia (Sheets, 1996). Boards of nursing began to establish written and practice examinations to measure competency; however, the practice acts were still permissive. Graduates of nursing-education programs not registered with the board were permitted to practice nursing, but they were not permitted to use the title "RN." The first mandatory licensure law was enacted by New York in 1938 (Weisenbeck & Calico, 1995). By the 1950s, mandatory licensure laws for the practice of nursing became widespread, requiring anyone who practiced nursing to be licensed by the state board of nursing. These mandatory licensure laws protected not only the title but also the scope of practice for nurses, resulting in greater public protection.

History of Advanced Practice Nursing Regulation

The 1960s set the stage for the expansion of nursing practice and the practice and regulation of APNs. The birth of the federal entitlement programs, Medicare and Medicaid, increased the number of individuals entitled to government-subsidized health care. With a predicted shortage of primary care physicians, the first formal nurse practitioner programs were opened (Safriet, 1992).

In 1971, Idaho became the first state to legally recognize diagnosis and treatment as part of the scope of practice for the advanced practice nurse. The regulation of APNs was accomplished through joint agreement of the state board of nursing and the state board of medicine for each permissible act of diagnosis and treatment. The model of regulation established in Idaho set a precedent for subsequent models for the regulation of APNs, that is, some form of joint regulation by the board of nursing and board of medicine. The joint regulation was designed to compensate for the broad definition of the practice of medicine and based on the determination that advanced practice nursing was a "delegated medical practice" requiring some oversight by physicians. Today the struggle continues between nursing and medicine to define the scope of practice of the APN as nursing practice and to determine which regulatory board should maintain oversight.

Since 1971, virtually every state has developed some form of legal recognition of the APN. Both the American Nurses Association (ANA) and the National Council of State Boards of Nursing (NCSBN) have proposed model rules and regulations for the regulation of advanced practice nursing. However, because the battles for regulation of APNs are fought in highly political state-by-state environments, there is a plethora of titles, definitions, criteria for practice, scopes of practice, reimbursement policies, and models of regulation that is difficult for policymakers to navigate and understand in today's rapidly changing healthcare delivery system.

Since 1988, *The Nurse Practitioner:The American Journal of Primary Health Care* has provided an annual survey of each state board of nursing and nursing organizations to gather information on the legislative status of advanced practice nursing. Significant strides have been made by many states in regard to APNs gaining sole authority for scope of practice with no requirements for direct physician supervision. As of 2006, 27 states reported that APNs had sole authority for practice with no requirement for physician collaboration, direction, or supervision. In 14 states, the board of nursing has sole authority in scope of practice for nurse practitioners, but the scope of practice includes a requirement for physician collaboration. Five states reported that the scope of practice is authorized jointly by the board of nursing and the board of medicine (Phillips, 2006). All states now allow some form of prescriptive authority (Pearson, 2002).

Methods of Professional Credentialing

Regulation of the health professions is achieved through various methods of credentialing. The method selected is determined by the state government and is based on at least two variables: (1) the potential for harm to the public if safe and acceptable standards of practice are not met, and (2) the degree of autonomy and accountability for decision making by the professional. The least restrictive form of regulation to accomplish the goal of public protection should be selected (Gross, 1984; Pew Health Professions Commission, 1994).

The term *restrictive* as used in this context means the degree to which the model restricts an individual who has not met the prescribed criteria in the law and the explicit authority of the administrative agency from practicing within the scope of practice of the profession. Four methods of credentialing are used in the United States. Each of the methods is based on the regulation of the individual provider. The methods are described separately, moving from the most restrictive to the least restrictive method of credentialing.

Licensure

Licensure is "granting permission by a competent authority to do an act which, without such permission, would be illegal, a trespass, a tort, or otherwise not allowable" (Black, Nolan, & Nolan-Haley, 1992, p. 920). The licentiate is "one who has obtained a license or authoritative permission to exercise some function, esp. to practice a profession"

(Garner, 2004, p. 940). Licensure is the most restrictive method of credentialing and requires anyone who practices within the defined scope of practice to obtain the legal authority to do so from the appropriate administrative agency of the state.

Licensure implies competency assessment of the professional at the point of entry into the profession. A licensing examination is administered and ongoing continuing education or competency assessment by the legal authority is conducted to provide some assurance that acceptable standards of practice are met. Licensure offers the public the greatest level of protection by restricting use of the title and the scope of practice to the licensed professional who has met these rigorous criteria. Unlicensed persons cannot call themselves by the title identified in the law, and they cannot lawfully practice any portion of the scope of practice.

The administrative agency holds the licensee accountable for practicing according to the legal, ethical, and professional standards of care defined for the profession to the extent to which the laws and rules require. Disciplinary action may be taken against licensees who have violated provisions of statute or regulation, through administrative disciplinary procedure that assures due process. Most of the health professions are regulated by licensure because of the high degree of potential for harm to the public by individuals who are not qualified to practice the profession.

Registration

Registration is the "act of recording or enrolling" (Garner, 2004, p. 1310). Registration provides for a review of credentials to determine compliance with the criteria for entry to the profession and permits the individual to use the title "registered." Registration serves as title protection, but does not preclude individuals who are not registered from practicing within the scope of practice, as long as they do not use the title.

Registration does not necessarily imply that any competency assessment has been conducted prior to the registration. Some state laws may have provisions for removing incompetent or unethical providers from the registry or marking the registry when a complaint is lodged against a provider. Removing the person from the registry may not necessarily provide public protection because the individual may continue to practice as long as the title is not used. Some types of practitioners engage in practice, never having been placed on a registry; an example is the lay midwife who never implies to the public that he or she is a registered nurse midwife and who does not use the title "nurse" midwife. States are required to maintain a registry of unlicensed assistive personnel who practice in long-term care facilities as a result of the Omnibus Budget Reconciliation Act of 1987.

The title "registered nurse" was formulated in the early days of nursing regulation when the state boards registered nurses. Though nurses have been subject to licensure requirements for many years, the term *registered* has historical significance and has never been changed.

Certification

Certification is the "formal assertion in writing of some fact" (Black et al., 1992, p. 227), that is, providing a certificate. As applied to nursing regulation, certification is a voluntary process that may involve completion of required requisite education or competency assessment usually conducted by proprietary professional or specialty nursing organizations denoting that the individual has achieved a level of competence in nursing practice beyond the entry-level competence measured by licensure.

Certification, like registration, is a means of title protection. *Certification* is a term that may be used by both governmental agencies and proprietary organizations. When certification is awarded by proprietary organizations, it does not have the force and effect of law. However, in some states, certification is a regulated credential; states may offer a "certificate of authority" to practice within a prescribed scope or may offer certification to assistive personnel, such as dialysis technicians. When choosing a provider, astute consumers may inquire as to whether a provider is certified as a means of assuring a level of preparedness to practice. Employers also use certification as a means of determining eligibility for certain jobs or as a requirement for promotions within the agency. Some states have promulgated regulations that require an APN to be certified by a specialty nursing organization to be eligible to practice in the advanced role.

Recognition

Recognition is a process of "ratification or confirmation" (Black et al., 1992, p. 1271). As applied to nursing regulation, **official recognition** is a method of regulating APNs used by several boards of nursing that implies the board has validated and accepted credentials for the specialty area of practice. Criteria for recognition are defined in the practice act and may include requirements for certification. Official recognition is the least restrictive method of credentialing.

Professional Self-Regulation

Self-regulation occurs within a profession through the desire of members of the profession to set standards, values, ethical frameworks, and safe-practice guidelines beyond the minimum standards defined by law. This voluntary process plays an equally significant role in the regulation of the profession, as does legal regulation. The definition of professional standards of practice and the code of ethics for the profession are examples of **professional self-regulation**. The members of national professional organizations set standards of practice for specialty practice and determine who can use selected titles by administering certification examinations. Continuing education requirements as well as documentation of practice competency are often required for periodic recertification. The standards are periodically reviewed and revised to reflect current practice. Legal regulation recognizes professional standards as the acceptable standard of practice when making decisions regarding what constitutes safe and competent care.

Even though professional organizations can develop standards, they have no legal authority to ensure compliance with the standards. Legal regulation provides a mechanism for monitoring and enforcing compliance with standards of practice. Legal regulation and professional regulation are two sides of the same coin, working together to fulfill the profession's contract with society.

Regulation of Advanced Practice Nurses

Advanced practice nursing regulation has been the focus of the Advanced Practice Task Force of the National Council of State Boards of Nursing (NCSBN) for two decades. The evolution of APN practice across the United States has resulted in a patchwork of titles, scopes of practice, and regulatory methods. To bring some uniformity to the regulation of APNs, the NCSBN convened the Advanced Practice Task Force. Through the years, the task force has developed position papers for consideration by state boards of nursing in a quest for greater standardization and to strengthen the public protection mandate held by boards.

National nursing certifying agencies play an important role in the professional regulation of APNs. Specialty nursing organizations develop verification examinations to measure the competency of nurses in an area of clinical expertise. Most boards of nursing require the APN to be certified in the clinical specialty area appropriate to the educational preparation to legally practice in the role. The regulatory body has the authority to accept certification examinations if the examination meets the criteria predetermined by the board. The board may not "surrender regulatory authority by passive acceptance without evaluation of the examination content, procedures and scoring process" (National Council of State Boards of Nursing, 2002). To be legally defensible for licensure purposes, the certification examination must meet certain psychometric standards. The foundational basis for regulatory sufficiency is the examination's ability to measure entry-level practice; that it is based on a job analysis that defines job-related knowledge, skills,

The State Regulatory Process | **101**

and abilities; and that it is developed on psychometrically sound principles of test development.

The NCSBN and the national nursing specialty organizations collaborated to establish criteria that boards of nursing could use in the evaluation of certification examinations (Canavan, 1996). The Requirements for Accrediting Agencies and Criteria for APRN Certification Programs were developed in 1995 and updated in 2002 (National Council of State Boards of Nursing, 2002). The criteria can be located on the NCSBN Web site at www.ncsbn.org.

The national organizations that prepare certification examinations for APNs include the following:

■ American Academy of Nurse Practitioners
■ American Association of Nurse Anesthetists Council on Certification
■ American College of Nurse-Midwives Certification Council
■ American Nurses Credentialing Center
■ National Certification Board of Pediatric Nurse Practitioners
■ National Certification Corporation for the Obstetric, Gynecologic, and Neonatal Nursing Specialties

The NCSBN Advanced Practice Nursing Task Force has also sought to bring greater standardization to APN regulation in an effort to increase mobility of APNs. In 2000, the NCSBN Delegate Assembly passed the Uniform Advanced Practice Registered Nurse Licensure/Authority to Practice Requirements. These requirements include (1) an unencumbered RN license; (2) graduation from a graduate-level advanced practice program by a national accrediting body; (3) current certification by a national certifying body in the advanced practice specialty appropriate to educational preparation; and (4) maintenance of certification or evidence of maintenance of competence (National Council of State Boards of Nursing, 2002). Adoption of these uniform requirements by boards of nursing will facilitate the ease with which APNs can become a part of the multistate regulation model.

The State Regulatory Process

The Tenth Amendment of the U.S. Constitution reserves all powers not specifically vested in the federal government for the states. One of these is the duty to protect its citizens (police powers). The power to regulate the professions is one way the state exercises its responsibility to protect the health, safety, and welfare of its citizens. State law provides for administrative agencies to assume the responsibility for regulation of the professions. These agencies have administrative, legislative, and judicial powers to make and enforce the laws.

Administrative agencies have sometimes been called the fourth branch of government because of their significant power in the daily execution and enforcement of the law. They are given referent authority by state and federal governments to promulgate rules and regulations, develop policies and procedures, and interpret laws to implement the agency mission.

Boards of Nursing

Each state legislature designates a board or similar authority to administer the practice act for the profession. The board's powers, duties, and composition are defined by the law. Traditionally, there are three major duties for licensing boards: (1) control entry into the profession through examination and licensure; (2) monitor and discipline licensees who violate the scope and standards of practice; and (3) monitor continuing education and/or competency of licensees to protect the public from unsafe or poor quality practice. In most states, boards of nursing have the additional duty to establish criteria for review and approval of nursing education programs that lead to licensure as a registered nurse (RN) or licensed practical nurse (LPN), and to set criteria for recognition of and prescriptive powers for APNs.

There are 61 boards of nursing in the United States and its territories. Each board of nursing is a member of the National Council of State Boards of Nursing. Some states have separate boards for licensing RNs and LPNs. As members of the NCSBN, the boards have the privilege of using the national licensure examination and meeting together to discuss matters of common interest (National Council of State Boards of Nursing, 1997).

Composition of the Board of Nursing

Generally, boards are composed of licensed nurses and consumer members. In most states, the governor appoints the members. At least one state, North Carolina, conducts elections for the board vacancies. Nurses who are interested in serving as board members often gain appointment to those positions through the helpful endorsements of their professional associations, as well as the support of their district legislators.

Some state laws designate that nurses from specific educational and practice settings, as well as APNs, must be represented on the board of nursing. In other states, the criteria for appointment only require licensure in the profession and a residency requirement. Information on vacancies on the board of nursing can be obtained from the board office or the governor's office. Knowing the composition of the board and when vacancies occur is important to allow the profession to exercise political influence in gaining the desired representation on the board. Information related to serving on boards and commissions is found later in this chapter.

Board Meetings

All state government agencies function within open meeting or "sunshine" laws that permit the public to observe or participate in the discussions of the board. Boards may go into closed "executive session" when necessary. Rules for executive sessions are specified in the APA and must be adhered to by the agency. The board may meet in executive session for certain reasons, including discussion of personnel matters, obtaining legal advice, contract negotiation, and disciplinary matters. Boards usually "report out" of executive session when public session resumes. All voting is a matter of public record and occurs only in open public session.

Board meetings may vary in the degree of formality. Most states' APA requires the board to post notice of meetings and the agenda in a public place usually 30 days prior to the meeting. Sometimes the notice of meeting is published in major state newspapers. The agenda is public and available on request from the board office or from its Web site.

Participants in the board meeting include the board members, the board staff, and legal counsel for the board. Legal counsel advises the board in matters of law and jurisdiction. Some boards may have "staff" counsel, but many states receive advice from their representative from the state attorney general's office, known as an "assistant attorney general," or AAG. Staff or other invited guests may present reports during the meeting. Individuals may provide testimony to the board on matters of interest.

In making decisions, board members must consider several factors, including implications for the public welfare, national standards of care, impact of the decision on the state as a whole, and the legal defensibility of the decision. First and foremost, the board must act only within its legal jurisdiction. All actions of the board are a matter of public record. Most boards of nursing publish newsletters that summarize the major actions of the board during each meeting. Licensees may request to be placed on the mailing list for the newsletter if one is not automatically received.

Monitoring Competency of Nurses: Mandatory Reporting

The most critical role of the board of nursing is assuring public safety. Most nurse practice acts (NPAs) have mandatory reporting provisions that require employers to report violations of the NPA. Licensed nurses also have a moral and ethical duty to report unsafe and incompetent practice to the board of nursing. The NPA defines those acts that are considered misconduct and provides for a system of due process to investigate complaints against licensees. Procedures for filing complaints, conducting investigations, and issuing sanctions for violations are enumerated in rules and regulations of the NPA.

The licensed nurse is accountable for knowing the laws and regulations that govern the practice of nursing in the state of licensure and adhering to the legal, ethical, and professional standards of care. Some NPAs include standards of practice in the regulations. Other states may refer to professional or ethical standards established by professional associations. The employing agency also defines standards of practice through policy and procedures that must be followed by each nurse employee.

A nurse who holds a multistate license (one license that permits a nurse to practice in more than one state as long as the state is entered into a multistate compact) is held accountable for knowing and abiding by the laws of the state in which the practice occurs in addition to the home state of licensure. Multistate regulation is discussed in more detail later in this chapter. Ignorance of the law is not an excuse for misconduct. Most boards of nursing now have the complete NPA online on their Web sites, as does the National Council of State Boards of Nursing (see www.ncsbn.org).

Promulgating State Regulations

Government agencies have the authority and duty to promulgate regulations to amplify its statute. As discussed earlier in this chapter, a law may provide overarching parameters, but the details of the processes required to implement the law are written into the regulations. The APA of each state specifies the process for the promulgating regulations, including how the public is notified of proposed regulations and its opportunity for public comment. It is important that the APN becomes familiar with the APA to know when and how to provide comment. State processes differ; some states have designated commissions or committees responsible for review and approval of regulations; other states submit regulations to the general assembly or to committees of the legislature. Certain elements are common to the promulgation of regulations. These include (1) public notice that a new regulation has been proposed, or of a proposal to modify an existing regulation; (2) opportunity to submit written comment or testimony, and in addition the opportunity to present that testimony verbally at a rules hearing; and (3) publication of the final regulation in a register or state bulletin.

In some states a fiscal impact statement is required. This statement estimates the cost of compliance with the regulation. Also, in some states, the rule promulgation process requires oversight by a commission of legislators whose role it is to ensure that the regulatory agency promulgating the rules does in fact have the authority to do so, does not exceed the scope of its rule-making authority, and does not draft rules that would conflict with its own statute or that of any related discipline. For example, in the case of nursing, legislative commissions would cross-check the statutes and rules regulating other health professions.

Monitoring State Regulations

Administrative agencies promulgate hundreds of regulations each year. Regulations that affect advanced nursing practice could be promulgated from a variety of agencies. Knowing which agencies are most likely to have the authority to put forth regulations that affect health care and professional practice, as well as monitoring the legislation and regulations proposed by those agencies, is important to protect the scope of practice of APNs.

The most obvious agencies the APN should consider tracking are the licensing boards of other health professions, such as medicine, pharmacy, counselors and therapists, and other health professionals. In this rapidly changing healthcare environment, numerous conflicts occur over scope of practice issues, definitions of practice, right to reimbursement, and requirements for supervision and collaboration.

When reviewing regulations, there are several points that are important to consider. Exhibit 4–1 provides some key questions to consider when analyzing a regulation for its impact on nursing practice.

Exhibit 4–1 Questions to Ask When Analyzing Regulations

1. Which agency promulgated the regulation?
2. What is the source of authority (the statute that provides authority for the regulation to be promulgated)?
3. What is the intent or rationale of the regulation? Is it clearly stated by the promulgating agency?
4. Is the language in the regulation clear or ambiguous? Can the regulation be interpreted in different ways by different individuals?
5. Are there definitions to clarify terms?
6. Are there important points that are not addressed, that is, omissions?
7. How does the regulation affect the practice of nursing? Does it constrain or limit the practice of nursing in any way?
8. Is there sufficient lead time to comply with the regulation?
9. What is the fiscal impact of the regulation?

Consider the following situation and how the proposed regulations would affect the practice of the APN.

EXAMPLE: Assume the board of pharmacy has drafted the following definition of the practice of pharmacy. The practice of pharmacy includes, but is not limited to, the interpretation, evaluation, and implementation of medical orders; the dispensing of prescription drug orders; initiating or modifying the drug therapy in accordance with written guidelines or protocols previously established and approved by a practitioner authorized to independently prescribe drugs; provision of patient counseling as a primary healthcare provider of pharmacy care.

If this definition was included in the pharmacy practice act requiring that anyone who "initiated or modified a drug therapy in accordance with written guidelines or protocols" must be licensed as a pharmacist by the board of pharmacy, how would this affect the practice of nursing and, especially, the APN? This is but one example of numerous definitions of scope of practice that are promulgated that has significant overlap with the advanced practice of nursing. A solution to this dilemma would be to negotiate for the addition of an exemption for APNs in the pharmacy practice act.

In a growing managed care market, it is also critical for APNs to be aware of regulations that mandate benefits or reimbursement policies and to lobby for inclusion of APNs. Several states have promulgated open-panel legislation known as "any willing provider" and "freedom of choice" laws. These bills mandate that any provider who is authorized to provide the services covered in an insurance plan must be recognized and reimbursed by the plan. Insurance company lobbyists as well as business lobbyists oppose this type of legislation. As managed care contracts are negotiated, APNs must ensure that services of the APN are given fair and equitable consideration. Other important areas include workers' compensation participation and reimbursement provisions and liability insurance laws.

APNs achieved landmark success in 1997, with grassroots **lobbying** efforts, to gain Medicare reimbursement for all nurse practitioners, regardless of location of practice. Prior to 1997, Medicare reimbursement for nurse practitioners was restricted to those nurse practitioners who provided services in specific geographic locations and who practiced with physician supervision.

In summary, state agencies that govern licensing and certification of healthcare facilities, administer public health services (public health, mental health, alcohol and drug abuse), govern reimbursement, as well as the health professions licensing boards, are all agencies that could promulgate regulations that would have implications for the practice of the APN.

Serving on Boards and Commissions

One way to participate actively in the regulatory process is to seek an appointment to the state board of nursing or other board or commission that affects health policy. Active participation in the political process, especially during times of rapid change and reform, will ensure the voice of APNs is heard in setting the public policy agenda.

When seeking appointments to boards and commissions, select an agency whose mission and purposes are consistent with your interest and expertise. Because most board appointments are gubernatorial or political appointments, it is important for the APN to obtain endorsements from legislators, influential community leaders, and their professional associations.

Letters of support should document the APN's contributions to employment and community service. Delineate involvement in local, state, and national organizations. The letter from the employer should indicate a willingness to provide the time to fulfill the responsibilities of the position during the term of office. In addition, a personal letter from the APN who is seeking appointment to the governor that expresses interest in serving on the board should be offered, including the rationale for volunteering for service on the particular board or commission, evidence of a good match between one's expertise and the role of that board or commission, and expression of a clear interest in serving the public. A resume or curriculum vitae should be attached. Letters should emphasize desire to serve over self-interest; appointment decisions should be based on how much the individual can offer the board or commission in serving the public good. This kind of public service requires a substantial time commitment; it is wise to speak to other members of the board or call the executive director or administrator of the agency to determine the extent of that commitment.

The Federal Regulatory Process

Many forces have contributed to the federal government becoming a more central figure in the regulation of the health professions. The most significant factor is the advent of the Medicare and Medicaid programs. The federal initiatives that have grown out of these programs are largely focused on cost containment (prospective payment) and consumer protection (combating fraud and abuse) (Jost, 1997; Roberts & Clyde, 1993).

With the "graying" of Americans, the cost of administering the Medicare program is skyrocketing, with predictions of bankruptcy if substantive changes are not made in either the criteria for eligibility or the methods of reimbursement. Numerous changes to the system are expected in the coming years.

One of the most significant changes occurred in July 2001 when the Centers for Medicare and Medicaid Services (CMS) was created to replace the former Health Care Financing Administration (HCFA). The reformed agency provides an increased emphasis on responsiveness to beneficiaries and providers, and quality improvement. Three new business centers have been established as part of the reform: Center for Beneficiary Choices, Center for Medicare Management, and Center for Medicaid and State Operations (Centers for Medicare and Medicaid Services, 2001).

The practice of APNs has also been influenced by changes in the Medicare reimbursement policy. In 1997 legislation was passed in Congress calling for Medicare reimbursement of APNs regardless of setting and went into effect in January 1998. These regulations provide direct reimbursement to APNs for providing Medicare Part B services that would normally be provided by a physician. These services are not restricted by site of geographic location as services have been in the past. Under this legislation, APNs can see both new and continuing patients without restriction. Reimbursement rates are set at 80% of the lesser of the actual charge or 85% of the fee schedule amount for the physician (American Academy of Nurse Practitioners, 2003). APNs must secure a Medicare provider number to be eligible for reimbursement.

The evolution of government has changed the relationship between the state and federal regulatory systems. Responsibilities once assumed by the federal government have been shifted down to the state level, such as administration of the Medicaid programs and management of the welfare program. The impetus guiding this change is that states are better equipped to make decisions about how best to assist their citizens and the sentiment against creating federal bureaucracy and increasing the tax burden. Even though states have primary authority over regulation of the health professions, federal policies also have an enormous effect on healthcare workforce regulation. All the policies related to reimbursement and quality control over the Medicare and Medicaid programs are promulgated by the U.S. Department of Health and Human Services and are administered through its financing agency, the CMS. Other federal statutes that have a regulatory impact on healthcare providers and that the APN should be familiar with include the following:

- Clinical Laboratory Improvement Amendments of 1988 (CLIA 88)
- Occupational Safety and Health Act of 1970 (OSHA)
- Mammography Quality Standards Act of 1987 and 1992 (MQSA 87 and 92)

- Omnibus Budget Reconciliation Act of 1987 and 1990 (OBRA 87 and 90)
- Americans with Disabilities Act of 1990 (ADA)
- North American Free Trade Agreement of 1993 (NAFTA, effective date January 1, 1994)
- Telecommunications Act of 1996
- Health Insurance Portability and Accountability Act of 1996 (HIPAA)

The Veterans Administration hospitals and the Indian Health Services both are regulated by the federal government, as are the uniformed armed services. Individuals who are employed in these services must be licensed in at least one state and are subject to the laws of the state in which they are licensed and the standards of care and policies established in the federal system. The Supremacy Clause of the U.S. Constitution gives legal superiority to federal laws (Braunstein, 1995). When a federal law or regulation is promulgated, it takes precedence over any state law. State laws in conflict with federal laws cannot be enforced. At times, the courts may be asked to determine the constitutionality of a law or regulation to resolve jurisdictional disputes.

The Commerce Clause of the U.S. Constitution limits the ability of states to erect barriers to interstate trade (Gobis, 1997). Courts have found that the provision of health care is interstate trade under antitrust laws. This finding sets the stage for the federal government to preempt state licensing laws in the practice of professions across state boundaries, if it chooses to do so.

The impact of technology on the delivery of health care, such as "telehealthcare" or "telecare," allows providers to care for patients in remote environments and across the geopolitical boundaries defined by traditional state-by-state licensure. This raises the question as to whether the federal government will intercede in standardizing licensing requirements across state lines to facilitate interstate commerce, usurping the state's authority. Licensing boards are beginning to identify ways to facilitate the practice of telehealthcare, at the same time preserving the power and right of the state to protect its citizens by regulating the professions at the state level. One innovative approach to nursing regulation, **multistate regulation**, is discussed later in this chapter.

Promulgating Federal Regulations

The federal regulatory process is a two-step process established by the federal Administrative Procedures Act. A notice of proposed rulemaking (NPR) is published in the proposed rule section of the **Federal Register** that informs the public of the substance of the intended regulation and provides information on how the public may participate in providing comment, attend meetings, or otherwise participate in the regulatory process. The second step involves careful consideration of public comment by the agency and amendment to the regulation, if warranted. The final regulations are issued by the agency through publication in the rules and regulations section of the *Federal Register* and become effective 30 days after publication (see Exhibit 4–2).

Emergency Regulations

Provisions for promulgating emergency regulations are defined at both the state and federal levels. Emergency regulations are promulgated if an agency determines that the public welfare is immediately adversely affected. Emergency regulations may take effect immediately upon publication, are generally temporary, are effective for a limited time (usually 90 days, with an option to renew), and must be followed with permanent regulations that are promulgated in accordance with the APA process.

Exhibit 4–2 Federal Rule-Making Process

Congress authorizes law that provides authority for rule promulgation

↓

Advance notice of proposed rule-making
(Optional)

↓

Proposed rule published in the *Federal Register*
(Comment period specified, informal hearings optional)

↓

Final rule published in the *Federal Register*

↓

Rule becomes effective in 30 days after publication

↓

Final rule updated in code of federal regulations
(Updates done on a quarterly cycle by agency title)

Source: Goehlert, R. U., & Martin, F. S. (1989). Federal administrative law. *Congress and Law Making: Researching the Legislative Process* (2nd ed.). San Francisco, CA: ABC–CLIO, pp. 82–83.

Locating Information

The *Federal Register* is the bulletin board or newspaper of the federal government. It is published daily, Monday through Friday, except for federal holidays and is updated daily by 6 a.m. It contains executive orders and presidential proclamations, rules and regulations, proposed rules, notices of federal agencies and organizations, sunshine act meetings, and corrections to previous copies of the *Federal Register*. Each document in the *Federal Register* begins with a heading that includes the name of the issuing agency, the Code of Federal Regulations title, and a brief synopsis of the contents. After the heading, a preamble is published that contains the type of action, summary of action, deadline for comments, address to which the comments may be sent, a contact person, and other supplementary information (Goehlert & Martin, 1989). The *Federal Register* may be accessed online via the Governmental Printing Office Web site at www.gpoaccess.gov/fr/index.html.

The Code of Federal Regulations (CFR) is a compilation of all final regulations issued by the executive branch agencies of the federal government. The CFR consists of 50 titles that represent broad subject areas. The CFR is updated annually in sections. Each quarter, one section of the CFR is updated according to a schedule that includes all regulations that have been passed since the prior printing. Consequently, there is never a publication that has all the regulations passed in it for the year. An index that helps in locating rules by agency name and subject headings is published and revised semiannually (Goehlert & Martin, 1989). The Code of Federal Regulations is online at the Government Printing Office (GPO) Web site at www.gpoaccess.gov/cfr/index.html.

Each state government publishes similar documents that identify the proposed regulations, notices, final regulations, and emergency regulations. The publication is usually called the State Register or the State Bulletin. The publication cycle can be obtained by calling the state legislative printing office or the state legislative information system office. Copies of these documents are usually available in the local libraries and may be available online on the state's governmental Web site.

The myriad of proposed regulations promulgated by agencies at the state and federal levels is so expansive that it is to the APN's advantage to belong to the appropriate professional organizations, most of which employ lobbyists whose business it is to track legislation. Specialty organization newsletters and journals, legislative subscription and monitoring services, and bulletins that summarize proposed regulations may be used to monitor these processes. Subscription services track legislation for an agency or organization and provide an abstract including the substance of bills and regulations and the progress through the legislative or regulatory process. Both free and subscription legislative information services are available online. Examples of online services include the following:

■ State Net: Information and intelligence for the 50 states and Congress, located at www.statenet.com
■ Thomas Legislative Information: Sponsored by the U.S. Library of Congress, located at http://thomas.loc.gov
■ GPO Access: Located at www.gpoaccess.gov

In addition, numerous private services are available and can be found by searching the Internet. Several nursing and healthcare associations also feature relevant updates and information on current legislative and public policy issues (see Exhibit 4–3).

Exhibit 4–3 Selected Web Sites of Interest

URL	Summary of Content
http://www.statenet.com	Legislative and regulatory reporting services from all 50 states and Congress. A subscription service that provides comprehensive and timely information on legislation.
http://thomas.loc.gov	Thomas Legislative Information System. Sponsored by the U.S. Library of Congress. Summarizes bills, provides full text of bills and the Congressional Record, information on the legislative process, and U.S. government Internet resources.
http://www.ahrq.gov	Agency for Healthcare Research and Quality. Information on healthcare research, evidence reports, clinical practice guidelines, consumer health information; hyperlinked to U.S. Dept. of Health and Human Services (DHHS).
http://www.ctel.org	Center for Telemedicine Law. Information on the latest findings in the regulation of telemedicine, proceedings of national telemedicine task force, state-by-state updates on telemedicine legislation.
http://www.nursingworld.org	American Nurses Association. Access to all ANA services; access to *Online Journal of Issues in Nursing*; jointly prepared with Kent State Univ.
http://www.ncsbn.org	National Council of State Boards of Nursing. Information on all National Council services and committee activities, access to state nurse practice acts, information on progress of multistate regulation.

Exhibit 4–3 Selected Web Sites of Interest—continued

URL	Summary of Content
http://www.hhs.gov	U.S. Dept. of Health and Human Services. Access to all agencies within the department, that is, ACHPR, CDC, CMS, HRSA, NIH, and so forth. Consumer information and policy information.
http://www.hschange.com	The Center for Studying Health Systems Change. A Washington, DC–based research organization dedicated to studying the nation's healthcare systems and the impact on the public.
http://www.nurse.org	State-by-state display of advanced practice nursing organizations, links to related sites that contain legislative and regulatory information, NP Central (a comprehensive site for APN CE offerings, salary information, job opportunities).
http://www.nursingethicsnetwork.org	Nursing Ethics Network. A nonprofit organization committed to the advancement of nursing ethics. Site contains ethics research findings and online inquiry.
http://www.acnpweb.org	American College of Nurse Practitioners. Comprehensive site featuring latest trends and issues affecting APN practice and regulation.
http://www.aanp.org	American Academy of Nurse Practitioners. Comprehensive site featuring latest trends and issues affecting APN practice and regulation.
http://www.cms.hhs.gov/hipaa	Centers for Medicare and Medicaid Services. Latest legislative and regulatory information on reimbursement, HIPAA implementation.
http://www.hhs.gov/ocr/hipaa	Office of Civil Rights. Fact sheets, sample forms, FAQs on HIPAA implementation along with related links and educational materials.
http://www.iom.edu	Institute of Medicine. Provides objective information to further science and health policy. A leading and respected authority on health issues. Access to published reports.

Providing Public Comment

There is a small window of opportunity for public input into the development of regulations. Most comment periods are a minimum of 30 days from the date of the publication of the proposed rule. Sometimes an NPR will provide for a longer period of time to submit comments if the agency anticipates the issue will be one of strong public interest or will be controversial in nature. It is very important that the APN is vigilant in tracking when the comment periods are set.

Public hearings may be held by an agency on a proposed rule, but are not required unless the APA establishes criteria for when a public hearing must be held by the agency. Generally the agency is required to hold a hearing when a request is made by a specified number of individuals or agencies. Written comments received by the agency are made a part of the permanent record and must be considered by the agency's board or commission members prior to the publication of the final rule. A final rule can be challenged in the courts if the judge determines that the agency did not comply with the APA or ignored public comments.

The *Register* names the individual in the agency who can be contacted to submit comments. It is best to place the comments in writing to ensure inclusion in the public record. It is permissible to call the agency and provide comments orally if time is of the essence. Faxing comments or providing an electronic copy may also be an option if the comment period is near expiration. It is of utmost importance that the deadline posted in the *Federal Register* is met because agencies can rightfully disregard comments received after the deadline.

When providing public comment in writing, or testimony at a hearing, it is important for the APN to:

- Be specific regarding whether the regulation is supported or opposed. Give examples using brief scenarios or experiences when possible.
- Have credible data to back the position, such as statistics. Use research findings that can be explained in common language; avoid medical jargon.
- Know what the opposition is saying and respond to these concerns.
- Convey a willingness to negotiate or compromise toward mutually acceptable resolutions.
- Demonstrate concern for the public good, rather than self-interest.
- Be brief and succinct. Limit remarks to one or two pages or 5 minutes for oral testimony.

Regulatory agencies charged with public protection are more likely to address concerns that are focused on how the public may be harmed or benefited rather than concerns that seem like turf protection and professional jealousy. Demonstrate support for your position by having colleagues who represent a variety of organizations and interests submit comments. This is a powerful method to employ; it is important to demonstrate the degree of concern because the number of comments received is one way the agency measures support or nonsupport for the regulation.

Lobbying and Political Decision Making

Lobbying is the act of influencing a governmental entity to achieve a specific legislative or regulatory outcome. Anyone can lobby, and it has been demonstrated that the grassroots lobbyists can achieve the most effective lobbying efforts (DeVries & Vanderbilt, 1992). Grassroots lobbyists are neighborhood constituents who have the power to elect officials through their vote. Grassroots lobbying efforts take organization and a commitment on the part of the constituent to be well informed on the issue being considered and to respond when called.

Professional nursing organizations have become increasingly more aware of the strength in grassroots lobbying efforts and have made concerted efforts toward educating their members regarding ways to communicate with legislators and regulatory agencies. The "Aunt Mary Network," a method of linking legislators with a nurse who is a relative or friend, has proved very successful (Pruitt, Wetsel, Smith, & Spitler, 2002). Legislative workshops are excellent forums to teach nurses how to exert their political influence to shape public policy in the interest of consumer welfare.

It is important to be aware of state ethics laws as they relate to lobbying. There are strict reporting requirements in most ethics laws in a state along with restrictions that apply to the use of funds and gifts. Participating in organized lobbying efforts is critical to successful outcomes. There is no substitute for visibility in the legislative and regulatory process. Building trusting relationships, demonstrating interest and concern for the public good, and providing information on issues important to the profession are all things that can be done through regular participation in the legislative and regulatory process. It is best not to wait until there is an important bill or regulation pending to begin developing relationships with legislators, and just as important, the legislator's staff and staff of administrative agencies. Contact with legislator offices to convey interest in the activities and issues of the agency and volunteering to serve on committees and task forces help to develop name recognition, credibility, and trust. There are several key points to developing a successful lobbying plan:

■ The importance of unity within the profession. Divisiveness within the ranks of the profession is a sure road to defeat and fuels the opposition's fire. At a minimum, if a group cannot agree to support the initiative, work toward a compromise so that the group will not openly oppose the cause. Seek and define a base of support external to the profession. Identify groups and individuals who have something to gain if your cause is successful, that is, consumers and other licensed professionals.

■ Timing is everything. There are times and windows of opportunity for a political agenda to be moved forward. Sometimes it is just as important to wait for a favorable climate. At the same time, be aware of the environment and know when the time is right to avoid missing a critical window of opportunity. During periods of reform, unfreezing occurs and there is a stronger propensity for changes to be made.

■ The regulatory process is an evolving process. Do not be discouraged if regulations do not include all the aspects supported by the nursing community. Amendments to regulations can be made at a later time. Sometimes success comes one step at a time.

Identify who the proponents and the opponents are on a particular issue, and recognize that all have the same goal—to influence the governmental entity in their favor. Understanding that there are many tactics that can be employed to influence the regulatory and legislative process will enhance success in the process. The American Nurses Association Government Affairs Web site includes an "RN Activist Tool Kit," which has information on a variety of ways that nurses can become involved and stay involved in government affairs (American Nurses Association, 2007). Another effective strategy in influencing legislative and regulatory outcomes is attendance at board and committee meetings. Listening to the dialogue and understanding the issues and concerns of the regulators can provide invaluable insight into what strategies need to be employed.

Strengths and Weaknesses of the Regulatory Process

The regulatory process is much more ordered than the legislative process in that the administrative procedures act in each state and at the federal level directs the process that must be undertaken. There is guaranteed opportunity for comment and public input. The regulatory process has built-in delays and time constraints that slow down action. On the other hand, the regulatory process also is much more controlled by administrative agencies and can often become tedious and complex in detail of implementation. Regulations may not always be written by individuals who are knowledgeable about the substance or impact of new or revised rules, making the public input process especially important.

One power that may be provided to administrative agencies is to interpret regulations. It is especially important to be aware that existing regulations may be misinterpreted by the staff or board of an agency, resulting in a new meaning being imposed rather than the original intent of the regulation.

New interpretations to existing statutes and regulations may occur over time. For this reason, it is especially important to review opinions and/or declaratory rulings of the board, attorney general opinions, and opinions of the court. Official opinions carry the force and effect of law even though they are not promulgated according to the APA. There is a fine line between the duty to interpret existing laws and regulations and establishing new laws or standards without complying with the APA. The courts have revoked several board rulings requiring boards to promulgate new regulations according to the APA. In some states, such as Ohio, official opinions interpreting statute or regulation are only generated by the attorney general's office or the courts. However, regulatory boards may offer interpretive guidelines or other documents to facilitate public understanding and compliance.

Current Issues in Regulation and Licensure

Regulation in a Transforming Healthcare Delivery System

The current system of regulation of healthcare professionals is based on the regulation of the individual provider and the employment setting. Questions have been raised as to whether this system is the best means of public protection or whether the system has become a means of protecting the profession and creating monopolies for services (Gross, 1984; Pew Health Professions Commission, 1994). As new healthcare occupations and professions have emerged, there has been increasing professional debate about which tasks can be accomplished by which professions. Overlapping scopes of practice have naturally emerged among nursing, medicine, pharmacy, social work, physical therapy, occupational therapy, and other licensed health professions. Overlapping scopes of practice are appropriate when competency and education to perform the acts are substantially equivalent. However, restrictive practice acts have made overlapping scopes of practice a battlefield for debate, a debate with which APNs are very familiar.

The Pew Health Professions Commission (1995) has suggested that the current century-old regulatory system is out of sync with the nation's healthcare delivery and financing structures and in need of major reform. The web of laws and regulations created by bureaus, agencies, boards, and legal departments makes it difficult for the public and those regulated to participate in what Dower and Finocchio (1995) call an "exclusionary scheme" (p. 2). The Pew Health Professions Commission suggests that states review the regulatory process in light of the following criteria:

- Does regulation promote effective health outcomes and protect the public from harm?
- Are regulatory bodies truly accountable to the public?
- Does regulation respect consumers' rights to choose their own healthcare providers from a range of safe options?
- Does regulation encourage a flexible, rational, and cost-effective healthcare system?
- Does regulation allow effective working relationships among healthcare providers?
- Does regulation promote equity among providers of equal skill?
- Does regulation facilitate professional and geographic mobility of competent providers? (Dower & Finocchio, 1995, p. 1)

Workforce regulation has a tremendous impact on the cost and accessibility of health care. Restrictive scopes of practice limit the ability of comparably prepared providers to provide care. Concurrently, employers have expanded the use of unlicensed assistive personnel (UAP) who infringe on the scope of practice defined for the licensed nurse. Boundary disputes within and across disciplines flourish— between nursing and allied health providers, allied health providers and medicine, nursing and medicine, dental hygienists and dentists, and nurses and UAPs.

The Pew Task Force on Health Care Workforce Regulation has challenged the state and federal government to respond to the complex issues regarding the education and regulation of the health professions. The task force has offered 10 recommendations to make the state regulatory system more responsive to the evolving healthcare system (see Exhibit 4–4).

The creation of super boards with a majority of consumer representatives is one suggestion the Pew Health Professions Commission has advocated. Gross (1984) advocates for increasing competition among providers and giving the consumer more choice. Gross suggests one alternative to individual licensure of professionals would be to regulate dangerous procedures, or those procedures that, when inadequately

Exhibit 4–4 Ten Recommendations for Reforming Healthcare Workforce Regulation

1. Use standardized and understandable language for health professions regulation and its functions to clearly describe them for consumers, provider organizations, business, and the professions.

2. Standardize entry-to-practice requirements and limit them to competence assessments for health professions to facilitate the physical and professional mobility of the health professions.

3. Base practice acts on demonstrated initial and continuing competence. Allow and expect different professions to share overlapping scopes of practice. Explore pathways to allow all professionals to provide services to the full extent of their current knowledge, training, experience, and skills.

4. Redesign health professions boards and their functions to reflect the interdisciplinary and public accountability demands of the changing healthcare delivery system.

5. Educate consumers to assist them in obtaining the information necessary to make decisions about practitioners and to improve the board's accountability.

6. Cooperate with other public and private organizations in collecting data on regulated health professions to support effective workforce planning.

7. Require each board to develop, implement, and evaluate continuing competency requirements to ensure the continuing competence of regulated healthcare professionals.

8. Maintain a fair, cost-effective, and uniform disciplinary process to exclude incompetent practitioners to protect and promote the public's health.

9. Develop evaluation tools that assess the objectives, successes, and shortcomings of their regulatory systems and bodies to best protect and promote the public's health.

10. Understand the links, overlaps, and conflicts between the healthcare workforce regulatory systems and other systems that affect the education, regulation, and practice of healthcare practitioners and work to develop partnerships to streamline regulatory structures and processes.

Source: Pew Health Professions Commission. (1995). *Task Force on Health Care Workforce Regulation: Policy considerations for the 21st century.* San Francisco, CA: UCSF Center for the Health Professions, pp. 3–8.

performed, would cause irremediable consequences. This system of regulation has been implemented in Ontario, Canada. The Ontario model of regulation regulates 13 dangerous procedures and determines which professionals may engage in these procedures based on demonstrated competency and education. This model is under study by those groups interested in alternatives to the current regulatory system and could be the next frontier of debate in reforming healthcare regulation.

There is a window of opportunity to achieve significant reform in the regulation of the health professions in the 21st century. Advanced practice nurses must be open to the concept of new regulatory models that may emerge. Regulation will determine who will have access to the patient, who will serve as the gatekeeper in a managed care environment, who will be reimbursed, and who will have autonomy to practice. APNs must be visible participants throughout the political process to shape a dynamic and evolving system that is responsive to the healthcare environment and ensures consumer choice and protection.

Multistate Regulation

Technology has transformed the healthcare delivery system and is challenging the state-by-state regulatory and licensing system. Mergers, acquisitions, and buyouts of healthcare systems have produced giant conglomerates that operate across state lines. Care is coordinated by case managers who may be located in distant states. The Internet and e-mail afford patients hundreds of disease specialty home pages on the World Wide Web sponsored by institutions and voluntary associations. Over the past decade, a variety of telemedicine services has emerged, serving both patients and healthcare providers. United HealthCare's Web site, called Optum Online, offers nursing online services. Individuals submit questions, and then nurses research answers and provide personalized information within 48 to 72 hours (Gobis, 1997).

Although states have done much over the years to facilitate interstate mobility of nurses, there are still cumbersome licensure processes that make seamless transitions across geopolitical boundaries difficult or impossible. The confusion is prominent especially in the regulation of APNs. Not only is there a variety of methods used to regulate APNs, ranging from second licensure to official recognition, titles vary from state to state, as do the scopes of practice and even the jurisdiction for regulation (i.e., nursing, medical, or joint boards). The NCSBN definition of Uniform Advanced Practice Registered Nurse Licensure/ Authority to Practice Requirements will promote standardization of APN regulation to allow APNs to participate in multistate regulation as well as compete in a global market.

Moving to a multistate regulatory system has advantages for the profession and must be carefully executed state by state to ensure that the mission of the boards to protect the public is achieved.

To that end, the NCSBN delegate assembly adopted the **mutual recognition** model of multistate regulation in 1997. Mutual recognition is a method of licensure in which boards voluntarily enter into an **interstate compact** to legally recognize the policies and processes of a licensee's home state to permit practice in the remote state without obtaining an additional license. If a violation of law occurs, the state in which the violation occurs is responsible for disciplinary action (National Council of State Boards of Nursing, 1998).

To implement the mutual recognition model of nursing regulation, each state legislature must sign the interstate compact into law. Advanced practice nurses initially were not a part of the interstate compact agreement. With the move toward adoption of the Uniform Requirements for Licensure/Authority to Practice, APNs will be able to participate in the multistate regulation process. The APN must reside in a state that has already joined the interstate compact and subscribed to the uniform requirements. The multistate license does not, however, include prescriptive authority. Prescriptive authority must be sought independently in the state of practice.

Given the climate in the federal government related to the business of health care and the concept that this business is interstate commerce, a number of states have quickly moved to preserve state regulation of the professions while facilitating interstate practice. As of January 2007, 20 states are participating as "compact states," and 2 additional states are in process and expect to be participating within the year (National Council of State Boards of Nursing, 2007).

The Future of Advanced Practice Nurse Regulation

Much has been written in this chapter on the problems and issues related to the regulation of APNs. However, not all of the problems associated with the full utilization and practice of the APN are external to the profession; some of the problems have been created within the profession. The proliferation of APN educational programs with numerous specialty areas that have limited scopes of practice has created much of the public confusion regarding the role and scope of practice of the APN. Multiple educational pathways to achieve APN certification and legal credentialing have complicated the regulatory process further (O'Malley, Cummings & King, 1996). The numerous titles used for APN practice are confusing not only to the public but to regulatory agencies such as the Centers for Medicare and Medicaid Services that establishes national reimbursement policies. Clear definitions of APN role and title, educational requirements, and scope of practice must become a regulatory priority.

Credentialing APNs has been a major source of debate at the national level. Should this level of provider be licensed rather than officially recognized? Should there be a core competency examination developed at the national level for APN credentialing? Do certification examinations developed by the specialty nursing organizations meet the legal defensibility of an entry-level licensure examination? Who is an APN? Should there be a minimum education requirement for use of the title? These are all questions that continue to be raised in forums between specialty nursing organizations and licensing agencies. Until the role of the APN is clearly understood by consumers and policymakers, APNs will continue to be underutilized and undervalued.

Two important issues related to the future of advanced practice nursing regulation that require monitoring by APNs include the NCSBN initiative to consider state board of nursing regulation of APNs in the future, and the related matter of the direction in which future APN education is moving, the practice doctorate.

The NCSBN 2006 draft Vision Paper *The Future Regulation of Advanced Practice Nursing* has been the subject of debate among advanced practice nursing organizations and the American Association of Colleges of Nursing (AACN) (American Association of Colleges of Nursing, 2006; National Council of State Boards of Nursing, 2006). The Vision Paper proposes sole regulation of advanced practice RNs (APRNs) by boards of nursing in 10 years, and identifies nurse anesthetists, nurse midwives, and nurse practitioners (not clinical nurse specialists) as APNs. An NCSBN APRN Advisory Panel will be reviewing feedback obtained during stakeholder meetings during FY 2007, and the next steps will be influenced by this stakeholder response.

Parallel to new directions in regulation of APNs is the new direction in advanced clinical nursing education. In an effort to respond to the changes in national direction for health professions education and credentialing, the AACN Board of Directors endorsed a Position Statement on the Practice Doctorate (DNP) in Nursing (American Association of Colleges of Nursing, 2004), which calls for a new level of educational preparation for advanced practice nursing roles to the doctorate level from the masters level by the year 2015. The AACN cites the need for change in graduate nursing education as a response to the increasing complexity of the nation's healthcare environment and cites national calls to action from the Institute of Medicine (IOM), the Joint Commission on the Accreditation of Healthcare Organizations (JCAHO), and the 2005 National Institutes of Health (NIH) report calling for the development of nonresearch clinical doctorates in nursing. Two AACN task forces have been initiated to address questions related to nursing education, certification, regulation, and practice raised by the development of DNP programs. As of July 2007, 46 DNP programs are currently enrolling students nationwide, and the AACN reports that more than 190 others are under development at U.S. nursing schools (American Association of Colleges of Nursing, 2007).

Reimbursement

Significant breakthroughs are being made in reimbursement policy for APNs, largely as a result of the formation of grassroots lobbying efforts and coalitions of APN specialty nursing organizations. With the passage of federal legislation in 1997 allowing APNs to bill Medicare directly for services, APNs have had the opportunity to increase consumers' access to care. The managed care markets value efficiency and effectiveness in providers. APNs are learning how to cost out services in the competitive market to win contracts and demonstrate cost-effective, quality-care outcomes to patients.

In managed care contracts where reimbursement is capitated, the amount of reimbursement is not as important as knowing whether the services can be provided for the capitated fee. Research studies are needed to document the cost of care and demonstrate nursing interventions that reduce the use of costly healthcare services over time. Studies that demonstrate the value-added activities of nursing intervention, cost-benefit analysis of interventions, and patient satisfaction with care are emerging in the literature and can be very useful in negotiating contracts for patient populations. Understanding the business aspects of healthcare financing and creating successful practices are new roles for entrepreneurial APNs who are managing the health care for a group of clients. It is a role in which APNs are gaining more comfort and experience.

Impact of the Nurse Shortage on Regulation and Licensure

Supply and demand projections substantiate that the shortage of nurses and other healthcare providers will continue well into 2015. The factors driving the shortage include a growing aging population who will consume more healthcare services, the aging of the nursing workforce resulting in a large cohort of nurses retiring from the profession, and the inability of nursing to attract men, minorities, and young people into the profession. Even though there have been numerous initiatives at the state and federal levels to reverse this trend, the nurse shortage continues to fuel policy on work environment issues across the nation.

Several issues bear monitoring during this period of a declining nursing workforce. They include the following:

1. Delegation and supervision of unlicensed assistive personnel (UAP). Practice for UAPs will continue to be debated and expanded as the shortage of licensed staff make it difficult to meet all the care demands of the public. Providing safe and effective care while delegating care to UAPs will place additional responsibilities on the licensed nurse.
2. Mandatory overtime legislation. Research has shown that fatigue affects the mental acuity of an individual, leading to more errors in judgment and in medical errors that could result in harm to the patient. The Institute of Medicine (IOM) has published findings that

link medical errors to the number and educational level of nurses employed as well as to fatigue of the staff (Institute of Medicine, 1999). Employers have used the concept of patient abandonment to force employees to remain on duty against their will, threatening staff who leave the employment setting with patient abandonment that would result in a report to the licensing board. Laws have been passed in several states that preclude an employer from requiring staff to work beyond their scheduled assignment against their will.

3. Staffing ratios. In some states, the nurses have organized to pass legislation to implement staffing ratios that guarantee a nurse-to-patient ratio dependent on the acuity of the patient. Staffing ratios have both positive and negative implications. Although the regulations for staffing ratios may require a set number of nurses to be employed, the minimum ratios imposed by law may be seen by the employer as the maximum number that must be employed, thereby placing a cap on hiring and negatively affecting the quality of care.

4. Foreign nurse recruitment. There is often an attempt to increase the recruitment of foreign-educated nurses when there is an acute nurse shortage in the United States. Legislation is often introduced during these periods of time to relax the standards for licensure and to accept competency examinations that are not equivalent to the National Council Licensure Examination (NCLEX). The nursing community must be vigilant to these attempts to lower the standards for licensure and thus prevent discrimination against U.S.-educated graduates.

5. Proliferation of new nursing education programs. Nationally, colleges, universities, and other accredited and legitimate public and private educational institutions are finding that the business of nursing education is becoming more attractive; there are more qualified applicants for nursing programs then there are seats. However, proprietary organizations are also seeing nursing education as an opportunity for profit, without consideration of the infrastructure and support systems necessary to carry out a quality program. State Boards of Nursing are being challenged to strike a balance between an open marketplace and a desire to protect the stretched interests of existing programs that are struggling to maintain a cadre of qualified faculty and ensure clinical placements for their students.

Other trends and issues will surface over the next several years that may affect the regulation of nurses and APNs. It will be increasingly important to stay abreast of legislative and regulatory initiatives and to affiliate with professional organizations to preserve and protect professional standards.

Conclusion

Today is an era of rapid transformation in almost every aspect of life. Change is constant, and it rapidly forces adaptability and flexibility on the part of all individuals. Changes in the delivery of health care are transforming the practice and regulation of the APN. Today the APN must develop skills to capitalize on the chaos in the healthcare system and create opportunities for the advantage of the profession rather than fear the future. One way to capitalize on the times is to become politically astute and learn to shape public policy through working with coalitions of nurses, other providers, and consumers to advocate for quality health care at an affordable cost.

Knowing how to navigate the regulatory process will give the APN the tools needed to become a confident spokesperson. Seeking and finding information on the status of issues critical to the APN, such as reimbursement, scopes of practice, and licensure issues, keeps the APN knowledgeable about how best to influence outcomes. Participating in professional nursing organizations provides a forum for building strong coalitions and gaining power in the political process. Each APN has the ability to make a difference.

Discussion Points and Activities

1. Contrast the major differences in the legislative and regulatory processes.
2. Describe the major methods of credentialing. List the benefits and weaknesses of each method from the standpoint of public protection and protection of the professional scope of practice.
3. Discuss the role of professional organizations in regulating professional practice.
4. Describe an ethical dilemma that you have recently experienced. What principles were in conflict with each other? Which principle ruled in your decision? Why?
5. Obtain a copy of a proposed or recently promulgated regulation. Using Exhibit 4–1, analyze the regulation for its impact on nursing practice.
6. Assume the board of nursing has promulgated a regulation requiring all APNs to have 20 contact hours of continuing-education credit in pharmacotherapeutics each year to maintain prescriptive authority. Write a brief (no more than two pages) testimony supporting or opposing this proposed regulation.
7. Describe the federal government's role in the regulation of health professions. Do you believe the role will increase or decrease over time? Explain your rationale.
8. Discuss the pros and cons of multistate regulation. Based on your analysis, defend a position either for or against multistate regulation.

9. Prepare written testimony for a public hearing defending or opposing the need for a second license for APNs.

10. Contrast the board of nursing and the national or state nurses association vis-à-vis mission, membership, authority, functions, and source of funding.

11. Identify a proposed regulation. Discuss the current phase of the process, identify methods of offering comments, and submit written comments to the administrative agency.

12. Download at least one resource from one of the Web sites listed in Exhibit 4–3 and evaluate it according to reliability of the author, last update, and appropriateness of data. Share the resources with colleagues.

13. Evaluate the board of nursing in your state using the criteria for review of regulatory agencies developed by the Pew Health Professions Commission (1995).

14. Identify the states that have implemented nurse staffing ratios. List some of the obstacles the state has encountered in the implementation phase.

References

American Academy of Nurse Practitioners. (2003). *Medicare reimbursement fact sheet.* Washington, DC: Author. Available online at: www.aanp.org

American Association of Colleges of Nursing. (2004). *AACN position statement on the practice doctorate in nursing.* Retrieved June 19, 2007, from: www.aacn.nche.edu/DNP/DNPPositionStatement.htm

American Association of Colleges of Nursing. (2006). *Nursing organizations respond to NCSBN's Draft 2006 APRN vision paper.* Retrieved June 19, 2007, from: www.aacn.nche.edu/Education/ncsbnvision.htm

American Association of Colleges of Nursing. (2007). *Doctor of nursing practice (DNP) programs.* Retrieved July 11, 2007, from: www.aacn.nche.edu/DNP/dnpprogramlist.htm

American Nurses Association. (2007). *Government affairs: RN activist tool kit.* Retrieved June 19, 2007, from: www.anapoliticalpower.org

Black, H. L., Nolan, J. R., & Nolan-Haley, J. M. (1992). *Black's law dictionary* (6th ed.). St. Paul, MN: West.

Braunstein, M. (1995). Homecare in cyberspace. *Computer Talk for Homecare Providers,* pp. 5–12.

Canavan, K. (1996). Credentialing agencies agree on outside review. *American Nurse,* 28(5), 6.

Centers for Medicare and Medicaid Services. (2001, June 14). *Fact Sheet: The new Centers for Medicare and Medicaid services.* Retrieved June 19, 2007, from: www.hhs.gov/news/press/2001pres/20010614a.html

DeVries, C. M., & Vanderbilt, M. W. (1992). *The grassroots lobbying handbook.* Washington, DC: American Nurses Association.

Dower, C., & Finocchio, L. (1995). Health care workforce regulation: Making the necessary changes for a transforming health care system. *State Health Workforce Reforms,* 4, 1–2.

Garner, B. A. (2004). *Black's law dictionary* (8th ed.). St Paul, MN: West.

Gobis, L. J. (1997). Licensing and liability: Crossing the borders with telemedicine. *Caring, 16(7),18–24.*

Goehlert, R. U., & Martin, F. S. (1989). Federal administrative law. *Congress and law making: Researching the legislative process* (2nd ed.). Santa Barbara, CA: ABC-CLIO.

Gross, S. (1984). *Of foxes and hen houses.* Westport, CT: Quorum.

Institute of Medicine. (1999). *To err is human: Building a safer health system.* (Report of the IOM). Available online at: www.iom.edu /CMS/8089/5575.aspx

Jost, T. S. (1997). *Regulation of the health professions.* Chicago: Health Administration Press.

National Council of State Boards of Nursing. (1997). Using nurse practitioners certification for state nursing regulation: An update. *Issues, 18(1).*

National Council of State Boards of Nursing. (1998, April). *Multi state regulation task force communiqué.* Chicago: Author.

National Council of State Boards of Nursing. (2002). *Regulation of advanced nursing practice position paper.* Retrieved June 19, 2007, from: https://www.ncsbn.org/1993_Position_Paper_on_the_Regulation_of_Advanced_Nursing_Practice.pdf

National Council of State Boards of Nursing. (2006). *Draft—Vision paper:The future regulation of advanced practice nursing.* Available online at: https://www.ncsbn.org

National Council of State Boards of Nursing. (2007). *Participating states in the NLC (nurse licensure compact).* Retrieved June 19, 2007, from: https://www.ncsbn.org/158.htm

O'Malley, J., Cummings, S., & King, C. S. (1996). The politics of advanced practice. *Nursing administration Quarterly, 20(3),* 62–69.

Pearson, L. J. (2002). Fourteenth annual legislative update. *Nurse Practitioner: The American Journal of Primary Health Care, 27(1),* 10–52.

Pew Health Professions Commission. (1994). *State strategies for health care workforce reform.* San Francisco: UCSF Center for the Health Professions.

Pew Health Professions Commission. (1995). *Report of task force on health care workforce regulation (executive summary).* San Francisco: UCSF Center for the Health Professions.

Phillips, S. J. (2006). Eighteenth annual legislative update. *Nurse Practitioner, 31(1),* 6–38.

Pruitt, R., Wetsel, M., Smith, K., & Spitler, H. (2002). How do we pass NP Autonomy Legislation? *Nurse Practitioner: The American Journal of Primary Health Care, 27(3),* 56–65.

Roberts, M. J., & Clyde, A. T. (1993). *Your money or your life:The health care crisis explained.* New York: Doubleday.

Safriet, B. J. (1992). Health care dollars and regulatory sense: The role of advanced practice nursing. *Yale Journal of Regulation, 9,* 2.

Sheets, V. (1996). Public protection or professional self-preservation. *NCSBN Monograph, 3.*

Weisenbeck, S. M., & Calico, P. A. (1995). *Issues and trends in nursing* (2nd ed.). St. Louis, MO: Mosby.

5

Policy Design

Patricia Smart, PhD, RN, FNP-BC

Key Terms

➤ **Fire alarms** Signals built into a policy that alerts policymakers that the design, implementation, or evaluation phase is in danger of failing.

➤ **Fuzzy/crisp charges** Degree of clarity of objectives and directions for implementation in a mandate, regulation, or law.

➤ **Participation** Extent to which individuals in the target population join in government programs.

➤ **Policy link** Connection between policy ideas and their implementation.

Introduction

The purpose of this chapter is to examine the component of the policy process that involves the "tools" that government uses to get people to do what they might not ordinarily do. It is well recognized that the scope of government's involvement in social issues in the United States has increased rapidly during the last 75 years. Federally funded healthcare programs such as Medicare and Medicaid have made a major impact on how health care is implemented by providers and perceived by the public. As noted by Comer (2002), government involvement in health care has occurred at the state and local levels through program administration, educational preparation, licensing, and regulation of practice.

The United States has one of the most sophisticated healthcare systems (although challengers call it a "sick care system") in the world in terms of technology and preparation of healthcare professionals. Yet in many of the health indices designed to evaluate the overall health of a country, the United States rates comparatively low. For example, as found in *Healthy People* 2010, life expectancy in the United States for females is 78.9 years, while in many other developed countries such as Japan, France, Canada, and England a female's life expectancy is 82.9 years, 82.6 years, 81.2 years, and 79.6 years, respectively. Infant mortality also is an important measure of a nation's health. *Healthy People* 2010 notes that in 1995, the United States ranked 25th among industrialized countries in infant mortality. Furthermore, new cases of low birth weight and very low birth weight, both of which contribute to infant mortality, have increased in the United States (U.S. Department of Health and Human Services, 2002).

Frequent failure of solutions to many social problems and tactics to restrict government spending have combined to raise questions about the effectiveness of social programs. Efforts to restrict spending continue to be in the process of debate with no resolution in sight. Ulbrich (2003) comments on American ambivalence regarding expanding the role of government, particularly in the area of health care. She notes that an underlying basis from which all discussions and arguments regarding the role of government in health care are formed is the belief that personal financial risks should be individually assumed. These risks are associated with earning a living and managing one's income and assets wisely as opposed to shared responsibility through government.

Policies are usually designed to influence behavior and, as noted earlier, get people to do what they ordinarily might not do. As noted by Longest (2002), health policies address health concerns through laws, regulations, or programs that focus on health determinants including behavioral choices, physical environment in which people live and work, and social factors. Although many studies regarding the policy process have been conducted, few have examined the process of policy design in issues of health care. The focus of most policy studies has been on the implementation of effective programs, and data have been gathered on statistical outcomes. This author argues that design considerations also should be a component to be considered during all phases of the policy process to promote policy success. For example, in the agenda-setting phase, the social issue must be stated in such a way that it will capture the attention of lawmakers and framed so that government response will be feasible and adaptable. During the implementation phase, the design of the policy provides guidance and also provides an overall picture of the plan by specifying the intended outcomes. During the evaluation phase (included in the design), the program objectives are clearly identified and measurable or it would be difficult to determine that the focus is on an outcome that addresses the original issue

The Policy Process

The *policy process* is the act of addressing or ignoring publicly perceived problems. Leichter (1979) notes that policy is contained in legislative enactments including budgets, court mandates, and executive orders. According to Thompson (1981), the policy process "involves a complicated interaction among government institutions, actors, and the particular characteristics of substantive policy areas" (p. ix). Heclo (1978) notes that "a policy, like a decision, can consist of what is not being done" (p. 134).

Policies that address social problems in the United States usually are formulated by a combination of legislators and aides, the executive branch, courts, and special-interest groups. Professional experts are often asked to serve as panel members or consultants or to serve on committees that provide input to policymakers. Advanced practice nurses (APNs) are asked to serve on committees that relate to health care. For example, nurse leaders were invited to sit at the table during the early 1990s when Hillary Clinton was proposing a national plan to change existing healthcare policies.

The proliferation of participants in policy formation makes systematic program design focused on outcomes difficult to achieve. Social problems are usually intractable and difficult to solve. As noted by Safriet (2002), most social issues are not brought to the attention of policymakers until there is a crisis with multiple causative factors. Decision making with regard to relevant factors that relate to or have an impact on perceived social problems often is conducted hastily because of lack of information, constituency impatience, and lack of expertise (Dryzek, 1983).

Review of Policy Research

Implementation

Much of the research contributing to an understanding of the policy process is found in implementation literature. Although the design of a policy affects the implementation phase, many studies have ignored environmental factors existing in the design phase that would have impact on policy implementation. For example, attitudes and expectations of policymakers are often different from the attitudes and expectations of policy participants. Policy success or failure is seen by many policy scholars as occurring only in the implementation phase of policymaking. It is important to understand how the pitfalls can produce a negative impact on policies and programs. APNs are in a position to play a key role in the design of health policies and must have knowledge of ways to improve the probability of success.

Pressman and Wildavsky (1973) note the complexity of implementation and difficulty in achieving policy success when many branches and divisions of government attempt to work together. For example, multiple veto points among multiple policy actors often act to obscure the original intent of policies. *Veto points* are those areas of vulnerability in the policy process where decisions might be made that could undermine the original intent of the policymakers and, therefore, need to be addressed in the design phase. For example, in the process of obtaining a state's recognition for prescriptive authority for APNs, the proposal (beginning of the policy) was examined critically by many interested groups, including physicians, pharmacists, and health insurance agencies. At any point, members of these groups could recommend amendments that could, at best, alter or, at worst, "shoot down" the proposal, thus avoiding the potential of sabotage during the implementation process.

Bardach (1977) identifies several factors required for sound implementation. He looks at relationships among implementation actors and labels the activity process among policy players as "game playing." He identifies activities such as bargaining and negotiating among players that make a tremendous impact on policy success and failure. Bardach also notes that a good policy must begin with a design that incorporates scenarios that can anticipate games and "**fire alarms**." For example, in some states, APNs have to be willing to allow a representative from the board of pharmacy or the board of medicine to be on the governing board that regulates nursing at the advanced level.

Others researchers (Elmore, 1979–1980; Mazmanian & Sabatier, 1983; Van Meter & Van Horn, 1975; Lipsky, 1980) identify variables, including policy form and content and organizations and their resources and people. Their work provides major contributions to the study of the policy process in the development of frameworks from which to conduct scientific inquiry and theory building. Additional studies (Goggin, Bowman, Lester, & O'Toole, 1990; Durant & Legge, 1993) provide mechanisms to address questions of conceptualization and measurement.

Agenda Setting

Many scholars focus on how a perceived problem reaches the government agenda in the process of policymaking. For example, Kingdon uses the Cohen and colleagues' description of the decision process (Cohen, March, & Olsen, 1972) as a loose collection of ideas that emerge from "organized anarchies." Kingdon (1995), writing about the public decision-making system in the United States, adds the notion of independent streams that he labels the policy stream, the political stream, and the problem stream. He contends that a choice opportunity occurs when the person with a problem and the person with a solution come together. He describes this rather cavalier, fluid activity as decision making in the realm of policymaking, and the outcomes as a function of how the streams happen to combine.

On the other hand, Dryzek (1983) argues that a modicum of reasoning should be introduced into the policy process. He asserts that haphazard, loose coupling of ill-defined streams will not produce policies with the properties of adaptation, homeostatic capability, and feedback that are necessary to withstand policy analysis and revision. Dryzek further argues that the type of policy designed for specific problems depends on the complexity and uncertainty of the policy and the lack of feedback to the policymakers.

Ingraham (1987) also rejects the notion that policymaking takes place in a "garbage can." The garbage can metaphor refers to a process of decision making that consists of separate streams of problems, solutions, participants, and choices that couple and uncouple to produce alternative solutions to problems (Kingdon, 1995). Ingraham states that more rigorous studies should be conducted to examine the critical components of the policy process. She says that the most notable omission has been the effort to "determine the exact nature of the problem and its causes, the potential range of solutions and the most appropriate strategy for achieving desired outcomes" (p. 613). Ingraham also notes that the problem-solving nature of public-policy design has rarely been examined.

Policy Links

During the 1980s, political scientists studied the content of policy with the intention of providing a clearer understanding of the link between policy design and policy outcome (**policy links**). Their efforts hold importance for APNs whose roles often require interpretation and implementation of policies. To improve the likelihood of policy success, APNs must be able to critically analyze policy content; that is, what the original intent of the policy is, and if the policy is designed in such a way as to assure the intended outcome. Dryzek (1983) argues that efforts to analyze the policy process should place more emphasis on the study and utilization of policy design. Schneider and Ingram (1990) also argue for a closer look at design and proposed a framework to examine behavioral assumptions and attributes of policy content that can be employed by APNs to conduct the work of government.

Government policies are subject to a wide scope of interpretation that depends on who brings problems to national attention and which legislative group attaches itself to problems and solutions. Jones (1984) maintains that often a policy is not the direct result of a perceived public problem because the problem itself is not stated clearly. He insists that it is fairly standard for policies to be vague to allow flexibility in implementation and administrative discretion at the program level. Jones notes further that policy formulation often follows a haphazard path that may proceed without a clear problem definition. This author agrees that policy formulation is often haphazard and argues that policy formulation rarely includes a clear, well-thought-out design. An opportunity exists for APNs who recognize the value of vagueness. Rather than waiting for clear directives, the nurse must learn and become comfortable with ambiguity because it allows discretion and flexibility in decision making and action, thereby enhancing the ability to individualize management.

The Design Issue

Scholars have begun to analyze the link between policy design and implementation. Mandates that often are not clear in intent or purpose, or that are unclear regarding implementation, often are handed down by legislators and are difficult to conceptualize and implement. The result of unclear mandates often results in a mismatch between congressional intent and bureaucratic behavior. For example, federal money that is allocated to states for harm-reduction programs, such as smoking cessation during pregnancy, may reach a segment of the target group that may not need it. Many college-educated women will not smoke during pregnancy, yet the private healthcare providers have access to as much federal money to develop an antismoking program as their public agency counterparts.

Several scholars have noted that rather than focusing on implementation, the original intent of a policy should be spelled out and reflected in the design of the policy. Linder and Peters (1987) state in their study that policy design was a reason for policy failure. Describing some programs as "crippled at birth," these scholars note that the best bureaucracies in the world may not be able to achieve desired goals successfully if a particular policy that may be excessively ambitious is used (i.e., the problem is too complex for a single policy). Also, if there is a misunderstanding of the nature of the problem, inappropriate policies may be formulated. Linder and Peters propose that implementation should be examined, but only as one of the conditions that must be satisfied for successful policymaking. They maintain that by shifting the focus of study to policy design, a more reliable and explicit answer can be found regarding policy success.

This author proposes that by examining the assumptions made by policymakers regarding **participation** of the target population, the process of development of policy, the tools used to develop a definition of the problem, and the match between policy development and outcome, policies relating to infant mortality and low birth weight can avoid some of the factors that may contribute to the policies being "crippled at birth." Policy design can be conceptualized as a process that can occur at both the policy formulation and implementation phases or as a blueprint approach that shapes policy (Linder & Peters, 1990). Policy formulation and design have been recognized as important links between problem identification and policy implementation. Design is perceived as a critical and vulnerable factor in the overall policy process.

Other scholars concur with Linder and Peters. Ingraham (1987) argues that a systematic analysis of program design, rather than analysis using the garbage can model, could enhance policy success by allowing the option of considering alternative strategies and providing causal links culminating in theory building. She focuses her work on two areas of policy design.

The first area is related to the level of design; that is, the extent to which a program has been structured consciously and systematically and the extent to which several elements of design content and process are examined. For example, what is the range of solutions that was considered, how is strategy chosen, and is the match between strategy and available resources examined? Ingraham (1987) argues that the lowest level of design activity is the simplistic two-step process involving direct transference of political rhetoric to a program with absence of design considerations. She notes that Lowi (1960) suggests that many liberal policies of the past suffered from this translation and notes further that more conservative rhetoric and policies suffer because of lack of design considerations as well.

Ingraham (1987) also examines the location of design activities as her second focus on policy design. Her posture is that policy formulation and design no longer take place exclusively in the legislative arena. Instead, activity is seen more often in many different locations in the policy system. She notes that input from experts outside the legislative body requires a greater effort toward clarifying goals and objectives and requires negotiation and bargaining. Ingraham identifies several variables that may influence both level and focus of policy design, including problem intractability, goal consensus, commitment to solution, and alternatives. She maintains that continued identification and elaboration of factors influencing policy design are necessary to understand the policy process further. Advanced practice nurses should heed Ingraham's advice by staying abreast of societal and environmental changes that could affect health policy. For example, the recurrence of tuberculosis has become a major public health concern. With earlier detection, many individuals could have been protected against the recent recurrence, and the national economic impact would have been less.

Often there are mismatches between legislative intent and bureaucratic outcomes. Bureaucrats often receive "**fuzzy**" (as opposed to "**crisp**") **charges** with vague marching orders (Lerner & Wanat, 1983, p. 500). Fuzzy charges can be a problem with a program in general or may refer to more micro factors such as determining which clients are eligible for services. One major consequence when executing fuzzy mandates is the need to interpolate a workable mandate from the vague charge. This results in "conceptual satisficing" (p. 505) because of lack of time to explore all alternatives fully. These scholars contend that a continuous line of fuzzy mandates often requires extensive organizational shifts with subsequent changes in bureaucratic outcomes. For example, many contend that the *Roe v. Wade* (1973) decision by the U.S. Supreme Court in which the court contended that a woman has the right to decide what happens to her body has been abused by a society that has used the decision to support broader issues of contraception.

Upon reviewing the current policy literature, it is apparent that the design phase of the policy process continues to be an area where few policy scholars choose to focus their efforts. However, there are a few policy studies that are looking at design when examining social policy. For example, in a study conducted to examine policy-instrument utilization to promote electricity-efficient household appliances and office equipment, Varone and Aebischer (2001) determine that the political climate in which a policy is implemented is a critical factor to be considered when choosing instruments. In summary, policy design is an integral component of implementation. An understanding of policy tools or instruments chosen for policy design and the underlying assumptions of policymakers during the design process is critical to an understanding of the overall policy process.

Policy Instruments

Some policy scholars have directed their attention to instruments chosen by policymakers in developing policy, the process by which strategy is chosen, and have identified factors that influence policy design. Sardell (1990) notes that the definition or framing of an issue is critical to the nature of activity on the issue, the type of groups that become involved, and the development of specific policies. Thus, the study of instruments or tools by which the government achieves desired policy goals has allowed researchers to examine policies in relation to their intent and to begin to infer predictive capabilities of tools.

Originally, many scholars argued that this method of analysis eliminated or reduced significantly the aspect of political practice and political community. The idea has become somewhat modified and acceptable to most scholars. Linder and Peters (1990) note that most instrument research efforts focus on the presumed merits of tools, as opposed to the heuristics and decision-making routines employed by those who choose the instruments or tools.

Other scholars have noted the dearth of information regarding the decision-making process and policy content in the design phase. Dryzek (1983) contends that the fit of policies to their environments usually is related directly to the complexity of the problem and that complex and uncertain circumstances often lead to avoidance of policy analysis. In other words, the more complex the problem and subsequent policy, the less likely that analysis will occur. He notes that most policy-design analysis focuses on methods of alternative selection or how the selections should be made. Design quality would be improved with the shift of analytical focus toward the generation of alternatives. That is, by exploring the various alternatives and the potential for success, greater enlightenment of the intricacies of the problem would be experienced. He examines which factors lead to decisions reached by policymakers toward instrument choice (i.e., the content of the decision-making process).

Dryzek also argues that strategic thinking that involves the consideration of the cultural, institutional, physical, and biological environments should be conducted. By encompassing these components, a tendency toward following standard operating procedures is avoided. Such considerations lay the groundwork to enhance the decision-making abilities of future generations. Advanced practice nurses can exert great influence in helping policymakers understand the components. For example, a nurse can provide information on health beliefs and practices of diverse cultural groups that can assist a legislator in designing an appropriate program or policy.

Two scholars proposed a framework for studying policy based on "policy tools." Schneider and Ingram (1990) offer a framework to analyze implicit or explicit behavioral theories found in laws, regulations, and programs. Their analysis uses government tools or instruments and underlying behavioral assumptions as variables, which guide policy decisions and choices. Their contention is that target group compliance and utilization are important forms of political behavior that should be examined closely. Combined with process variables such as competition, partisanship, and public opinion, Schneider and Ingram argue that the tools approach moves policy beyond considering the standard analysis and improved frameworks. They note that policy tools are substitutable and often states use a variety of tools to address a single problem. To understand which tools are most productive, emphasis should be placed on using them in conjunction with a particular policy design. APNs use their knowledge of policy tools to make suggestions and recommendations to government leaders who are designing policies and programs.

Policy Design Model

Schneider and Ingram (1990) state that public policy almost always attempts to get people or enable people to do things they would not have done otherwise. These scholars describe policy tools as those methods chosen by policymakers to overcome barriers to policy-relevant actions. Large numbers of people in different situations are involved in policymaking. Actions required by these players include compliance with policy rules, utilization of policy opportunities, and self-initiated actions, which promote policy goals.

Schneider and Ingram list several reasons they suggest may affect the failure to take actions needed to ameliorate social, economic, or political problems: (1) lack of incentives or capacity; (2) disagreement with the values implicit in the means or ends; or (3) the existence of high levels of uncertainty about the situation that make it unclear what people should do or how to motivate them. Schneider and Ingram describe five specific policy tools used by governments in designing policy. They identify five broad categories of tools, which include authority, incentives, capacity building, symbolic and hortatory, and learning.

Authority tools are used most frequently by governments to guide behavior of agents and officials at lower levels. Authority tools are statements backed by the legitimate power of government that grant permission and prohibit or require action under designated circumstances. An example of an authority tool is a law, regulation, or mandate that requires women to qualify under regulated criteria for prenatal services.

Incentive tools assume individuals are utility maximizers and will not be motivated positively to take action without encouragement or coercion. These tools rely on tangible payoffs (positive or negative) as motivating factors. Incentive policy tools manipulate tangible benefits, costs, and probabilities that policy designers assume are relevant to the situation. Incentives assume individuals have the "opportunity to make choices, recognize the opportunity, and have adequate information and decision-making skills to select from among alternatives that are in the best interests" (Schneider & Ingram, 1990, p. 516). An incentive tool, for example, may be coupons for free public transportation to prenatal clinics to encourage pregnant women to seek care. If the APN assumes that lack of transportation is a barrier to access prenatal care, the outcome from an attempt to use this particular incentive may fail.

Capacity-building tools provide information, training, education, and resources to enable individuals, groups, or agencies to make decisions or carry out activities. These tools assume that incentives are not an issue and that target populations will be motivated adequately. For capacity-building tools to work, populations must be aware of the risk factors the tools possess and how these tools can help. Capacity-building tools focus on education. For example, information may point out the risks of smoking and drugs on a fetus, and information on such risk factors is distributed to the target population. The underlying assumption is that information about the cessation of smoking is considered valuable, and that pregnant women will stop smoking if they have correct information.

Symbolic and hortatory tools assume that people are motivated from within and decide whether to take policy-related actions on the basis of their beliefs and values. An example of this type of tool is a poster directed at adolescents that uses an adolescent model to issue advice or a warning. Such tools seek to gain the attention of the target population (adolescents) through use of peer imagery. Slogans also are symbolic and are used so that consumers link a positive or negative outcome to a particular behavior.

Learning tools are used when the basis upon which target populations might be moved to take problem-solving action is unknown or uncertain. Policies that use learning tools often are open-ended in purposes and objectives and have broad goals. A needs assessment of the target population may be conducted by a task force. This type of survey provides knowledge and insight for policymakers and is an example of a learning tool. For example, if a community program related to addressing childhood obesity is to be proposed, a needs assessment must be conducted to determine what information is going to be needed before a proposal is drawn up for presentation to the county council.

Policy tools are important resources for the APN because they can enhance efforts to provide accurate information so that the patient can make informed decisions. For example, educational pamphlets relating to health promotion behaviors such as dietary considerations for the diabetic can be sent home with the patient. This will reinforce information received from the care provider and help the patient adhere to a fairly complicated change in lifestyle.

Behavioral Dimensions

In addition to understanding the types and the roles of tools in developing policy, the nurse in advanced practice must understand behavioral assumptions and the political context in which tools exist. The political climate in which social problems are addressed often prescribes the choice of tools to be implemented. Various tools are used when addressing similar social problems. Often these tools are interchanged and many times result in differing outcomes when used by different agencies, states, or countries. In the United States, for example, liberal policymakers are inclined to use capacity-building tools when developing policy for the poor and minority groups, whereas conservative policymakers might use the same types of tools in developing policy applicable to businesses.

Schneider and Ingram (1990) report that a shift in focus to the behavioral dimensions of policy tools permits comparative analysis across policy types, which yields information about the effectiveness of alternative tools when particular circumstances of the policy arena are held constant. The two researchers propose that the concept of policy-tool choice in policymaking can be used to compare the behavioral assumptions of policy from different states and countries, particularly on like issues that have shown contrasting results.

Health care is fraught with a multitude of factors that are difficult to identify and control. One of the most elusive factors inhibiting policy success is the ability to predict consumer behavior and participation in a program. Another factor that exacerbates the problem of control is the introduction of policies designed to control healthcare costs. Recently, the main shift in the health policy agenda has been from access to cost containment. Cost containment policies threaten to jeopardize access to health care and its quality. For example, healthcare staff power has decreased, and the most sophisticated technology is available to only a few. Not only are the poor at risk for not receiving adequate health care, but the situation affects the middle-income sector also.

Child health is an area in which the paradoxes of health policy are seen very clearly. Industrialized nations provide high technology and specialized services to those with acute conditions, while often misdirecting the focus away from primary care and the social factors that increase medical risks. The United States ranks first in the world in its ability to save the lives of premature and very small infants, yet ranks 15th in the proportion of babies born at low birth weight (Sardell, 1990) and, currently, ranks 25th in infant mortality (U.S. Department of Health and Human Services, 2002). Despite this country's ability to save these special-care infants initially, neonatal mortality (death up to 27 days after birth) and postneonatal mortality (death from 28 days to 1 year) affect the United States profoundly.

Although the infant mortality rate has declined over the past 20 years, the overall rate in the United States for infant mortality is still 7.2%. In addition, one can anticipate that with budget crises and the lack of resolution regarding access, the infant mortality rate will not improve and may, in fact, increase as a result of less than adequate prenatal visits. Rather than expanding national health insurance coverage as would most liberal-democratic countries, the United States, with its bias against public solutions, allowed employment-based insurance to expand to the point where the state could merely fill main gaps with welfare-oriented safety nets. According to Sardell (1990), studies conducted at local levels in the 1960s and 1970s found that reductions in neonatal mortality were related to the introduction of neonatal intensive care services, the availability of family planning services, Medicaid services, and the legalization of abortion.

Miller (1988) was commissioned by the U.S. Institute of Medicine to study outreach for prenatal care. He compared rates of low birth weight and infant mortality in 10 European countries with the United States. All of the nine European nations whose rates of low birth weight were lower than that of the United States had national standards for prenatal care with organized community services at the local level and national financing and monitoring of these services. In all 10 countries, services were provided to all women, regardless of income and with minimal financial barriers to care. Incentives were offered for women to seek prenatal care, such as paid leave for prenatal classes or visits, transportation to services, early reservations for delivery, and children's allowances. Furthermore, home visits were routinely made after delivery in every cited European country. Although most states and counties in the United States have begun to offer home visits, it is the result of an insurance-driven mandate of 24-hour stays in the hospital for uncomplicated vaginal deliveries and 72-hour stays for women who deliver by cesarean.

Conclusion

Policy design is an integral component of implementation. The choice of policy tools and the underlying assumptions of policymakers during the design process are critical to an understanding of the overall policy process. Scholars concur that a shift of research focus from implementation to design is an important step for further research.

Case Study in Policy Design

This case study in policy design examines government health policies related to pregnancy outcomes. A comparison was made between one U.S. southern state and the Netherlands using factors such as political culture, economies, policy background, government response, and policy participation. Although the state and national levels of government are different, they are appropriate for comparative analysis because of their bicameral political structures.

Infant Mortality: Comparative Issues

One of the most important issues facing nations today involves pregnant women and their infants. The problem of infant mortality has been on the government agenda of the United States for decades, and policies have been designed and implemented to relieve this problem. However, infant mortality and its causes and consequences in the United States remain a critical social issue, and the country lags behind most industrialized nations in solving the problem. A major cause of infant death is low birth weight (2500 grams or less). Even though the infant mortality rate is improving, the problem of low birth weight is becoming more prevalent. Low birth weight costs both lives and money. According to the former federal Office of Technology Assessment, the U.S. healthcare system spends between $14,000 and $30,000 per low-birth-weight child, mainly in intensive care costs during the infant's first year. Lifelong costs for the low-birth-weight infant have been estimated at $250,000 per child (Singh, 1990). A major contributor to low birth weight and subsequent death is unplanned pregnancy. At particular risk for unplanned pregnancy is the adolescent.

Prenatal Care

Experts recognize that early and adequate prenatal care is one of the most important factors in preventing low birth weight; however, more than 24% of American women do not receive adequate prenatal care (Lee & Estes, 1990). The question emerges as to why a significant portion of American women living in a country with a highly developed and sophisticated healthcare system are not receiving prenatal care needed to prevent low birth weight and potential death of their infants.

The study revealed several disturbing facts regarding policymaking in the United States in general and in South Carolina specifically. In the area of political culture, differences were evident. Even though South Carolina and the Netherlands are pluralist societies with democratically derived leadership and bicameral legislatures, many factors contribute to very different approaches to policymaking. The Constitution of the United States leads to a system of checks and balances that has led to a federal legislature that, even when dominated by the same party as the executive, has considerable autonomy and may be divided strongly on a given issue.

This diffusion of power makes it difficult to enact and implement policies. The structure of federalism (a system of government that allows each state considerable room for decentralized development in terms of adapting to unique human and environmental circumstances) offers opportunities for bolder programs in states than at a national level. Because of the growth of regulatory activities, policymaking has become even more complex with more interdependency and conflict.

APNs in the United States often work in settings where even small policy changes involve multiple disciplines or departments and actors. For example, in a primary care setting, such as a family-planning center, a policy change relating to Medicaid payment would affect patient recordkeeping for the social worker, dietitian, physician, and business manager as well as the nurse. The APN must be prepared to assume a leadership role in the collaboration of the various disciplines in providing comprehensive care to the patient.

This study found the Dutch government is centralized with little discretion allowed to lower-level administrators in municipalities. This is the result of clear, specifically stated policies that limit administrative and management flexibility. More recently, however, the Dutch government has become more decentralized with more political discretion and power being assumed at the local levels.

As noted by Lijphart (1977), the Netherlands has managed to overcome potential problems caused by cleavages through exceptional cooperation and coordination among elite members of each segment in the policymaking process. Elite members are those who have the greatest influence in policymaking. For example, popular legislators, intellectuals, and business leaders are often considered elites. Political changes have occurred in the Netherlands, however, that have brought more average citizens into positions of political power. This factor will have an effect on the decision-making process of policymaking as well as the various tools used to address social problems.

The South Carolina policymaking system, on the other hand, is fraught with cleavages and turf issues that have affected policymaking in critical areas. An excellent example of this is seen in the problem of infant mortality. This study suggests that the polarization over the issue of infant mortality before it becomes a problem (preventing unplanned pregnancies) has kept South Carolina in the top ratings in ratios of infant mortality per one thousand live births.

Economies

The gap between equality and distribution of income is greater in the United States than in the Netherlands. Income in the Netherlands falls within a close range. Sardell (1990) notes that access to health care among the poor and unemployed is a long-standing concern of proponents of maternal and infant care. However, despite an unemployment rate that exceeds that of South Carolina, prenatal services are provided to all Dutch women, regardless of income, with minimal financial barriers to care.

Policy Design Factors Related to Prenatal Care in South Carolina and the Netherlands

The purpose of this case study was to determine which policy design factors, if any, produce desired outcomes in the area of prenatal health care. This study examined and compared policymaking instruments related to infant mortality and low birth weight in South Carolina and the Netherlands. South Carolina's infant mortality rate of 10.5% is significantly higher than the 8% infant mortality rate in the Netherlands. If factors related to policy design addressing infant mortality are found to affect design outcome, these factors may be isolated to determine degree of impact. Exhibit 5–1 provides an overview of the findings.

The policymaking tools developed by Schneider and Ingram (1990) are described as instruments that can be substituted for one another and are often used in conjunction and cooperation with one another. Policymaking tools may conflict with one another. For example, the law in South Carolina requires that health care must be provided for pregnant women who are within 185% of the poverty level. Yet, incentive tools such as funding are limited, and the reimbursement process is cumbersome and not prompt. Thus, most private physicians providing prenatal care are not willing to serve this population. Each of the tools has the capacity to allow institutions to achieve the same policy purpose, yet this utopian outcome does not often occur. Policy variables, policy players, demographics of the target population, and policy influence were shown to play a significant role in outcome differences.

The findings from both sites were described under four headings:

1. Policy background, which relates to the way each government perceives the problem and describes the approach taken by each site in problem resolution

Exhibit 5–1 Findings: Policy Design Factors Related to Prenatal Care

South Carolina	The Netherlands
Infant mortality perceived as a problem.	Infant mortality perceived as a problem.
Anecdotal and discretionary approach.	Universal approach to policy design.
Individual, independent initiatives.	Overall policy.
Abortion policy, family planning, and sex education programs restricted, limited, and conservative. Policymaking slow and incremental.	Abortion policy, family planning, and sex education programs easily accessible, available to all, and liberal. Policymaking slow and incremental.
Reactionary response. Addresses infant mortality as a medical issue, rather than a social problem with medical consequences.	Preventive response. Addresses infant mortality from a holistic approach, which includes social and environmental factors.
Narrow focus on issue of infant mortality as well as family planning, sex education, and abortion. Has leaders who consider these topics politically risky.	Broad, sweeping changes 20 years ago on family planning, sex education, and abortion. Has political leaders who support and endorse these topics.
Process variables: Factional political and public environments. Strong partisanship exists. Cleavages and gaps exist among players and target population. Public opinion is fragile. Interest group strength is minimal. Policy analysis and evaluation are not priorities. Political support is apathetic with few exceptions.	Process variables: Homogeneous and consociational political and public environments. Harmonious relationships exist among political elites. Public support policies are in place. Strong special interest lobbyists at work. Statistical data gathered and communicated. Political support consistent and proactive.
Assumptions regarding target group behavior: Co-production is uncoordinated, not encouraged, and there is no joint tenancy; compliance is minimal; utilization is below expectations, and political support is apathetic with a few exceptions.	Assumptions regarding target group behavior: Co-production is organized and joint tenancy is encouraged; compliance is responsive; utilization is sought and maximized; and political support is strong and proactive.
Tools: Findings support that Schneider and Ingram's defined policymaking tools (1990) are comparable to those used in the Netherlands. Focus of tools is retrospective.	Tools: Findings support that Schneider and Ingram's defined policymaking tools (1990) are utilized and are consistent with those used in South Carolina. Focus of tools is retrospective.
Social indicators and demographics appear to have minimal impact.	Social indicators and demographics appear to have minimal impact.

2. Government responses, which describe the direction taken by each government in addressing prenatal care as a deterrent to infant mortality and the effectiveness of governmental response (this section also discusses policies and initiatives of each site with applicable policy tools used for decision making and implementation)
3. Policy-process variables, which relate to the components that affect the policymakers' decision making
4. Policy participation, which discusses policy participation

Policy Background

Policy background examined aspects of problem identification. In South Carolina, Dery's (1984) description of problem identification was found to be applicable. Dery notes that the way a problem is defined determines how difficult it appears to policymakers to address and to discover solutions. If information relating to causative factors affecting a problem is not identified, available, communicated to, or understood by policy decision makers, the problem usually appears to be so complex and insurmountable that problem solving is ignored or attention is focused on smaller components of the problem that are more easily addressed. Current approaches to the problem of infant mortality in South Carolina are described by a majority of respondents in this state as fragmented, undefined, and lacking a specific plan.

Most subjects described the issue of infant mortality as a problem that encompasses a multitude of social and economic factors rather than merely a singular, unique problem. Interviewees related that the causes of infant mortality are intertwined with many socioeconomic factors such as poverty, lack of education, and poor self-esteem. Each of these factors alone encompasses many seemingly unsolvable issues that affect the others.

The study showed that, on average, 12% of pregnant women in South Carolina were known to visit a prenatal healthcare provider no more than five times during their pregnancies and, therefore, received less than adequate prenatal care. Seven percent of white women did not receive adequate care and more than 18% of "black and others" received less than adequate care.

Key policymakers commented about the lack of a cohesive, comprehensive policy addressing infant mortality. This lack was noted by most informants to be a result of policymakers' unwillingness to make broad sweeping changes in the way they historically have addressed this issue. Most informants described change in policy as being slow and incremental.

Most informants described the communication infrastructure between researchers and decision makers as poor, and direct communication of information regarding problem factors as being transmitted rarely. In addition, the many layers of bureaucracy proved to be a formidable barrier to clarity of facts regarding issues and problems.

Data providers in South Carolina expressed a lack of clarity regarding what information decision makers were requesting. Data providers did not believe that decision makers were always clear on what information they needed. On the other hand, informants in the Netherlands perceived that they were able to resolve communication problems effectively.

For example, when studies were conducted to examine factors affecting pregnancy outcome, Dutch decision makers communicated effectively the areas that they wanted included in the study and data providers designed the study to those specifications. When the study revealed that unwanted pregnancy affected pregnancy outcomes, the information was communicated directly and explained to decision makers who developed policy immediately to address unwanted pregnancy. The policy designed and implemented by Dutch policymakers was a nationwide effort at reducing unwanted pregnancies. This effort included the introduction of formal sex-education classes to begin in the fifth and sixth grades and to continue throughout the high school program. Church leaders and the media became committed to providing accurate, objective information regarding reproductive anatomy, birth control, and prevention of sexually transmitted diseases. There is no teen pregnancy "problem" in the Netherlands.

Most informants in South Carolina noted the lack of a "bold thinker" in the policymaking body with a special interest in infant mortality. Kingdon (1995) noted that bold thinkers and charismatic leaders provide the energy and direction to address problems through methods and plans not tried before. As noted by Schneider and Ingram (1990), the presence of a bold thinker provides the impetus to explore different ways to address problems. APNs can provide the bold thinking to explore innovative ways of addressing many of the health problems existing today.

Informants in the Netherlands agreed that the issue of infant mortality was recognized to be a multifaceted arena, as in South Carolina, and was not perceived to be a singular, isolated issue. However, the Dutch related that when the issue became a part of managed health care, fragmentation of services, access to care, participation, and utilization of care ceased to become relevant issues. Dutch informants stated that sex education was taught in all schools during the fifth and sixth grades. In addition, issues relating to reproduction, birth control, and prevention of sexually transmitted disease were openly discussed by the parents, churches, and the media. The same, factual information was consistently provided to young people. Key informants in the Netherlands noted that sex is discussed as a knowledge issue rather than a moral one.

In the Netherlands, as in South Carolina, there are multiple political actors who were involved in addressing infant mortality. As a pluralist society, many political factions exist with cleavages between factions. As described by Lijphart (1984), Dutch politics have the unique characteristic of being able to overcome major disputes because political elites from each faction work together to reach a consensus regarding programs. For example, policymaking actors were able to overcome factional cleavages regarding moral issues surrounding unwanted births to consider the overall good for society by the prevention of unwanted births.

The solution process in South Carolina was noted to be an anecdotal approach to finding solutions for social problems. For example, an infant, who spent the first 3 weeks of life in a neonatal intensive care unit as a result of premature birth and subsequent problems related to low birth weight, was described as unable to go home on the scheduled date because the home was without heat. Financial support had to be obtained from a social agency to enable the mother to take the infant home. Although this method of solving an immediate problem is recognized by policymakers and providers as a less than desirable way to handle a crisis, all respondents stated that it was the feasible thing to do at the time. Subjects noted consistently that crossing financial boundary zones occurs frequently and exacerbates the original problem of murky functional areas. This appears to intensify the difficulty in clearly identifying and subsequently addressing the problem of infant mortality.

Solutions to problems in South Carolina often are localized and are not communicated to other areas in the state that may be attempting to address the same issue. Lack of communication results in a "reinvention of the wheel" approach to resolution and likely assures that solutions chosen will continue to be case specific. This anecdotal approach to problem solving is very different from the universal approach to problem solving used by the Dutch.

Interviewees in the Netherlands related that solutions chosen are universally applied. All Dutch women have access to prenatal health care, counseling, and information about pregnancy alternatives. All pregnant women who use the healthcare system are assessed uniformly and consistently using identical criteria and are referred to appropriate services on an equal basis. Those with risk factors are provided care consistent with the risk. All Dutch women have access to the same social services. There are no eligibility criteria to gain access. Specific problems, such as lack of resources to pay for health services, do not arise because basic healthcare insurance is available to all.

Each initiative has its own set of objectives and goals that are described as rather vague. Furthermore, most initiatives have not been evaluated to determine effectiveness. Although the 5-year trend in infant mortality has shown steady improvement, respondents were not able to identify which initiatives were instrumental in the improvement rate. They felt that clarification of the issue was needed to establish a policy with overall-encompassing objectives that could be evaluated. This lack of action on studying causation of improvement rates keeps the state focused on addressing social problems, including infant mortality and lack of prenatal care. These problems appeared easier to address anecdotally than through an overall policy. In contrast, the Netherlands uses policy types that are described as effective and consistent.

Government Response

This research found that governments in both countries used tools similar to those described in Schneider and Ingram's framework (1990), although the policy environments differed a great deal. Policies and initiatives developed and implemented by policymakers were analyzed by applying policy tools used in the conceptualization and implementation of the policy. As noted by Schneider and Ingram, "Policy tools are used to overcome impediments to policy relevant actions" (p. 510). Successful realization of policy goals requires active participation by the target population. However, if policymakers are not cognizant of motivating and deterring factors affecting the decision-making process of the target group, incorrect assumptions regarding participative behavior can result in an ineffective policy.

Although data relating to government responses to the problem of infant mortality revealed that policymakers are informed regarding beliefs and values of the target population, government-designed policies to address infant mortality have not been successful in reducing the rate of infant mortality. Although key informants in South Carolina were unable to identify a specific policy that addresses infant mortality, several initiatives established by the executive branch were discussed. The initiatives are implemented by the Department of Health and Environmental Control and are available only to those pregnant women who qualify on the basis of financial status. These initiatives employ tools such as providing free bus passes for prenatal patients to the prenatal clinic, which may help in achieving initiative goals, although specific goals relating to specific tools are not clearly stated or specified.

One of the more encompassing initiatives is a federally funded grant project that places an emphasis on identifying barriers to prenatal care and posing solutions to remove the barriers. Various tools were chosen by policymakers to aid in accomplishing the goal of improving access for pregnant women to prenatal health care. An example is a program in which private physicians agree to provide prenatal care for a certain number of patients who qualify for nationally funded prenatal care. This program is entitled Partnership for a Healthy Generation.

Although total compliance for participation in the Partnership for a Healthy Generation is not mandated by law for the target population or for localities, access to federal and state financial support for prenatal health care is accompanied by certain expectations of the state. An example of an authority tool used by South Carolina is found in the requirements stipulated by this policy. To receive government-funded coupons that provide free food, medication, infant care (including immunizations), and free maternal care, the pregnant woman must apply through the local health department. Eligibility is determined through a qualification process, including a thorough history relating to sexual activity, marital status, and educational status. Initially, the process took approximately 6 weeks. The initiative's goals were to decrease the process to 2 to 3 weeks. If the patient has been identified as being at high risk (through past obstetric history, family history, or current disease), the process is often hastened further. In the Netherlands, there is only one system of health care. All patients, wealthy and those on welfare, seek prenatal care from the same healthcare providers. There is no qualifying process to receive prenatal care.

Another initiative in South Carolina is the High Risk Channeling Project that channels high-risk pregnant women into appropriate levels of care. This regulatory project determines which healthcare provider and which hospital setting a pregnant woman uses during her pregnancy. The Netherlands also has a high risk channeling policy in which pregnant women, who are considered at high risk, are referred to an obstetrician. The pregnant women who are not considered at risk are seen by family practitioners and midwives.

The area of family planning reflected the widest gap in the choice of tools. Several initiatives exist in South Carolina that address family planning. All initiatives are activated through local and individualized programs with no single program providing a clear and consistent framework to be followed by other programs. Family-planning health professionals are not allowed to enter the schools to provide counseling. Students are encouraged to visit health departments to receive family-planning advice and are urged to inform their parents of their visits. Although sex education is taught in the state-funded schools, each county may present the package in any form it chooses. Most key policymakers, who are informed about the content of the sex-education curriculum practices around the state, report that it is often a very brief (15-minute) discussion each semester that covers broad concepts. In contrast, Dutch schools mandate a comprehensive sex education to all students beginning in the fifth grade. In addition, a government-funded family-planning service is available through all general practitioners and midwives. The government is supported in these efforts by the majority of the Dutch citizens and most of the clergy.

Policy-Process Variables

Policy-process variables may make a major impact on the success or failure of a policy or program. Process variables include partisanship, public opinion, interest group strength, homogeneity between policymakers and the target population, and influence of policy analysis.

In South Carolina, partisanship affected decisions on policies addressing maternal and infant health. Schneider and Ingram (1990) note that Democrats are disposed more favorably than are Republicans toward capacity-building tools or positive inducements for populations such as the poor. However, Democrats in South Carolina have traditionally been politically conservative. Therefore, most policies relating to family planning, unwanted pregnancies, and infant mortality have been conservative in nature. The Netherlands, in contrast, is noted for its ability to provide an arching relationship among political elites to provide harmony and stability. Lijphart (1977) notes that the Netherlands is "a dramatic example of the survival of a nation state as a stable democracy despite extreme social pluralism" (p. 103).

Public opinion regarding policies that address unwanted pregnancies in South Carolina is polarized. The divisions between those who favor open, factual, and consistent information regarding sexuality and sex education and those who feel that such an environment would foster more promiscuity and unwanted pregnancies are also reflected in the legislature.

In the Netherlands, public opinion is strongly and cohesively in favor of open communication between adolescents and the community at large regarding unwanted pregnancies. Statistics show that the results of unwanted pregnancies—infant mortality and elective abortions—are at a much higher rate in South Carolina than in the Netherlands. A gap also exists in South Carolina between policymakers and the target population. Most informants state that this gap contributes to relative lack of public support and the weakness of special-interest groups lobbying for prenatal care. Quite the opposite exists in the Netherlands. Political support is apathetic and inconsistent in South Carolina, yet is supportive, consistent, and proactive in the Netherlands.

Policy Participation

The success of a policy or program is highly dependent upon whether the target population perceives the services provided by the program to be valuable enough to warrant participation. Policy participation in this study revealed that co-production (assumption of the values and involvement of establishment of goals) of a policy is not coordinated in South Carolina, but that Dutch citizens are very involved with policy design and formulation. All Dutch citizens use the same healthcare system and, therefore, have more interest. Utilization of services in South Carolina is poor, which informants suggest is the result of very little input regarding policy formulation from the target population. Dutch women fully participate in family-planning and prenatal healthcare programs.

Conclusion

The nursing profession is undergoing rapid change in educational and training programs and in tasks and roles that nurses assume. Beginning as a helping profession with a hospital-based background, nursing education in the United States has moved to university settings that offer bachelor and advanced degrees.

Baccalaureate-prepared nurses currently represent 32% of the total number of nurses in the country and the number is rising. The number of baccalaureate nurses returning to universities for advanced education in nursing through master's and doctoral degrees also is growing. Nurses in advanced practice are taking their rightful places as providers of quality nursing care in diverse settings.

As a component of advanced practice nursing, active participation in the policy process is essential in the formulation of policies designed to provide quality health care to all individuals. To be effective in the process, APNs must understand how the process works and the points at which the greatest impact might be made. The design phase of the policy process is the point at which the original intent of a solution to a problem is understood. APNs can be extremely effective in this phase as policy tools are considered and selected.

Discussion Points and Activities

1. Identify a health policy and the tools used by the institution/agency to implement the policy.
2. Using your understanding of the behavioral assumptions underlying the tools, determine the potential for success or failure. Identify policy variables that will affect success or failure.
3. Identify a policy (rule/regulation/etc.) that has been in use for several years yet has had little success. Identify the variable that may be inhibiting success and offer possible solutions. Write or call your legislator to express your concerns (using data) and offer a proposal for revision. Explain why your proposal may increase success of the policy implementation and outcome.
4. How does the political climate affect the choice of policy tools and the behavioral assumptions made by policymakers?
5. Submit an article for publication to a refereed journal about a clinical problem based on the policy design process.

References

Bardach, E. (1977). *The implementation game: What happens after a bill becomes a law*. Cambridge, MA: MIT Press.

Cohen, M., March, J. G., & Olsen, J. P. (1972). A garbage can model of organizational choice. *Administrative Science Quarterly, 17*, 1–25.

Comer, M. E. (2002, May). Factors influencing organized political participation in nursing. *Power, Politics, and Policymaking, 3*(2), 97–107.

Dery, D. (1984). *Problem definition in policy analysis.* Lawrence, KS: University Press of Kansas.

Dryzek, J. S. (1983). Don't toss coins in garbage cans: A prologue to policy design. *Journal of Public Policy,* 3(4), 345–368.

Durant, R. F., & Legge, J. S., Jr. (1993). Policy design, social regulations and theory building: Lessons from the traffic safety policy arena. *Political Research Quarterly,* 46(3), 641–657.

Elmore, R. F. (1979–1980). Backward mapping: Implementation research and policy decisions. *Political Science Quarterly,* 94(4), 601–616.

Goggin, M. L., Bowman, A. O'M., Lester, J. P., & O'Toole, L. J., Jr. (1990). *Implementation theory and practice: Toward a third generation.* New York: Harper Collins.

Heclo, H. (1978). Issue networks and the executive establishment. In A. King (Ed.), *American political system.* Washington, DC: American Enterprise Institute.

Ingraham, P. W. (1987). Toward more systematic consideration of policy design. *Policy Studies Journal,* 15(4), 611–628.

Jones, C. O. (1984). *An introduction to the study of public policy* (3rd ed.). Monterey, CA: Brooks Cole.

Kingdon, J. W. (1995). *Agendas, alternatives, and public policies.* Boston: Little, Brown.

Lee, P. R., & Estes, C. L. (1990). *The nation's health.* Sudbury, MA: Jones and Bartlett.

Leichter, J. M. (1979). *A comparative approach to policy analysis: Health care policy in four nations.* New York: Cambridge University Press.

Lerner, A. W., & Wanat, J. (1983). Fuzziness and bureaucracy. *Public Administration Review,* 43(6), 500–509.

Lijphart, A. (1977). *Democracy in plural societies.* New Haven, CT: Yale University Press.

Lijphart, A. (1984). *Democracies.* New Haven, CT: Yale University Press.

Linder, S. H., & Peters, G. B. (1987). Design perspective on policy implementation: The fallacies of misplaced prescriptions. *Policy Studies Review,* 6(3), 459–475.

Linder, S. H., & Peters, G. B. (1990). Research perspectives on the design of public policy: Implementation, formulation, and design. In D. Palumbo and D. J. Calista (Eds.), *Implementation and the public policy process: Opening up the black box.* New York: Greenwood Press.

Lipsky, M. (1980). *Street-level bureaucracy.* New York: Russell Sage Foundation.

Longest, B. B., Jr. (2002). *Health policymaking in the United States* (3rd ed.). Chicago: Health Administration Press.

Lowi, T. (1960). *The end of liberalism.* New York: Norton.

Mazmanian, D. A., & Sabatier, P. A. (1983). *Implementation and public policy.* Dallas, TX: Scott, Foresman.

Miller, C. A. (1988). Prenatal care outreach: An international perspective. In Institute of Medicine, *Prenatal Care: Reaching Mothers, Reaching Infants.* Washington, DC: National Academy Press.

Pressman, J., & Wildavsky, A. B. (1973). *Implementation: How great expectations in Washington are dashed in Oakland; Or, Why it's amazing that federal programs work at all.* Berkeley: University of California Press.

Safriet, B. J. (2002). Closing the gap between can and may in health-care providers' scopes of practice: A primer for policymakers. *Yale Journal on Regulation,* 19, 301–334.

Sardell, A. (1990). *The U.S. experiment in social medicine: The community health center program.* 1965–1986. Pittsburgh: University of Pittsburgh Press.

Schneider, A., & Ingram, H. (1990). Behavioral assumptions of policy tools. *Journal of Politics,* 52(2), 510–529.

Singh, H. K. D. (1990). Stork reality, why America's infants are dying. *Policy Review, 2*, 391–398.

Thompson, F. J. (1981). *Health policy and the bureaucracy: Politics and implementation*. Cambridge, MA: MIT Press.

Ulbrich, H. (2003). *Public finance: In theory and practice*. Mason, OH: Thomson.

U.S. Department of Health and Human Services (USDHHS). (2002). *Healthy People 2010*. Washington, DC: National Academies Press.

Van Meter, D. S., & Van Horn, C. (1975). The policy implementation process: A conceptual framework. *Administration and Society, 6*, 455–488.

Varone, F., & Aebischer, B. (2001). Energy efficiency: The challenges of policy design. *Energy Policy, 29*, 615–629.

6

Policy Implementation

Marlene Wilken, PhD, RN

Key Terms

➤ **Environmental factors** A broad category of nonstatutory variables in the implementation process that includes socioeconomic conditions; public support; attitudes, resources, and commitment of constituency groups; and leadership of implementing officials.

➤ **Implementation games** Refers to a variety of strategies and maneuvers used to achieve control by agencies and groups involved in the implementation process.

➤ **Policy implementation** The process of putting a policy or program into effect.

➤ **Policy structure** The ability of statute to shape policy implementation based on several elements such as clear, consistent objectives; causal linkages between interventions and objectives; funding; hierarchical integration of agencies; behaviors of agency officials; and access by outsiders.

➤ **Tractability** A component of policy implementation that addresses the ease or degree of manageability of a problem. Elements include technology, diversity, target groups, and extent of behavioral change.

Introduction

The phenomenon of implementation has been studied for years in academia. **Policy implementation** is usually studied from either the top-down or bottom-up perspective. Either way, the implementation process is a participatory endeavor, taking place in specific and varied democratic processes. When the word implement is used as a verb, it must have an object to indicate what is being implemented. The object becomes a policy, and for some scholars and researchers the subject of study becomes policy implementation. Implementation implies action and has start and end points. The success or failure of implementation is judged against the specific policy goals. Implementation is about who participates, why and how they participate, and with what effect. Authors Hill and Hupe (2002) suggest that implementation should be considered in the context of organizational behavior or management. "Seldom is there a perfect fit between the problem defined by the policy makers, the design of the policy aimed at alleviating the problem, and the implementation delivered by the policy" (p. 5).

In this chapter, several policies that involve nurses and other health professionals are examined in the context of organizational behavior and/or management. We have all been involved in situations where policy goals/outcomes were evaluated as successful, partially successful, or not successful. Implementation is an ongoing cycle including problem identification and problem solving (Palumbo & Calista, 1990).

Those who study policy implementation provide several reasons why gaps occur in policy implementation and result in less than optimal policy success. Others offer recommendations to policymakers to help ensure policy success. The following list is a summary of the key elements to be considered when making policy and examining policy implementation. Policy:

- needs to be relevant, feasible, and based on sound theory with appropriate rationale that will correctly identify the design conditions and desired effect of the target groups
- objectives need to be clear and consistent or, at a minimum, identify criteria for resolving goal conflict
- should provide the persons in charge of implementation sufficient jurisdiction and leverage points over the target groups to help reach the desired goals
- must maximize the likelihood that the implementing officials and target groups have sufficient resources to comply
- needs to be examined periodically to ensure there is ongoing support from outside and within the agency/organization and that conditions have not changed over time that affect implementation (Mazmanian & Sabatier cited in Hill & Hupe, 2002)

Implementation involves private agencies and groups that are often contractors for carrying out policies; the target groups themselves; and the socioeconomic, cultural, and political conditions in the environment in which polices are supposed to operate (Palumbo & Calista, 1990). These groups plus other nonstatutory variables such as public attitudes and resources, commitment and leadership of officials are known as **environmental factors**.

Policy Implementation Players

There are many reasons why policy implementation continues to be a major stumbling block in the policy process. The majority of problems that interfere with policy implementation are people problems that are often referred to as political problems. The bottom-up perspective examines the individuals who interact with the consumer, and political scientists refer to these players as "street-level" bureaucrats.

Nurses are implementers faced with many of the same issues related to policy implementation as street-level bureaucrats. A variety of dilemmas can occur when interacting with clients. Implementers practice coping strategies such as negotiation and may find themselves in circumstances not foreseen, being confronted with rules that are often vague but within which they are compelled to act. They see themselves required to interpret the policy involved in a creative but justifiable way. Sometimes they are working with scarce resources. How often have you heard someone say or even think to yourself, "If they would just come down here and see how it is in the real world they wouldn't make policies that are impossible to carry out!" As a result, implementers may decide to alter the policy/procedure based upon their perception of shortcomings in the policy. These perceptions of policy shortcomings may be based on a desire to enhance their professionalism, strengthen leadership, and perhaps restructure their organization (Hill & Hupe, 2002). **Policy structure** shapes the way that a statute or program is implemented; philosophical or pragmatic differences between agency officials and street level bureaucrats often alter original legislative intent.

In the top-down model, administrators and other top-level players can have a significant impact on policy implementation. Personal attitudes and perceptions come into play during policy implementation. When the results of a policy are determined to be disappointing or even worse, administrators are often quick to blame the implementers. When policymakers find out that the policy they wrote yields disappointing results, they may be inclined to take additional measures in hopes of ensuring tighter control of the implementation. Both often add more (internal) rules and regulations. Successful policy can lead to more of the same policies with the idea that if this policy worked well, adding additional policies may improve further.

Bardach (1977) reports that control is at the core of implementation maneuvers, or **implementation games**. Control can be exercised in a variety of ways with the end result being decisions about withholding or delivering elements of the policy. Types of maneuvers involve the diversion of resources, deflection of goals, dilemmas of administration, and the dissipation of energies. The diversion of resources manifests itself in several ways. Organizations and individuals who receive government money tend to provide less in the way of exchange services for that money. Playing the budget game is another diversion. Persons responsible for the budget do what they can to win favor in the eyes of those who have power over their funding. Therefore, the incentives shaped for implementers by those who control their budgets influence what the implementers do with respect to executing policy mandates. When implementers perform in a less effective manner, there is a larger share of the task left undone and this provides an opportunity to ask for more money. Sometimes implementers do not have the necessary resources for compliance, such as the know-how or supplies.

During the implementation phase, goals often undergo some change. This deflection of goals can be the result of (1) some feeling that the original goals were too ambiguous; (2) goals that were based on a weak consensus; (3) goals that were not thought out sufficiently; (4) an organization that realizes the program will impose a heavy workload; (5) a program that takes the organization into controversy; or (6) required tasks that are too difficult for the workers to perform. The agency will try to shift certain unattractive elements to different agencies. If nobody wants the responsibility, consumers get the runaround and each agency involved can claim it is not their problem.

Playing the dissipation of energy game wastes a great deal of implementers' time in avoiding responsibility, defending themselves against others, and setting themselves up for advantageous situations. Some may use their power to slow or stall the progress of a program until one's own terms are met. This action can lead to delay, withdrawal of financial and political support, or the total collapse of a program.

The presumption that once regulations and policies are enacted they are largely followed turns out to be unwarranted in many cases. Compliance with the rules of a program can be far from what the policymakers envisioned. There is little in the implementation literature to address how to improve compliance, but building staff capacity to detect and correct noncompliant actions and having staff work with individuals to induce compliance are mentioned (Deleon & Deleon, 2002).

When policy implementation is examined or evaluated, one question that begs discussion is the notion of "good enough." Is 100% compliance realistic? If not, what measures need to be taken to get closer to an acceptable compliance rate? Does the policy need to be reexamined? What are the implementers doing and reporting? Is this a policy, person, or systems problem? Do the measures of success need to be reconsidered or redefined?

Conclusion

Problems with policy implementation are widespread in the United States. During the implementation process, various forces try to change the policy, and implementation does not go according to plan. These forces involve individuals, groups, organizations, and sometimes the governmental bodies that are responsible for implementation. The entire nursing community and other health professionals can affect implementation in both positive and negative ways.

Control is at the heart of the implementation process. Manifestations of control can take many forms including diversion of resources, deflection of goals, dilemmas of administration, and the dissipation of energies. Even the best policy will not ensure successful implementation, and one certainty of implementation is that it is unpredictable.

Case Study: Advanced Practice Nurses and Pain Management

Trossman (2006) examined the outcomes of the Joint Commission on Accreditation of Healthcare Organizations (JCAHO) related to pain management. She indicates that when the JCAHO pain assessment and management standards were developed in 2001, some thought that pain management changes would be implemented at a fast pace nationwide. Such was not the case because nurses have been slow to embrace the changes. There are several reasons why the JCAHO standards are still not being implemented fully in many organizations.

The first reason stated by the president of the Illinois Nurse's Association (INA) is the "misconception about pain medication and addiction . . . with many health care providers defining dependency and addiction the same way, though they are vastly different" (Lucy cited in Trossman, 2006, p. 29). Another INA member believes healthcare facilities should adopt policies that prevent placebo use because it sends the message to patients that healthcare professionals "do not actually believe a patient is experiencing pain" (Wentz cited in Trossman, 2006, p. 29).

A third barrier to effective pain management policy is the limitation of prescriptive authority for advanced practice registered nurses (APRNs). Some states do not allow APRNs to prescribe Schedule II and III controlled substances. When the APRN is the primary care provider, not being able to prescribe scheduled drugs can leave the patient with ineffective pain management.

Another barrier to providing pain management is the clinician's fear of being investigated by the Drug Enforcement Agency (DEA). Although only a small number of nurses have been disciplined for improperly prescribing, the message has been disseminated among APRNs and some are now concerned about possible consequences of using their prescriptive authority in prescribing scheduled drugs for pain management (Trossman, 2006).

In 2004, the DEA withdrew a Web site developed to address interdisciplinary education guidelines for healthcare professionals to address pain management. The Web site was canceled as a result of intervention in the policy at the federal level. Attorney General John Ashcroft, appointed by President George W. Bush, determined that the educational Web site was at odds with what the president believed to be the traditional hard-line law enforcement. Despite this setback, some believe that the DEA may be reviewing some of the rules and considering a change that would allow APRNs to write sequential prescriptions for Schedule II drugs (Trossman, 2006).

To address the issues noted previously, the American Nurses Association (ANA) House of Delegates passed a resolution in 2006 to promote strategies that would address improving pain management for APRNs. Support would assist professional APRNs to meet the needs of clients in addressing pain, the fifth vital sign. Nurses should support legislation that allows for APRNs to prescribe Schedule I and II drugs in states not currently allowing such prescriptive authority and ensure that APRNs are not discriminated against when prescribing or administering controlled substances. In addition, APRNs need to support consumer and professional education on pain management, which includes the primacy of pain management over fear of addiction.

At the systems level, ANA has collaborated with the American Society for Pain Management Nursing (ASPMN) to provide a Scope and Standards of Practice document and a certification exam on pain management. ANA continues to address pain management issues at the federal level. You can get involved by visiting the Web sites of the American Alliance of Cancer Pain Initiatives (www.aacpi. wisc.edu), the Power Over Pain Campaign (www.painfoundation. org/poweroverpain), and American Society for Pain Management Nursing (www.aspmn.org) (Trossman, 2006).

Discussion Points and Activities

1. What are the attitudes presented from constituency groups related to pain management?
2. What games are being played in an effort to control the implementation of the pain management standards?
3. What can the APN do to improve the management of pain from a policy perspective?

Case Study: Lead Poisoning in Children

In 1998, states were mandated to screen for blood lead levels (BLLs) on all children ages 1 to 2 years enrolled in Medicaid programs. The *Healthy People* 2010 objectives for childhood lead poisoning are to eliminate elevated blood lead levels in children. A Superfund site, contaminated with lead, is located in Douglas County, Nebraska. Superfund sites are hazardous waste sites that are part of the U.S. Environmental Protection Agency's (EPA's) Superfund Program. The blood lead level screening data in 2002 for Douglas County indicated that 437 (4.6%) of the 9521 children screened in 2002 had elevated BLLs (> 10 µg/dL) (Wilken, Currier, Abel-Zieg, & Brady, 2004).

A survey was conducted to examine the blood lead screening rate for children ages 12 to 18 months, on Medicaid, who were seen in any of four health clinics located in the Omaha lead site between 1999 and 2002. Data were analyzed for compliance rates between pediatricians and family practice providers. Documented mandated blood lead screenings were present in 78.9% records. A comparison of the screening rates for each clinic found one free-standing clinic at 100% documentation and the others at 72%. No significant differences were found when comparing screening rates of pediatric and family practice providers.

The findings demonstrated missed opportunities to meet the federal mandate. A second study was done to identify which factors make lead screening programs successful and which elements contribute to missed opportunities. Federally qualified healthcare centers were selected in locations near EPA-designated Superfund lead sites across the United States. Seventy-five percent of clinics indicated that policies, procedures, or protocols were in place regarding blood lead level screening. Self-reported compliance rates ranged from 75% to 96% with 69% of the clinics indicating that there were no concerns with BLL screening compliance rates. Approximately 62% of clinics indicated periodic chart reviews were conducted to assess compliance rates (Wilken & Currier, 2006).

Reasons given for improvements in compliance rates were staff education, standing orders, state mandates, and periodic chart reviews. Most clinics (74%) reported no accrediting/oversight agency requests for BLL compliance rates. *Oversight* is a term used by federal or voluntary agencies that implies a "watchful supervision and management" of programs and agencies. Oversight addresses the accountability of programs, and without accountability provided by oversight, the importance of compliance may be undervalued, leading to a gap in policy implementation.

Other reasons cited for gaps in implementation of BLL screening included lack of pediatric insurance, lack of standing orders necessitating provider orders before BLL screenings can be performed, and lack of awareness of need for BLL screenings. Parents are also blamed for the low compliance rates for not seeking health care for their children. However, 25% of these children who were at the clinic to receive their measles, mumps, and rubella (MMR) vaccinations did not receive the mandated BLL screening. To improve compliance rates, staff education, protocols, and chart audits appear to be needed. Federal oversight or accountability provisions need to be in place to ensure that compliance rates are achieved, thus providing the "jurisdictional power" for effective policy implementation (Wilken & Currier, 2006). The **tractability** of the problem is often a serious factor for determining the ultimate success or failure of proposed solutions.

Discussion Points and Activities

1. Identify what you believe are the three strongest reasons why opportunities are missed for mandated blood lead level screening.
2. Who is accountable for the missed opportunities to screen children for blood lead level?
3. What can the APN do to improve the implementation rate of mandated blood lead level screening from a policy perspective?

Case Study: Back to Sleep and Nothing But Baby Campaigns

Sudden infant death syndrome (SIDS) is the leading cause of death for infants ages 1 month to 1 year. In 1994, the American Academy of Pediatrics, the U.S. Public Health Service, and the SIDS Alliance launched the Back to Sleep Campaign (BTS) in hopes of reducing cases of SIDS. The campaign message was clear and concise: Place infants on their backs or sides for sleep. The groups targeted to implement the message were parents, health professionals, and other care providers (Hein & Pettit, 2001). The most recent campaign related to SIDS is called Nothing But Baby. The message in this campaign is that a pacifier is the only item allowed to be in the crib with baby. Babies should be put in a sleep sack, which negates the use of blankets or other bedding items and nothing else but a pacifier is supposed to be in the crib.

Several research articles explore how the Back to Sleep and Nothing But Baby guidelines and policies have been implemented in a variety of settings. The groups targeted to implement the new guidelines included healthcare professionals, parents, and child care providers. The sites studied included public health clinics, private physician offices, HMOs, hospital clinics, and hospital nurseries.

Hein and Pettit (2001) explore two aspects of implementation: what information was provided to parents while they were in the hospital after the birth of their infant and how the infant was placed for sleep while in the hospital. Nurses working in obstetric units in Iowa hospitals were surveyed. The findings indicated that almost 90% of the nurses informed the parents that the back or side positions were acceptable for sleep, and 90% of the nurses reported using either the side or back position for infants in the hospital. One could conclude that nurses were implementing the policy successfully, but when nurses were asked why they used the side position they stated fear of aspiration in the supine position. The most recent research, however, indicates that fear of aspiration in the supine position is unfounded and that supine is the safest position.

The researchers recognized that parents may imitate what they see the nurses doing in the hospital. In this study, there was a high likelihood that parents saw their child sleeping in a side-lying position rather than supine. Another factor to be considered was that some parents will not or cannot read printed information. So, it was possible that parents related to what they saw or were told versus print material they were given to read. The study shows that how nurses implement policy has a strong effect on what parents see and do. The study also addresses the need for implementers to be kept up-to-date on changes in policy to improve patient safety (Hein & Pettit, 2001).

Another research study examined the association between the type of prenatal care site and the mother's choice of infant sleep position. Women who had given birth within the previous 60 to 180 days were surveyed as part of an ongoing public health surveillance project of the Oregon Office of Family Health. Respondents were asked to identify the sleep position used most of the time and the site where the women received most of their prenatal care (Lahr, Rosenberg, & Lapidus, 2005). The prenatal care site was strongly associated with the mother's choice of prone infant position. Women receiving prenatal care from private physicians and health maintenance organizations (HMOs) were at higher risk of choosing prone infant sleep positioning. Could this be a case of the implementers in private physician clinics and HMOs lacking sufficient information on best practices or a case of implementers exercising their own judgment as to what is best? According to the authors, "Prenatal care providers at health department clinics have apparently communicated the 'Back to Sleep' message more effectively than private physicians" (Lahr et al., 2005, p. 171). In addition, differences in the frequency or quality of medical advice might also have contributed to the observed racial disparities in the choice of infant sleep position. Further investigation is needed regarding why high-risk mothers are more likely to choose the prone position and identify more effective and culturally competent measures to reduce this choice.

Another study focused on Back to Sleep practices in 110 extended-hours and nighttime child care centers in 27 states. Twenty percent of SIDS occurs in child care settings, and millions of children in the United States have parents who work alternative shifts. The objective of the study was to determine if nighttime child care centers (1) follow Back to Sleep recommendations; (2) are aware of the need for a safe sleep environment; and (3) have written policies directing proper SIDS risk reduction practices (Moon, Weese-Mayer, & Silvestri, 2003). Results related to the sleep position indicated that infants were placed in the prone position at least some of the time in 20% of the child care centers surveyed, with one center using the prone position exclusively. Infants were placed on their side at least some of the time in 71 (64.6%) centers, 32 (29.1%) exclusively placing the infant on the side and 36 (32.7%) of centers using the supine position exclusively.

The sleep environment was also evaluated in the study and the findings indicated that infants sleep in uncluttered sleep environments (not even a blanket) in 18% of the centers. The remaining centers in the study had a range of items allowed in the crib including blankets, comforters, stuffed toys, pillows, bumper pads, wedges, and other unspecified items (Moon, Biliter, & Croskell, 2001).

Among the 43 (39.1%) centers that acknowledged having heard of the BTS campaign, only 26 (23.9%) recalled receiving any written information from BTS. The policy was changed to supine sleep in only 3 (11.5 %) of the 26 centers that received the

BTS mailings, and 5 (19.2%) reinforced current practice/stressed importance of nonprone sleep positioning with staff and parents. The rationale cited for sleep positions varied. Prone positioning was allowed as a result of previous experience, SIDS or safety-related recommendations, parental request, infant comfort/infant "slept better," and fear of choking. (Moon et al., 2003).

Written policies regarding sleep position were reported in 59% of the centers. Presence of written policy was not associated with avoidance of the prone position. State regulations requiring nonprone sleep position for infants were in place in 6 of the 27 states, affecting 11 centers in the study. Presence of state regulations was neither associated with the sleep position practice nor associated with the presence of a written policy (Moon et al., 2003).

Stastny, Ichinose, Thayer, Olson, and Keens (2004) assessed newborn placement practices of the mother and nursery staff and their interrelationship in the hospital setting. Goals of the study were to elucidate the motivations, behaviors, recommendations, and knowledge of nursery staff regarding infant placement, to characterize the infant placement behaviors of mothers of newborns, and to define how nursery staff influence the positioning choice of these new mothers. The investigators visited eight hospitals, which accounted for approximately 49% of the births in Orange County, California, in 2000.

Over a 7-week period, the researchers solicited nursery staff and mothers to answer a brief questionnaire. Although a majority of the sampled nursery staff (72%) identified the supine position as the placement that most lowers SIDS risk, only 30% reported most often placing the baby in the supine position, with most staff citing fear of aspiration as the motivation. Only 34% of the staff reported advising exclusive supine position to mothers, but 36% of mothers reported using the supine position exclusively. Maternal infant placement choice varied by both the advice and placement modeling from staff nurses, with 63% of the mothers observing their infants placed in nonsupine positions by nursery staff. A mother's race/ethnicity also affected her use of the supine position exclusively. The researchers concluded that evidence-based educational interventions using scientific data to promote supine positioning should be implemented (Stastny et al., 2004).

Nursing practice was examined in positioning healthy newborns for sleep in the hospital setting by Bullock, Mickey, Green, and Heine (2004). The study was composed of a convenience sample of 528 practicing maternal-child nurses in 58 Missouri hospitals. Although 96% of the nurses surveyed stated they were aware of the American Academy of Pediatrics (AAP) guidelines recommending "back-to-sleep," 75% of the nurses used a mix of side-lying and supine positions, and 45% were concerned about risk for aspiration if the infant was placed only on supine. The hospital policy on infant positioning was known to only 53% of the nurses, and 80% of those who knew of the policy stated that the policy included the lateral position as being acceptable practice. Nurses are the role models for new parents regarding infant sleep positioning, and according to the authors, it is clear that more education is needed for hospital nurses about newborn sleep position, hospital policies, and AAP guidelines.

Discussion Points and Activities

1. Identify ways to minimize the variation in interpretation of the Back to Sleep policy.
2. Determine how to handle the problem of individuals who are not following policy/procedures for the exclusive use of the supine position.

References

Bardach, E. (1977). *The implementation game: What happens after a bill becomes a law.* Cambridge, MA: MIT Press.

Bullock, L. F. C., Mickey, K., Green, J., & Heine, A. (2004). Are nurses acting as role models for the prevention of SIDS? *MCN: The American Journal of Maternal-Child Nursing, 29*(3), 172–177.

Deleon, L., & Deleon, P. (2002). What ever happened to policy implementation? An alternative approach. *Journal of Public Administration Research and Theory, 12*(4), 467–492.

Hein, H. A., & Pettit, S. F. (2001). Back to sleep: Good advice for parents but not for hospitals? *Pediatrics, 107*(3), 537–539.

Hill, M. J., & Hupe, P. L. (2002). *Implementing public policy : Governance in theory and in practice.* Thousand Oaks, CA: Sage.

Lahr, M. B., Rosenberg, K. D., & Lapidus, J. A. (2005). Health departments do it better: Prenatal care site and prone infant sleep position. *Maternal and Child Health Journal, 9*(2), 165–172.

Moon, R. Y., Biliter, W. M., & Croskell, S. E. (2001). Examination of state regulations regarding infants and sleep in licensed child care centers and family child care settings. *Pediatrics, 107*(5), 1029–1036.

Moon, R. Y., Weese-Mayer, D. E., & Silvestri, J. M. (2003). Nighttime child care: Inadequate sudden infant death syndrome risk factor knowledge, practice, and policies. *Pediatrics, 111*(4), 795–799.

Palumbo, D. J., & Calista, D. J. (1990). *Implementation and the policy process: Opening up the black box.* New York: Greenwood Press.

Stastny, P. F., Ichinose, T. Y., Thayer, S. D., Olson, R. J., & Keens, T. G. (2004). Infant sleep positioning by nursery staff and mothers in newborn hospital nurseries. *Nursing Research, 53*(2), 122–129.

Trossman, S. (2006, December). Issues up close: Improving pain management call to action. *American Nurse Today,* 29–30.

Wilken, M., & Currier, S. (2006). A follow-up look at blood lead level screening compliance. Unpublished manuscript.

Wilken, M., Currier, S., Abel-Zieg, C., & Brady, L. A. (2004, February 23). A survey of compliance: Medicaid's mandated blood lead screenings for children age 12–18 months in Nebraska. *BMC Public Health, 4*(1), 4.

Program Evaluation

Ardith L. Sudduth, PhD, RN, APRN-BC, FNP

Key Terms

➤ **Ethical evaluation** Assessment that follows the principles of good conduct and moral behavior.

➤ **Evaluation report** Compilation of the findings of the program evaluation study. Reports are presented in a variety of formats depending upon the needs of those requesting the evaluation. Common formats include written reports, electronic transfer, oral presentations with multimedia enhancements, films, and videotapes.

➤ **Outcome evaluation** Assesses the extent to which a program achieves its outcome-oriented objectives. It focuses on outputs and outcomes to judge program effectiveness, but may assess program process to understand how outcomes are produced.

➤ **Policy** The purposeful, general plan of action developed to respond to a problem that includes authoritative guidelines. The plan directs human behavior toward specific goals.

➤ **Program evaluation** Analyzes social programs to gain an understanding of how well the intervention designed to solve a problem is meeting the objectives and goals set forth in the program's design.

> **Program evaluation design** The method selected to collect unbiased data for analysis to determine the extent to which a social program is meeting its designated goals, objectives, and outcomes and to assess the social program's merit and worth.

> **Public policy** Provides a definitive course of action, or nonaction, developed by a governmental body that is goal directed.

> **Qualitative evaluation design** Evaluation methods that assist the evaluator to determine the subjective meaning of the program and its interventions to the individual participants.

> **Quantitative evaluation design** Methods characterized as the "scientific model" of collecting measurable, objective data with an emphasis on explanation based upon well-defined expectations and observable events.

> **Social programs** Solutions developed to help solve an identified problem of human beings.

> **Theory** Used to design a program and its interventions and to explain and predict broad phenomena observed after data analysis.

Introduction

Advanced practice nurses (APNs) such as nurse practitioners, school nurses, advanced practice critical care nurses, clinical nurse specialists, and others have become key figures in the provision of health care or healthcare management of persons enrolled in governmentally funded programs. Advanced practice nurses that are providing care in rural clinics or inner-city clinics usually are part of a program sponsored by the local, state, or federal government. When working with Medicare and Medicaid participants, APNs are participating in governmental programs. Programs funded by governments, nonprofit organizations, and most private foundations require that these programs be evaluated regularly to meet a variety of purposes, including ensuring that the program is being conducted as developed, that there is fiscal responsibility, that goals and objectives are being met, and increasingly, that the outcomes are examined. To assist the APN to meet the often mandated requirements for **program evaluation**, this chapter presents some of the components of policy and program evaluation including conditions of evaluation, ethical considerations, potential design choices, and a few suggestions for reporting the results and recommendations of the evaluation.

Advanced practice nurses are not strangers to evaluation. They have long used evaluation in many clinical settings including the evaluation of a patient's response to a nursing intervention, use of outcome-based clinical evaluations, evaluation of a management strategy, or a self-evaluation for promotion. The transition to using these skills to evaluate a program is a natural evolution of nursing practice. Understanding the process of policy and program evaluation can help the APN to contribute to the evaluation of social programs by bringing the unique perspective of nursing practice. The federal government has had a health-care **policy** for a long time that has included the funding of hospitals and health care for the elderly. Policies also have supported funded programs to prepare advanced practice nurses. Healthcare policies are constantly being modified and in some cases expanded. An example of expansion occurred in the Balanced Budget Act of 1997 that expanded reimbursement to allow nurse practitioners to bill Medicare directly for services provided.

To meet the healthcare needs of a population or to help solve a social problem in the community, the APN may decide to seek funding from a governmental agency, foundation, or other resource to develop a new or unique service. Funding resources, including governments and nonprofit companies, demand that the evaluation process be built into the proposal for funding (Fredericks, Carman, & Birkland, 2002). Often, it is the APN who studies the needs for a social program intervention, writes the proposal in collaboration with other interested parties, and works to develop the evaluation process.

Policy, Public Policy, and Social Programs

To start the discussion of the role of the APN in evaluation of a social program, it is helpful to start at the beginning and define policy. A policy may be defined as a purposeful, overall plan of action or inaction developed to deal with a problem or a matter of concern in either the public or private sector. A policy includes the authoritative guidelines that direct human behavior toward a set of specific goals and provides the structure to guide action. Policy provides guidelines to levy sanctions that affect the conduct of affairs (Hanley, 2002). Policies can be determined by the private or public sector and together can have a significant and long lasting impact on communities and individuals (Center for Health Improvement, 2004). It is also important to remember that public policies are a result of the politics and values of those determining the policy (Mason, Leavitt, & Chaffee, 2002). One example familiar to nurses is the policy manual found in hospitals and clinics, which have been approved by authoritative figures such as a board of directors.

Public Policy

Public policy is developed by governments and the courts. A public policy becomes a definitive course of action, or sometimes a nonaction, developed by a governmental body that addresses public concerns or public problems (Hanley, 2002). It is goal directed toward some end and does not occur by chance. Public policy is determined by legislative bodies as they make laws, by executive bodies as they administer the laws, and by judicial bodies as they interpret these laws (American Nurses Association [ANA], 1997). Governments create public policy by making decisions regarding a health issue, such as requiring all children to be immunized before entering school. It may also be a policy for the government to act negatively by adopting a laissez-faire, or hands-off, policy and do nothing about an issue. The decision to do nothing may be as important as the decision to do something. In either case, some groups will be affected. Public policy provides direction to assist decision makers. Consider the thousands of decisions made by the Food and Drug Administration regarding the safety and effectiveness of consumer goods sold in the United States that includes the safety of drugs, vaccines, and the safety, purity, and nutritive value of foods (Anderson, 1975; ANA).

Public policies may be considered to be either positive or negative. Most programs that deal with the welfare of children; provision of safe water, food, and drugs; and public relief in times of disaster are considered quite favorably by the general public. However, public policies can have a flip side in that they also can create problems. Depending on one's point of view and individual circumstance, Medicare and home health reform is cause for joy or sorrow. An example quite familiar to many APNs has been the changing policies regarding eligibility for home health visits. These changes have been a concern of patients, families, home health nurses, nurse practitioners, and other APNs because all affected parties have had to struggle to ensure that essential care is provided. Although the idea of cost containment has been welcomed by some, the stresses and difficulties that are being met by patients, families, and nurses have made some question the wisdom of these changes. It is important that the results of policy changes are carefully evaluated for the multiple outcomes that can be a result of what may appear to be a positive change.

Whereas public policy is developed by governmental bodies and officials, it is often influenced by multiple nongovernment persons and environmental factors. For example, in the 1960s, there was increasing concern about the access of affordable hospital care by the elderly. Families, labor unions, physicians, and many others were instrumental in creating the Medicare amendments to the Social Security Act. With the passage of these amendments, the federal government developed a policy of government assistance to provide hospital care to the nation's elderly. Over the years, numerous changes have been made to the initial amendments, many lobbied for by the ANA, but the overall goal of the federal policy of ensuring access to hospital and health care by the elderly and now other groups of citizens has continued.

Another important dimension of public policy is that it is not limited to a specific law or legislative proposal. Public policy is a dynamic, evolving phenomenon with an ability to adapt as the needs and desires of its citizens change. One cannot go to a book in the federal government and find a listing of "the" American healthcare policy. Healthcare policy changes over time. An example is the changing emphasis that has occurred over the past 70 years. In the 1940s and 1950s, the focus was on access to hospital care and Hill–Burton legislation provided funds for many rural hospitals. Medicare amendments were a further extension of access to health care. However, with the rising costs of the Medicare provisions, there has been a major push for cost containment since the 1970s with no end in sight (Jennings, 2001). Healthcare policy of the new millennium focuses not only on access, but on quality care provided at the lowest possible costs and determined by outcome evaluations. **Outcome evaluations** are those that focus on the benefits a program produces for the people who use the program (Thomas, Smith, & Wright-DeAguero, 2006). Trends in health policy will continue to be driven by major trends in the healthcare delivery system, which "is becoming more managed and consolidated, more cost and quality accountable, more consumer focused, and more communication and information technology driven" (Jennings, 2001, p. 224). Nurses can play an important role in the development of policies, including healthcare policy. In fact, the last revision of the ANA Code of Ethics for Nurses adopted in 2001 added a provision that states that nurses are "responsible for . . . shaping social policy" (Daly, 2002, p. 98).

Social Programs

Social programs are public policy made visible. After a problem has come to the attention of the appropriate governmental body, suggestions are made on how to solve the problem. After much deliberation, a solution or program is developed. If the matter is of sufficient concern to the legislative body and if the program has support, legislation is passed to authorize the development of the program and to fund it. Usually at the legislative level, the goals and objectives of a program are only general in nature. Specifics are frequently left to the developers of the program that provides some flexibility. Social policies and their effects on the health of individuals, families, and communities have been identified by the ANA Social Policy Statement as a part of nursing care and nursing research (Cohen & Milone-Nuzzo as cited in Reutter & Duncan, 2002).

During the decades of the 1980s and 1990s, federal legislators began to return control of some policies to state and local governments.

This allows states to determine how to use the resources with only minimal guidelines from the federal government. This shift of authority has increased the complexity of social programs and their evaluation because the policies are interpreted by multiple stakeholders such as state legislators, county boards of supervisors, and municipal governments and sometimes nonprofit, community organizations.

Program Evaluation

A **social program,** then, is the set of resources and activities that have been directed toward one or more common goals. The resources and activities vary from program to program and can be as small as a few activities, a small budget, minimal other resources, and managed by a staff of one or two. Some programs can be very large with extensive resource allocation, complex activities, and implemented at several sites or two or more levels of government.

Public policy has generated large numbers of programs intended to improve the lives of citizens in a very broad range of life, including health, education, environment, and social services that would have been unthinkable prior to the 1960s (Light, 2001). The growth of governmental programs at all levels of government has resulted in the need for program evaluation. The importance of program evaluation has also been underscored by federal legislation that mandates the process as well as supplying the funding needed to meet the evaluation requirements. The National Performance Review and the Government Performance and Results Act of 1993 (GPRA) was created to focus the evaluation process on accountability, performance measurement, and results (U.S. General Accounting Office, 2005). States, because of funding matches with the federal government, also require that programs be evaluated. This has become very evident in Louisiana, the author's state of residence. Following the devastating hurricanes Katrina and Rita, federal money was sent to the affected areas and programs quickly developed to assist the victims. Accountability for the funds and programs is now being mandated by both the federal and state governments.

Program evaluation has become a specialized field of inquiry and research. Evaluation provides information to assist others in making judgments about a program, service, policy, organization, or whatever is being evaluated. Evaluation is used to examine the programs to gain an understanding of how the human services policies and programs are solving the social problems that they were designed to alleviate (Westat, 2002). Program evaluation may be conducted for a wide variety of reasons, many of which are particularly adaptable to APN practice. Some of the very practical reasons that program evaluation may be conducted include the following (Posavac & Carey, 1992):

Determine the extent and severity of a problem

Choose among possible programs

Monitor program operations

Determine if the program has resulted in desired change (outcomes)

Document outcomes for program sustainability

Account for funds

Revise program interventions

Answer requests for information

Learn about unintended effects of program

Meet accreditation requirements

Determining the Extent and Severity of a Problem

Evaluation designs are used to determine if a problem is severe enough to establish a program to help solve it. In today's world of scarce resources, including time, money, trained personnel, and other valuable commodities, it is imperative that a well-documented program exists. Programs vie for resources, and the one that can show the best justification is the one most likely selected for implementation.

Choosing Among Possible Programs

Evaluation data may be used to help make difficult administrative decisions. Over the years, there has been an exponential growth in social programs. For example, in just the area of programs for children, it is reported that there are more than 17,500 organizations providing youth programs (Lerner & Thompson, 2002). All of these programs must compete with multiple other social programs in a community.

Often several excellent social programs have been established and are functioning in a community. When a request comes to add another program, difficult decisions must be made in these days of limited resources. A city may be sponsoring a homeless healthcare clinic, an after-hours sports program for inner-city youth, and a lunch program for the elderly. When it becomes apparent that a program to deal with school violence may need to be added, it may be that it will be added only if another program is eliminated. Program evaluation that provides systematic, reliable, and valid information will certainly assist the administrative staff in making difficult decisions. Unless there are good program evaluation data available, decisions are more likely to be made based upon perception, anecdotal evidence, or political pressure (Posavac & Carey, 1992).

Monitoring Program Operations

Monitoring a program has as its primary purpose the tracking and reporting of program outcomes that can provide feedback to the program sponsors and treatment team (Affholter, 1994). In general, new social programs are supported by authorizing legislation or private foundations. Rarely does the legislation or foundation specify in detail what the program is to be or how it is to be implemented. The details of program design and implementation are left to the agency or organization that has the authority to administer the program. Demonstration projects are one example of programs that are frequently established to meet general goals and objectives. They focus on a new approach to solve a problem and if the demonstration project is successful, additional programs may be funded in other locations.

Program monitoring is much easier when the program has been developed with clear, consistent, operational objectives that allow for direct and reliable measurement. The results of monitoring the program can help program managers pay particular attention to a specific performance problem or recognize outstanding achievements of the program. Data resources frequently used for program monitoring include direct observation by the evaluator, program records, surveys of program participants (and nonparticipants), and community surveys (Rossi, Freeman, & Lipsy, 2004). Some program sponsors have timely reports that must be submitted for evaluation. Other program sponsors will allow the recipient of a grant to alter the parts of the program sponsored by the grant as long as the intent is not changed. If a school APN developed a program to teach teenage fathers parenting skills and very few boys were enrolled in the program, the sponsoring agency might allow the program to be expanded to include teen mothers.

Determining If the Program Has Resulted in Desired Change

Legislative bodies, most nonprofit organizations, and philanthropic organizations request feedback about the program to determine if the program has achieved the stated goals. Organization officials want to know if the desired change has occurred, or in other words—what have been the outcomes of the program. This has become known as outcome-based evaluation. Outcomes are those benefits the participant receives from participating in the program. The United Way of America (http://www.unitedway.org/outcomes/) provides guidelines readily available on the Web for conducting outcome-based evaluation.

Outcome-based evaluation is used to determine if the services or activities provided by the program lead to observable, intended changes for recipients of the program. For example, the Centers for Disease Control and Prevention (CDC) Division of HIV/AIDS Prevention (DHAP) has developed a national data reporting system that requires all federally funded programs to comply with a standardized data collection system, evaluation guidance and training, and software support services to better determine if the HIV/AIDS prevention programs are meeting their goals as well as serving the needs of the clients and communities. (Thomas et al., 2006). The focus is on outcomes, including unintended effects to determine if the program has been effective. Outcome-based evaluation may also evaluate the program process to gain insight into how the outputs or outcomes have been achieved. (U.S. General Accounting Office, 2005). Systematic data collection for evaluation of goal attainment and fund management is much easier when the program design has included a detailed evaluation design.

Documenting Outcomes for Program Sustainability

Periodic evaluation of the social program, including management, program outcomes, and financial solvency, becomes essential when a program has been designed to be maintained over a long period of time. Careful and precise documentation must be developed to show that the program should be continued because it is achieving the targeted outcomes. Many programs sponsored by governments and other resources provide startup money, but expect that the program will be designed in such a way that the community, other interested parties, or the program itself will generate the financial, personnel, and other resources to keep it running long after the initial grant money has been used (Lapelle, Zapka, & Ockene, 2006). To ensure additional funding from the same source, or to enable a program to seek additional funding from different government or private agencies, the viability of the program must be established (Wallace, 2003). It is also wise for the staff to cultivate good political and public support for the program. Keeping interested persons fully informed of the achievements of the program requires additional work by the program staff, but it may be very important in retaining the funding and other support needed to sustain the program. The program staff, including the APN, cannot assume that political or public support will be there just because the program is doing a good job.

Accountability in Program Evaluation

Funding Agencies

Grant applications submitted to governmental resources and private foundations require that the program develop methods to ensure that the money being spent on the program is used as directed in the grant. Most government grants require at least an annual audit report be submitted regarding the use of funds. Some sponsoring governmental groups will make site visits to review financial records and to ensure that everything documented can be verified. However, some grant rules allow for the recipients of the grant to alter the use of funds with special permission of the granting agency. Some grants allow the principal program administrator to discuss the needs verbally, followed by written documentation of the request according to the agency policies and procedures.

Revising Program Interventions

Program evaluation provides valuable feedback to provide the essential information needed to make necessary revisions. Often several months to years can elapse between the development of an idea for a program and the receipt of funding or other resources allocated to the program. As time elapses, situations change, personnel are recruited with differing backgrounds, personalities, strengths, and weaknesses, or the program is administered differently from the original design. It is important to evaluate periodically to ensure that the program is progressing as designed and if change is needed, that revisions are made appropriately.

An excellent example of needing to change the interventions occurred when a cost-effectiveness evaluation was conducted on the program for preventing perinatal human immunodeficiency virus (HIV) transmission (Stoto, 2001). Based on clinical trials published in 1994 that indicated that proper treatment of HIV in the mother could reduce perinatal transmission, specialists in preventive medicine and public health recommended counseling all women at risk of AIDS on the benefits of testing and voluntary testing. This intervention was successful, but in 1996 Congress instructed the Institute of Medicine (IOM) to evaluate how successful states had been in reducing perinatal HIV transmission. Data revealed that only about 60% to 94% of women were offered HIV testing during pregnancy. After careful cost-benefit analysis, the IOM concluded that universal testing was cost effective and that universal testing was the best intervention for preventing HIV transmission in the perinatal period. In 1999, the American College of Obstetricians and Gynecologists and the American Academy of Pediatrics issued a joint statement that adopted the universal testing approach of the IOM. The Centers for Disease Control and Prevention (CDC) recommends universal HIV testing for all pregnant women; testing remains a voluntary decision by the pregnant woman (Centers for Disease Control and Prevention, 2001). This example demonstrates how evaluation can alter interventions and make a difference in a health policy.

Answering Requests for Information

Program evaluation and careful maintenance of records enable the project director to complete the large number of documents required by governmental agencies funding a social program. Periodic evaluation along with meticulous record keeping can provide a ready source for the data required. Otherwise, the person completing the surveys may find that he or she will be required to spend untold hours doing a manual search through the program files.

Learning About Unintended Effects of the Program

Program evaluations can also help discover any unintended effects of an intervention. As APNs know, medications can have good effects as well as negative side effects. Program evaluations are particularly valuable when systems have been built to detect unanticipated and unwanted outcomes of the treatment intervention (Posavac & Carey, 1992).

Meeting Accreditation Requirements

Many healthcare facilities are required to evaluate their facilities to meet accreditation standards, which usually have been authorized by legislation. While meeting these standards may not predict the effectiveness of the programs offered, it does imply that the program meets the standards set by an official accrediting body that serves to increase public trust. Advanced practice nurses in their more advanced roles as nurse practitioners, clinical specialists, etc., often are asked to assume a key role in preparing the accreditation self-report and to ensure that the agency and its programs meet the standards.

Theory: A Valuable Tool in Evaluation

The use of **theory** in program evaluation provides a map to guide the evaluation process. Advanced practice nurses have been using theory to guide their practice for many years, so the use of theory to guide evaluation of social programs is a normal extension of nursing knowledge and practice. Theory is defined in research and scientific inquiry as a set of interrelated concepts that explain and predict broad phenomena. A concept is an abstract idea about a part of the phenomenon. The concepts may include definitions, empirical facts, or propositions that are related to help explain and predict the phenomena observed. Theories do not have the simplicity of laws, nor do they have the same level of certainty. For example, a theory of illness held by ancients was that illness was the result of offending the gods; the belief that a special illness was the result of angering a particular god is a concept (Trussell, Brandt, & Knapp, 1981). An ideal evaluation theory would describe and justify why certain evaluation practices lead to specific results across the many situations that program evaluators must confront (Shadish, Cook, & Leviton, 1995).

The use of theory in developing a program and its evaluation is beneficial for evaluators and program administrators. A clear statement of theory gives direction (McEwen, 2007). When a social program is designed, those persons responsible for its development and implementation have some basic ideas of what they plan to achieve (outcome) and have some ideas on how they believe such a program will function to achieve the desired results (Clarke, 1999). Theory-based evaluations provide substantive theory about the problem and help define the conceptual relationship between program implementation and expected outcomes. Theories provide a vehicle to recognize the complexities of evaluation practice and integrate diverse concepts, methods, and practices.

Ethics and Evaluation

Program evaluation, by its very nature, evokes a sense of anxiety in most persons. Questions are asked such as: How does the program measure up? Are we doing a good job? What happens if the evaluator finds a problem with the program? Will the clients lose the service? Will I lose my job? How much information should I share with the evaluator? Will the evaluator be fair? From these questions, it can be seen that the role of the evaluator can create stress and the potential for ethical dilemmas for all involved in the evaluation process. Good program evaluation will plan for the potential for ethical conflict and develop strategies to avoid it or deal with the conflicts as they arise during the evaluation process.

Potential Areas of Ethical Conflict

Ethical issues must be considered whenever an evaluation design is planned or an evaluation is conducted by an evaluator. Posavac and Carey (1992) identify several major areas of ethical concern that include (1) the protection of the people treated; (2) the danger of role conflicts by providers; (3) threats to the quality of the evaluation; and (4) the discovery of any negative effects resulting from the evaluation. Put into a slightly different context by Sieber (1980), ethical dilemmas occur in three major areas: (1) conflict between the roles of researcher, administrator, and advocate; (2) conflict between the right to know and the right of privacy; and (3) conflict between the demands of the evaluator, political officials, and/or other significant stakeholders. Stakeholders are either individuals or organizations who are directly or indirectly affected by a social program's implementation or results and who believe they can make a difference to the outcomes (Rossi et al., 2004; Sikma & Young, 2003). Nurses have long recognized the need for ethical nursing care and developed a code of ethics that continues to be updated to reflect the changes in society and health care. The latest version now explicitly states the nurse's primary commitment "is to the patient, whether an individual, family, group, or community" (Daly, 2002, p. 98). The newest code reflects on the importance of the nurse's responsibility to participate as an equal in ethical debates.

Protection from Harm: An Ethical Priority

A central ethical concern is that the evaluation should not harm the participant or anyone else involved in the program. One of the first areas of evaluation is to determine if the program does any harm to someone receiving the program's intervention or if the program harms the program staff in any way. Neither the participants nor the members of the program staff should be harmed. One example of the ethical dilemmas faced in evaluating a health policy is that of newborn screening for specific metabolic disorders for early detection. Although this policy has been successful, the question of how ethical and clinical standards accommodate the rapid developments made possible by the continuing newly developed technologies (Green, Dolan, & Murray, 2006) has arisen. An unforeseen difficulty of a policy with no national standards allowed states to determine which tests were to be done and which tests not to do; thus, some states do fewer than 10 tests whereas others do more than 20. Another dilemma is who should pay for tests demanded by politically active and astute parents and others? Should the state test for abnormalities with no treatment? Some children may be identified to have anomalies that may or may not lead to disease— should they be "labeled" with these illnesses? As can be seen, although this testing program has been very successful, ethical dilemmas have arisen from the evaluation of the program.

In the process of evaluation, much information is collected to meet the requirements of either the program design or the persons that have commissioned the evaluation. An evaluator must use utmost care so that the program participants and staff do not have their privacy, anonymity, or confidentiality violated. This is particularly true since the passage of the Health Insurance Portability and Accountability Act (HIPAA) of 1996 that went into effect in 2003. The HIPAA rules also recognize the privacy and security issues associated with electronic patient information, which might be a data resource in a program evaluation (Cheung, Moody, & Cochram, 2002). A program evaluation researcher must maintain a high level of vigilance to ensure that privacy and security issues are not compromised in the process of data collection, data utilization, or data reporting.

Very real dilemmas can arise if courts subpoena an evaluator's records and these records contain information that might identify the program participant who has been guaranteed confidentiality. If such a problem arises, the evaluator would need to consult legal counsel. According to Hatry, Newcomer, and Wholey (1994), evaluators should continue cautiously and refrain from turning over subpoenaed information until the legality of such a request has been determined. Often group data are collected so that individuals are not identifiable.

Informed consent is a recognized component of all care provided by the APN and is a method frequently used to protect people from harm (Joel, 2006). Participants in the evaluation process should be informed of the evaluation, what it means, and offered a choice to participate or not participate. The APN, whether participating as the evaluator or as a member of the program staff, should be certain that confidentiality and privacy of participants and program staff have been secured in the design and implementation of the evaluation and its report.

Role Conflict: Potential for an Ethical Dilemma

There is potential for conflict at several levels in program development, implementation, and evaluation. The complexity of the institutional and political networks that have had to evolve in program development, funding, and evaluation in constantly changing political and institutional environments has a great potential for developing conflict and ethical dilemmas (Fredericks et al., 2002). Interested persons in the social program being evaluated may comprise many diverse groups of persons, including the politicians who sponsored the funding legislation, the designers of the program, the recipients, and supporting members of the community. These supporters are often called stakeholders because they have a vested interest in the program. Stakeholders may view the program very personally, as their "child," and may try to protect the program and the participants from outside scrutiny during the evaluation process and the sharing of evaluation results.

Most social programs are designed to implement a larger public policy. As a result there are many stakeholders who may become involved in the program evaluation process, including the political persons who first created the legislation to create the program, the administrators and other workers in the program, the recipients of the program, and the taxpayers funding the program. It is quickly apparent that many people have a stake in the success or failure of a program and, as a result, there is much opportunity for conflict. Ethical questions arise when some might wish a bad or even a mediocre program to continue when their jobs depend upon the program. Conversely, sometimes taxpayers want good programs ended to save tax dollars. Therefore, it behooves all evaluators to carefully determine the identity of the stakeholders, their concerns, and the very real pressures they could bring to bear upon the evaluator and the completed **evaluation**

report. After identifying potential conflicts, a plan can be developed that will avoid the pressure or at least keep it to a minimum.

When the evaluator is also the administrator of the program, there is much potential for ethical conflict. It is difficult to wear two hats at one time. If the evaluator is the administrator of the program, it is possible to have role conflict between the role of administrator and evaluator. As the administrator, the role is to ensure that the program runs smoothly with the least amount of interruption. The role of evaluator requires data to be collected to evaluate the program that may require record examination, interviewing recipients of the program, and discussing the evaluation with staff.

Objective Program Evaluation: An Ethical Responsibility

Objective evaluation needs to include a fair and accurate description of how the program succeeded or how it failed from the perspective of all who were affected by the program (Morris, 1999). If the evaluator does not provide a trustworthy evaluation and report it in a timely manner, this may be considered by some as unethical (Posavac & Carey, 1992).

Program evaluators must try to provide the best study possible by selecting the methods and evaluation tools that are most appropriate. Making a mistake in accurately identifying the outcomes of a program, for example, might either allow the program to continue when it should be eliminated or, conversely, the program may be canceled when it should be continued. In both situations, the ethical dilemma is readily apparent.

Another area of ethical concern is to ensure that the evaluation design fits the needs of those who have requested the information (Posavac & Carey, 1992). If the evaluator cannot provide the answers needed by the persons requesting the information, the evaluator must do the ethical thing and either decline to conduct the program evaluation or request that the evaluation tool be changed so that the evaluator can continue. For example, consider a program has been designed to help diabetics alter their lifestyles to prolong their lives. At the end of one year, the APN is asked to evaluate the program to determine if the program has made a difference in life expectancy. This would be an impossible task. Good program evaluation could not be done to answer this question because a 1-year period of time is not long enough to determine life expectancy. To agree to do an evaluation to answer this question would create an ethical dilemma. A better question, albeit a very limited one, might be to request the evaluation tool be revised to determine improved disease control as measured by hemoglobin A1C, lipid profiles, incidence of delayed healing, and other such parameters over the 1-year period as a measure of improved self-care.

An evaluator must also consider an ethical responsibility to provide a report promptly so that the results can be used while the program is being implemented. The design of the evaluation needs to be written with enough detail that the procedures used and the process of data analysis could be understood by the persons requesting the evaluation. The report must contain enough detail that later someone else could duplicate the evaluation or read the report and come to the same conclusions.

Reporting Negative Effects: An Ethical Requirement

An ethical dilemma occurs when the evaluator discovers that while many of the objectives of the program are being met, some aspects of the program may be having negative effects. The question becomes how to report these findings so that the data can be used by the program administrators to alter the program. If the negative effect is judged to be serious enough that the harm outweighs the benefits, the program should be ended or revised. An example of a negative result might be a program to establish transportation for the mentally handicapped. If the bus had big, bold letters on it that announced it was for the mentally handicapped, some might believe that this was demeaning. The program could be eliminated or altered so that the bus was not labeled and the program could continue.

Suggestions to Reduce Ethical Dilemmas in Program Evaluation

By the nature of social program evaluation, there is bound to be the potential for ethical dilemmas to arise. Some suggestions to reduce the incidence of an ethical dilemma include some of the following ideas:

The APRN can design an evaluation process that avoids ethical dilemmas. The APN should consent to provide program evaluation only after carefully studying the request and establishing clear guidelines for the study. The APN does not need to determine the "right and wrong" of observed phenomena, but instead must create a working environment that does not compromise or create ethical dilemmas (Morris, 1999).

Good communication is essential throughout the evaluation process but is invaluable when avoiding conflict and especially ethical conflicts. One suggestion that may be helpful is to establish written agreements between the evaluator, the program requesting evaluation, and any other significant stakeholders that have been identified in the evaluation design. A clause that provides a mechanism for either party to withdraw from the relationship should be included if issues that cannot be resolved develop as the evaluation is conducted (Sieber, 1980).

The evaluator must also be aware of his or her own strengths and weaknesses as well as strong belief systems. An evaluator that firmly believes that all people who are homeless are lazy probably should not be the person participating in the evaluation of a homeless shelter.

Ethical evaluation practice can be very challenging in the real-world settings of program implementation. Advanced practice nurses who become involved with a social program or its evaluation must continue to function with clear ethical principles just as in clinical practice. It is imperative that the APN recognize the potential for ethical conflict and develop plans to confront these issues to bring resolution to them. Any comments or questions that cast a shadow on the program can sometimes be taken quite personally by the stakeholders.

Suggestions to Avoid Conflict

Program evaluation is complex and involves multiple stakeholders ranging from highly powerful political and social leaders to the program implementers and their support staff to the recipients of the program. All of the persons involved are interested in the program at various levels. Five suggestions for program evaluators to assist in avoiding conflict were made by Smith and associates (as cited in Clarke, 1999, p. 17).

First, recognize the potential conflicts between multiple stakeholders and deal with them in a diplomatic, efficient manner. Attempt to identify the primary and secondary stakeholders. Failure to examine potential and actual conflicts can easily lead to problems throughout the evaluation process.

Second, involve the multiple interest groups in the design of the evaluation study. If each group "owns" a portion of the design and is engaged as active participants in the process, there is less chance the varying groups of stakeholders will splinter off or create additional tensions in the evaluation process. Likewise, this approach recognizes the importance of each group and allows for compromises as needed.

Third, keep the multiple stakeholders and members of the evaluation team informed about the progress of the evaluation. It is easier to maintain cooperation among divergent groups if the groups are kept current with the project and are given the opportunity to provide feedback from their perspective.

Fourth, ensure that all stakeholders understand the goals and objectives of the program as they have been developed. This helps the stakeholders better understand exactly what the program was established to accomplish and identify the objectives that have been met and those that have not been met.

Fifth, identify the political and organizational environmental conditions in which the evaluation is being conducted. These situational factors are important to understand throughout the evaluation process to develop the design, implement the evaluation project, and disseminate the results.

Program Evaluation Design Options

As discussed earlier, the environment in which program evaluation takes place often is complex and includes a large number of stakeholders who have been involved in some manner in the development and implementation of a social program. In designing a culturally sensitive evaluation, it is critical to the success of the evaluation from inception to completion that the stakeholders be involved in the process (Westat, 2002).

It is important to determine who holds the power to make decisions regarding evaluations, especially when there are multiple levels of stakeholders involved in the program. School-based programs are key examples of organizations with multiple stakeholders, all of whom interact with each other at varying levels. Federal, state, and local resources may be involved in significant ways with their multiple layers of decision makers. When an APN is asked to participate in the evaluation of a school-based health program, it would be essential that the APN consider the heads of the agencies sponsoring the program's priorities both politically and personally. Next, the school board and superintendent would be recognized as powerful decision makers. School principals, counselors, and teachers provide another layer of decision making. Parents have indirect authority because they can choose to allow their student to participate or not (Guzman & Feria, 2002). Students also influence the outcomes of the evaluation because they control the information that they share with the evaluator. Knowing the chain of command is essential when developing evaluation designs to ensure that decisions can be made to increase the likelihood of success of the evaluation process.

The earliest evaluation designs were based on the scientific approach that is founded on the principle of causation. The goal of quantitative evaluation is to collect sufficient data to rule out rival hypotheses by such means as control or comparison groups or by statistical adjustments (Polit & Beck, 2004). Quantitative evaluation methods seek to be precise and to identify all the relevant variables prior to the data collection. The method also seeks to minimize the role of the evaluator or data collector in the collection of the evaluation data.

The **quantitative evaluation design** continues to have merit. However, as the complexity of social programs was revealed, additional evaluation designs were needed to determine additional information about how a program was affecting the individual recipients of the program interventions. Evaluation designs began to incorporate the qualitative approach. The **qualitative evaluation design** approach has as its basis the belief that it is the quality or the subjective reality that has true meaning in the events, lives, and behaviors of individuals (Fine, Weiss, Weseen, & Wong, 2000). Qualitative data are used in much of life. It is qualitative reasoning that allows a reader to solve a mystery. The reader can conclude that "the butler did it" based upon data collected from a variety of sources and combining the information in a qualitative manner (Posavac & Carey, 1992).

Evaluators, using a qualitative approach, attempt to seek an understanding of the meaning of public policy, its attendant programs, and interventions from the perspective of the recipients of the program, the staff, community, and other significant persons (House, 1994). If an inner-city emergency room APN observed that many homeless persons used the waiting room as a shelter, he or she might approach the city to establish a shelter for the homeless. To establish a successful program, the design, implementation, and outcomes of the program would have to include not only the city's point of view, but also the needs and views of the homeless themselves. Qualitative issues, such as desire for autonomy by the homeless, can make or break social programs with the best of intentions.

To be successful in achieving an evaluation that is useful to the persons who have requested it and to be beneficial to the social program and its recipients, the design of the evaluation must receive careful planning. A good design is like a good road map when planning a car trip from San Francisco to New York. It helps to decide where you are going, how to get there, how long it will take, and how many side trips can be made on a limited budget. Details regarding qualitative and quantitative designs may be found in many research texts. It must be repeated that **program evaluation designs** must be able to provide effective, useful, reliable, and valid information as well as be able to be conducted within the many constraints of real life such as limitations of resources including time, money, personnel, and expertise.

Some down-to-earth suggestions by McNamera (1997–2006) seem particularly useful to the novice APN evaluator. His suggestions include the following:

1. Don't fear evaluation—remember the 80/20 rule: The first 20% of the work will produce the first 80% of the plan—and this is a very good start.
2. Remember that there is no perfect evaluation plan. Getting something done is better than waiting until every last detail has been identified.
3. Include a few interviews in evaluation methods. The stories provide powerful descriptions of the outcomes of the program.
4. Don't review just successes—failures also give valuable insights into the function and outcomes of the program.

5. Keep the evaluation data after the report has been written. These data may be useful as the program continues and changes over time.

Evaluation Reports: Sharing the Findings

After the social program has been evaluated, the results of the evaluation study need to be shared with those who have requested the evaluation, significant stakeholders, the staff of the program, the community, and/or sometimes the recipients of the program's interventions. Hendricks (1994) offers six principles of reporting that provide the best information to those who have requested the evaluation and enhance utilization of the report.

1. Mode of writing and content of evaluation of the report is the responsibility of the evaluator. It is the responsibility of the evaluator to present the results of the evaluation in the form of a report in a timely and appropriate manner. The evaluator must select a format to report the evaluation data, its interpretation, and final recommendations that will be useful to those who have commissioned the evaluation. The evaluation report must be developed to meet the needs of the program, its staff, and the sponsors of the program. The task of presenting a meaningful evaluation report is up to the evaluator(s).

   The results are reported factually and in an unbiased manner so that anyone can read the data and be able to come to a useful conclusion on one's own. A separate section of the report can include the interpretation of the data by the author of the report. Last, the recommendations are presented.

   When evaluation reports are completed before a program had been targeted for closing, evaluation reports that are given to the staff and program sponsors can provide useful insights into how well the program is meeting its goals and objectives and give guidance for ways to improve the program. Effective communication is essential if the evaluation report is to be accepted and used. Part of the evaluation plan should include plans for communication with members of the program and other interested persons (Posavac & Carey, 1992). When possible, communication meetings should be planned and scheduled at mutually acceptable times and intervals.

   Evaluators must recognize that sometimes people associated with the program are fearful of the results of an evaluation. To allay some of this fear and potential for poor utilization of the evaluation report, one technique used by evaluators is to first present the report as a draft report. The early presentations provide key persons in the program an idea of the results of the data, some of the interpretations of the findings, and potential recommendations. The early meetings about a draft offer opportunities for valuable comments and discussion between evaluator and program staff and sponsors. After all inputs from the significant readers of the report are taken into account, a final report can be written.

2. Provide multiple opportunities for reporting the evaluation reports. Some evaluation reports will be more useful if they are presented to multiple audiences. If the APN has been selected to be the evaluator of a homeless shelter, the more audiences that can learn of the successes and areas of needed improvement, the more likely the APN is to build support for the program. The APN may seek to report to community groups, healthcare providers, city council members, and so forth, to reach a larger audience regarding the results of the evaluation. Frequently, community projects need to keep many diverse interested groups informed so that they will remain supportive of a good social program that is meeting its goals and objectives.

3. Reports should be succinct, with the major points presented clearly. Writing long, in-depth reports may result in these impressive documents being left on shelves to gather dust or languish in a computer file. Short, powerful sentences work best to grab the attention of decision makers (Jennings, 2003). The inclusion of an executive summary that gives a brief summary of the main findings and recommendations is appreciated (Clarke, 1999).

    Reports are written for the sponsors and stakeholders and as much as possible technical terms need to be kept at a minimum. Complex statistical interpretations may need to be simplified, depending upon the audience. Often, simple, descriptive statistics are more meaningful to a lay audience.

    It is wise to avoid using jargon, whether evaluation or technical, in the discussion because the readers of the report may not be familiar with the terms and tend to skip over the report without really reading it. A glossary of terms may be helpful to the readers (Clarke, 1999). Many evaluators find that presenting findings in graph form is a useful method of communicating information in a condensed and visible form. Detailed, additional information that is important to the total evaluation process may be put in appendices for those interested in a more detailed and in-depth presentation.

4. Write the report to catch the interests of the audience. Whenever possible, the evaluator(s) will find that their evaluation report will have a wider audience if it can be written in a style that is appealing and/or compelling to the audience. It needs to address the

special interests and concerns of those persons who will be receiving the report. Usually, there are multiple audiences for a report such as the legislators who created the program, the administrator who is implementing it, the recipients, and frequently the community at large.

Tailoring the report to the audience is important. For example, a program was developed to improve water quality as a result of chemical pollution of the ground water. The APN has been involved in the program to assist families living in an area of contaminated ground water to learn to use only approved water for drinking and cooking. As a member of the evaluation team, the APN would recognize that the report would be written quite technically with charts, graphs, and statistics for the water pollution experts, but the report would be written or presented more simply to the local residents of the community. Also, in today's world the report may need to be prepared in multiple forms. A written report is the standard and usually required for documentation of the complete report. However, other forms of the report may be developed to reach a divergent audience such as video/DVD presentations, PowerPoint shows, or Web-based documentation in either a long or shortened form.

5. Give direction and provide guidelines for action in the form of recommendations. The recipients of most evaluation reports want to learn about what is good about the program and what areas need improvement. Recommendations for action often are best received if the program staff reports them in identifiable, practical, and achievable terms. Unusual or unexpected outcomes must also be reported. If unusual outcomes are presented in a value-free approach, with several suggestions for change, the needs for improvement will be more readily acceptable.

   The question can be asked, how specific should recommendations be? An absolute rule cannot be given to this question. In general, recommendations should always be presented as two or more options unless there is only one, very obvious, recommendation to be made. A specific topic with suggestions for the direction of change may be more effective because it gives those involved in the program direction and flexibility in choosing an approach or making a decision. It is also helpful if the suggestions include some indication of cost, acceptance, or the effects of the recommendations.

6. Use multiple communication techniques to disseminate results of the evaluation. Whenever possible, the evaluator should consider using multiple communication techniques to disseminate the results of the evaluation research. Written reports may be delivered in printed or electronic formats. Videotapes, personal briefings, and community meetings are just a few examples of other methods of

sharing the results of a programs evaluation. The technique(s) used should be appropriate to the audience or audiences.

Program evaluations may be used not only by those who have supported, developed, implemented, and/or utilized the program, but also by "policy entrepreneurs" who use the report as a resource to support new policy ideas (Cabatoff, 2000). A well-written report that defines the evaluation findings in clear, nonpartisan terms may be helpful to those engaged in seeking political support for changes in a broader public policy.

Conclusion

Advanced practice nurses have unlimited opportunities to participate or conduct public policy or program evaluation. Public policy is developed by governments and the courts. Public policy is determined by legislative bodies as they make laws, by executive bodies as they administer the laws, and by judicial bodies as they interpret these laws

Public policy is determined by governments and put into practice by the development of social programs. Most governmental and other agencies that sponsor social programs require that these programs be evaluated. Evaluation may take many forms, including studying the extent and severity of a problem, determining if the program is meeting its goals and objectives, conducting a financial audit, examining program outcomes, verifying program outcomes, and seeking information about needed changes in the program.

The tools for evaluation include the quantitative and qualitative methodologies used by social scientists, which are carried out with a rigor needed to meet the needs of the evaluation. Evaluation is expensive in time, money, skilled personnel, and other scarce resources, so it is imperative that the evaluation study be done skillfully and efficiently to meet the multiple needs of multiple stakeholders.

After an evaluation has been conducted, the results of the study must be communicated. Some of the important principles of providing an evaluation report that is meaningful and useful include presenting the report to multiple audiences, providing multiple opportunities for others to learn about the evaluation report, writing the report succinctly with the interests of significant others included, giving guidelines for change, and using multiple presentation approaches when needed.

Evaluation of social programs is valuable and can provide very useful information to the advanced practice nurse who is providing care through a funded or sponsored social program. Evaluation can present exciting challenges for the APN who participates in program evaluation and the presentation of the results.

Discussion Points and Activities

1. What are the advantages of having an advanced practice nurse design and implement an evaluation of a healthcare program?
2. Define how policy, public policy, and social programs may play a role in the advanced practice nurse's practice.
3. List the reasons an APN might be a participant or conduct a program evaluation.
4. Under what conditions might the APN use a quantitative evaluation design? Qualitative design? Combined quantitative and qualitative design?
5. Identify the conditions in program evaluation that might lead to ethical conflict.
6. How might the advanced practice nurse avoid ethical conflict when participating or conducting a program evaluation?
7. Draft a program evaluation report within the framework of the component parts.
8. Suggest several ways that the advanced practice nurse might improve utilization of an evaluation report by the sponsors of the evaluation.

References

Affholter, D. P. (1994). Outcome monitoring. In J. S. Wholey, H. P. Hatry, K. E. Newcomer (Eds.), *Handbook of practical program evaluation* (pp. 96–118). San Francisco, CA: Jossey-Bass.

American Nurses Association. (1997). *Legislative and regulatory initiatives for the 105th Congress.* Washington, DC: American Nurses Publishing.

Anderson, J. E. (1975). *Public policy-making.* New York: Praeger.

Cabatoff, K. (2000). Translating evaluation findings into "policy language." In R. K. Hoopson (Ed.), *New directions for evaluation: No. 86. How and why language matters in evaluation* (pp. 43–54). San Francisco: Jossey-Bass.

Center for Health Improvement. (2004). *Advocacy toolkit.* Retrieved July 16, 2007, from: www.chipolicy.org/pdf/advocacytoolkitnew.pdf

Centers for Disease Control and Prevention. (2001, November 9). *Recommendations and reports: Revised recommendations for HIV screening of pregnant women.* Retrieved July 16, 2007, from: www.cdc.gov/mmwr/preview/mmwrhtml/rr5019a2.htm

Cheung, R. B., Moody, L. E., & Cockram, C. (2002). Data mining strategies for shaping nursing and health policy agendas. *Policy, Politics, & Nursing Practice, 3,* 248–260.

Clarke, A. (with Dawson, R). (1999). *Evaluation research: An introduction to principles, methods and practice.* London: Sage.

Daly, B. J. (2002). Moving forward: A new code of ethics. *Nursing Outlook, 50,* 97–99.

Fine, M., Weiss, L., Weseen, S., & Wong, L. (2000). For whom? Qualitative research, representations, and social responsibilities. In N. K. Denzin & Y. S. Lincoln (Eds.), *Handbook of qualitative research* (2nd ed., pp. 107–131). Thousand Oaks, CA: Sage.

Fredericks, K. A., Carman, J. G., & Birkland, T. A. (2002, Fall). Program evaluation in a challenging authorizing environment: Intergovernmental and interorganizational factors. In R Mohan, D. Bernstein, & M. Whitsett (Eds.), *New directions for evaluation:*

No. 95. *Responding to sponsors and stakeholders in complex evaluation environments* (pp. 5–21). San Francisco: Jossey-Bass.

Green, N., Dolan, S., & Murray, T. (2006). Newborn screening: Complexities in universal genetic testing. *American Journal of Public Health, 96*, 1955–1959.

Guzman, B. L., & Feria, A. (2002, Fall). Forces driving health care decisions. *Policy, Politics, & Nursing Practices, 3,* 35–42.

Hanley, B. E. (2002). Policy development and analysis. In D. J. Mason, J. K. Leavitt, & M. W. Chaffee (Eds.), *Policy and politics in nursing and health care* (4th ed., pp. 55–69). St. Louis, MO: Saunders.

Hatry, H. P., Newcomer, K. E., & Wholey, K. E. (1994). Improving evaluation activities and results: An introduction. In J. S. Wholey, H. P. Hatry, & K. E. Newcomer (Eds.), *Handbook of practical program evaluation*. San Francisco: Jossey-Bass.

Hendricks, M. (1994). Making a splash: Reporting evaluation results effectively. In J. S. Wholey, H. P. Hatry, & K. E. Newcomer (Eds.), *Handbook of practical program evaluation,* (pp. 549–575). San Francisco: Jossey-Bass.

House, E. R. (1994). Integrating the quantitative and qualitative. In C. S. Reichardt & S. F. Rallis (Eds.), *New directions for program evaluation: 61. The qualitative-quantitative debate: New perspectives* (pp. 13–22). San Francisco: Jossey-Bass.

Jennings, B. M. (2003). A half-dozen health policy hints. *Nursing Outlook, 51,* 92–93.

Jennings, C. P. (2001). The evolution of U.S. health policy and the impact of future trends. *Policy, Politics, and Nursing Practice, 2,* 218–227.

Joel, L. A. (2006). *The nursing experience: Trends, challenges, and transitions.* New York: McGraw-Hill.

LaPelle, N., Zapka, J., & Ockene, J. (2006). Sustainability of public health programs: The example of tobacco treatment services in Massachusetts. *American Journal of Public Health, 96,* 1363–1369.

Lerner, R. M., & Thompson, L. S. (2002). Promoting healthy adolescent behavior and development: Issues in the design and evaluation of effective youth programs. *Journal of Pediatric Nursing, 17,* 338–344.

Light, R. J. (2001, Summer). Editor's notes. In R. J. Light (Ed.) *New directions for evaluation: 90. Evaluation findings that surprise* (pp. 1–2). San Francisco: Jossey-Bass.

Mason, D. J., Leavitt, J. K., & Chaffee, M. W. (Eds.). (2002). *Policy and politics in nursing and health care* (4th ed., pp. 1–18). St. Louis, Mo: Saunders.

McEwen, M. (2007). Overview of theory in nursing. In M. McEwen & E. M. Wills (Eds.), *Theoretical basis for nursing* (pp. 24–49). Philadelphia: Lippincott, Williams & Wilkins.

McNamera, C. (1997–2006). *Basic guide to program evaluation.* Retrieved July 16, 2007, from: www.managementhelp.org/evaluatn/fnl_eval.htm

Morris, M. (1999). Research on evaluation ethics: What have we learned and why is it important. In J. L. Fitzpatrick & M. Morris (Eds.), *New directions for evaluation: 82. Current and emerging ethical challenges in evaluation* (pp. 15–24). San Francisco: Jossey-Bass.

Polit, D. F., & Beck, C. T. (2004). *Nursing research: Principles and methods* (7th ed.). Philadelphia: Lippincott, Williams & Wilkins.

Posavac, E. J., & Carey, R. G. (1992). *Program evaluation: Methods and case studies* (4th ed.). Englewood Cliffs, NJ: Prentice Hall.

Reutter, L., & Duncan, S. (2002). Preparing nurses to promote health enhancing public policies. *Policy, Politics, & Nursing Practice, 3,* 294–305.

Rossi, P. H., Freeman, H. E., & Lipsy, M. W. (2004). *Evaluation, a systematic approach* (7th ed.). New York: Random House.

Shadish, W. R., Jr., Cook, T. D., & Leviton, L. C. (1995). *Foundations of program evaluation: Theories of practice.* Newbury Park, CA: Sage.

Sieber, J. E. (1980). Being ethical: Professional and personal decisions in program evaluation. *New Directions for Program Evaluation, 7,* 51–61.

Sikma, S. K., & Young, H. M. (2003). Nurse delegation in Washington State: A case study of concurrent policy implementation and evaluation. *Policy, Politics, & Nursing Practice, 4,* 53–61.

Stoto, M. A. (2001). Preventing perinatal transmission of HIV: Target programs, not people. In R. J. Light (Ed.), *New directions for evaluation: No. 90. Evaluation findings that surprise* (pp. 41–53). San Francisco: Jossey-Bass.

Thomas, C. W., Smith, B. D., & Wright-DeAguero, L. (2006). The program evaluation and monitoring evidence-based HIV prevention program processes and outcomes. [Electronic version]. *AIDS Education and Prevention, 18*(Suppl. A), 74–80.

Trussell, P., Brandt, A., & Knapp, S. (1981). *Using nursing research: Discovery, analysis, and interpretation.* Wakefield, MA: Nursing Resources.

U.S. General Accounting Office (GAO). (2005, May). *Performance measurement and evaluation: Definitions and relationships.* Retrieved July 16, 2007, from: www.gao.gov/new.items/d05739sp.pdf

Wallace, J. (2003). A policy analysis of the assistive technology alternative financing program in the United States. *Journal of Disability Policy Studies, 14*(2), 74–81.

Westat, J. F. (2002). *The 2002 user-friendly handbook for project evaluation.* National Science Foundation Directorate for Education & Human Resources, Division of Research, Evaluation, and Communication. Retrieved July 16, 2007, from: www.nsf.gov/pubs/2002/nsf02057/nsf02057.pdf

Online Resources

AcademyHealth. Provides links to 4000 health services researchers in health policy and 125 affiliated organizations. It fosters networking among a diverse membership. http://www.academyhealth.org

Agency for Healthcare Research and Quality (AHRQ). Provides links to multiple resources. http://www.ahrq.gov/

CDC Evaluation Working Group. Provides multiple links to program evaluation information. http://www.cdc.gov/eval/resources.htm

Free Management Library. Developed by Authenticity Consulting. Provides more than 675 online resources for program evaluation and personal, professional, and organization development, including many detailed guidelines, worksheets, and more. http://www.managementhelp.org/

Outcome Measurement Resource Network. Developed by United Way of America. http://national.unitedway.org/outcomes/

Resources for Methods in Evaluation and Social Research. Provides free resources for methods in evaluation and social research, including information on how to do evaluation research. http://gsociology.icaap.org/methods/

The Internet and Healthcare Policy Information

Ramona Nelson, PhD, RN–BC, FAAN

Key Terms

➤ **Bookmark** A browser function that saves the Uniform Resource Locator (URL) for an Internet site on the user's computer. The user can then return to the site by clicking the bookmark.

➤ **Blog** A user-generated online journal that provides for comments from readers. The term is a merger of *Web* and *log*.

➤ **Browser** A software application that displays information found on the Internet. Examples include Netscape and Internet Explorer.

➤ **Homepage** The starting point or first page for a Web site. This page usually provides an overview of what is available on the site.

➤ **Host** Any computer system connected to the Internet. A host is indicated by the domain name. With virtual hosting it is possible for a single computer to host several different domains.

➤ **Internet site** An Internet location usually consisting of a collection of documents.

➤ **Link** A word, phrase, graphic, or address that, when clicked, loads a related Web page.

➤ **Search engine** A computer program or group of programs that search a database relating to the term or group of terms selected by the user to locate information in the database. The Internet is a database of Internet sites and can be searched with a search engine.

➤ **Signature file** A user-created file that will insert a message at the bottom of an e-mail message identifying the sender.

➤ **Uniform Resource Locator (URL)** The resource locators used by the World Wide Web as addresses for information. The URL connects the user directly to a particular document or page.

➤ **User interface** Screens that are presented to the user when that user interacts with a computer program. If the set of screens presented to the user makes it easy for the user to interact with the software program, the program is referred to as user-friendly.

➤ **Web page** Refers to a site on the Internet that uses Hypertext Markup Language (HTML) as its interface. Web pages are viewed with a browser. A page may include graphics, text, sounds, and movies.

Introduction

With hands-on experience dealing with the realities of healthcare delivery, the advanced practice nurse (APN) understands the impact of current healthcare policies and the need for new healthcare policies. To be an effective advocate and leader for ensuring that health policies benefit patients, families, and communities the APN must understand the process for developing and implementing health policy. Knowledge of the policy process requires an understanding of the whole process—from agenda setting through policy and program evaluation. This knowledge makes it possible for the APN to provide the needed leadership both individually and collectively through professional and other interest groups. Leadership demands anticipatory performance in which the APN foresees health problems and solutions and initiates appropriate actions in the public sector. The nurse in advanced practice must know how to access data, to present information, and to build a case that will affect public officials and motivate the general public.

This chapter introduces the APN to key health policy **Internet sites** and the use of effective search strategies to search for healthcare policy data. These sites include those established and maintained by the various levels of government, universities, and organizations. In addition, the chapter explores how the Internet is changing the development of healthcare policy.

Information Literacy and Health Policy

The APN must be information literate, possessing the skills needed to access, evaluate, and use information resources. Increasingly, the needed resources are available through electronic databases and the World Wide Web. Electronic resources make it possible for expert nurses to expand their comprehension of a problem, frame an argument, suggest one or more solutions, recommend policy tools in designing those solutions, and construct evaluation models for determining success or for making administrative decisions about continuation, change, or termination of a program.

Information Literacy Defined

In 2000, the American Library Association approved information literacy standards for higher education. They defined *information literacy* as a set of abilities requiring individuals to "recognize when information is needed and have the ability to locate, evaluate, and use effectively the needed information" (Association of College and Research Libraries, 2000, p. 2). An information-literate person is able to:

- Determine the information needed
- Access the needed information
- Evaluate the accessed information
- Incorporate the information into what is already known
- Use the information in achieving a goal
- Access and use information ethically and legally

These standards apply to all graduates of a baccalaureate education program. They have been widely accepted and are now included in the accreditation criteria of most higher education accrediting agencies. An APN should be able to apply these standards in accessing and using health policy data in all steps of the health policy development process from agenda setting through policy and program evaluation.

Using the Internet to Locate Health Policy Information on the World Wide Web

As of July 2006, the Internet Systems Consortium (2007) reported there were 439,286,364 hosts on the Internet. A **host** is defined as a computer on a network; in this case, the network is the Internet. Each computer has its own domain name indicated by the **Uniform Resource Locator (URL)**. However, a single computer is able to provide a home for multiple hosts. This is referred to as *virtual hosting*, where a single computer acts like multiple systems [and has multiple domain names and Internet Protocol (IP) addresses]. Each host can include numerous Web sites. A

Web site consists of several **Web pages** that are meaningfully linked together. For example, if a user is connected to Slippery Rock University, the Internet address or URL for the host is http://www.sru.edu. At this site, there are several Web pages related to the university.

A *Web page* is the screen that is seen when the Internet site is accessed. A **homepage** is the first Web page of an Internet site, often thought of as a "front door" to the site. Traditionally, a homepage contains an introduction to the site, an overview of the resources available at the site, and connecting **links**. A homepage may have several links to Web pages that are part of the site or to Internet sites located elsewhere. When accessing a Web site from a **browser** search, the user may be on any of the pages in the Web site. It is often useful to look for the home page and assess the site before considering the use of a new resource.

A URL is the Internet address for a site on the Internet. It functions as a traditional post office address. Each host on the Internet has a unique URL. If the user already knows the URL of a site, typing this information directly into the browser will immediately access that site. For example, Duke University maintains an excellent health policy resource site. The URL is http://www.hpolicy.duke.edu. Typing this URL in the browser provides immediate access to the Duke University health policy homepage. The homepage links with several other Web pages on this site as well as other hosts and pages with health policy information.

Using Search Engines

If the nurse knows the topic he or she is interested in, but does not know specific sites, then a **search engine** and/or directory site is needed. The main function of a search engine site is to find Internet resources based on specific criteria, such as topic, date, or agency. These sites can offer both a search engine and/or a directory of related topics. The directories have information about sites and are organized by topics. The search engines provide the opportunity to look up references or sites based on key words. Search engine sites may offer both directories and online searches or only the online search function.

Search engines and directories are designed and maintained on the Internet by various companies. Each company that provides a search engine has its own URL. Some well-known examples include http://www.google.com, http://www.yahoo.com, and http://www.lycos.com. Several sites on the Internet maintain a list of search engines with links to the engines. Many university libraries maintain such sites. One example can be located at http://www.sru.edu/pages/3128.asp.

Directories are usually more useful at the beginning of a search when background information about a topic is needed or when one is not sure where to start. Although directories are usually organized by topics in hierarchical structures, there are no standards in how these are structured. For example, the topic health policy can be located under medicine, government, or community. Sometimes it is useful to browse the directories.

In addition, because users have become more comfortable with information organized in networked links, the hierarchical structure of the information on the Web site may not be obvious. In these cases, it is more useful to search the site with a search engine. For example, Yahoo.com has a directory on health located at http://health. yahoo.com. Much of the information is organized around specific diseases and health promotion. This directory can be searched by using the search term "health policy."

Although the overall functions offered by search engines are similar, each company has taken a different approach to offering these functions. Each of the search engines and Web pages located on the Internet requires time, effort, and money to maintain. Each of these companies or institutions that maintain a search engine expends this time, money, and effort for a reason. The search engine may be a commercial venture or it can be an attempt by a government agency to improve citizen access to information. The motivation behind the search engine has a major impact on how it is designed and functions. Each engine has a different **user interface**. That means that the screens will not be identical and the method of entering keywords will vary. Search engines can also vary in the type of information they provide, how they locate information, and how they present the information they have located. All of these sites contain tutorials and help pages that explain how to use their sites. Additional information on these variations can be found at http://www.internettutorials.net/.

Many people who prefer a specific search engine or site will bookmark the engine's URL. When a site is bookmarked, the URL is saved in the browser and the user will not need to remember or type the URL again. The bookmark function can be accessed through the main menu at the top of the browser. Each browser uses slightly different terminology and approaches to add **bookmarks**; however, all browsers provide an opportunity to organize bookmarks into folders. In most cases, if folders are not used to organize the sites, the bookmarks quickly become a long, disorganized list of sites, many of which no longer function.

On any Internet site you may receive a message that "the server is down or not responding" such as the one shown in Exhibit 8–1. This can happen if the site is busy or if the sponsor of the site is having technical problems. The best approach in this situation is to try visiting the site again a little later. Another problem is that Internet sites disappear or just reorganize, and previously located files can disappear.

Sometimes it is possible to locate the document if it still exists by searching the site. Other times, the document is gone forever. That is why it is a good idea to download or print a copy of documents you are planning to cite or use in future research.

Locating Search Engines

There are many different types of information on the Internet. These include Web pages, e-mail discussion lists, and people data. A general search

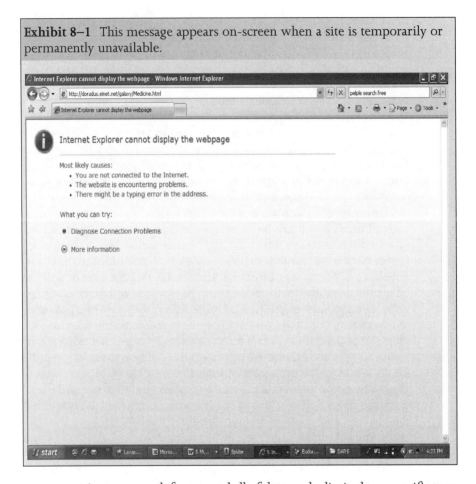

Exhibit 8–1 This message appears on-screen when a site is temporarily or permanently unavailable.

engine may search for any and all of these or be limited to a specific type of information. A search engine can also be designed to search a specific site. For example, the URL for the U.S. government is http://www.usa.gov/. This is the official Web portal for the U.S. government. The search engine on this site is designed to search for government-based information resources.

Another approach to locating and using general search engines is the use of meta-search sites. There are two types of meta-search sites. One provides a consistent interface to searching several different search engines. The Metacrawler search page located at http://www.metacrawler.com/ offers an example of this approach.

A second approach is to search using a number of search engines at once. One example of this type of site is Dogpile located at http://dogpile.com/info.dogpl/. Dogpile is a meta-search engine that searches other search engines such as Google, Yahoo!, MSN, and ASK. There are also sites that list sites of search engines. Box 8–1 lists several of these types of sites. Many of these sites include information about using search

Box 8-1 List of Search Engines
• http://allsearchengines.com/ • http://searchenginewatch.com/ • http://www.searchenginecolossus.com/ • http://www.beaucoup.com/ • http://en.wikipedia.org/wiki/List_of_search_engines

engines. A general or topic-specific search engine will search for Web pages; there are also search engines that search for specific types of information such as e-mail discussion lists, people data, and health sites.

E-Mail Discussion Lists

An e-mail discussion list is a virtual group of people with a common area of interest who communicate by means of an electronic distribution mail (e-mail) list. A virtual group exists on the Internet but not in the traditional spatial dimension. Individuals with an area of common interest join a list via subscription. After they have joined the list, members read messages posted to the list or send messages to other subscribers. Those who reply to e-mail discussion list messages should be aware that these messages are read by all subscribers. That is, replies should not be made unless the sender wants all list subscribers to read them. Subscribers also can send or post messages to individual members on the list by using the Internet e-mail address of the individual. In this way, a reader can respond specifically to another list member with some degree of confidentiality and without all members reading the response.

Like other groups of people each e-mail discussion list can have its own personality. A new user is often wise to lurk for a period of time before joining the discussion. One way to assess the nature of the group is to review the signature files of the participants. A **signature file** can be thought of as a mini bio or brief introduction to the person posting a message.

Box 8–2 lists Internet sites that can be used to search for lists focused on policy-related issues. Many of these sites also explain how the list works and the process for subscribing. The APN may want to search the different search engines using the keywords "health policy." If "health policy" does not produce a successful result, try searching for a list with just the term "policy."

With each of these search engines you will find several different discussion groups. The search engines will return overlapping, but different results. Some groups focus on specific areas of health policy whereas others are more general. If a specific e-mail discussion list looks interesting, it is usually possible to learn more about the list before subscribing. Exhibit 8–2 shows an example of the kind of information that can be available.

Box 8-2 Search Engines for Finding E-Mail Discussion Lists

- http://www.lsoft.com/catalist.html
- http://tile.net/lists/
- http://groups.yahoo.com/
- http://lists.topica.com/dir/

People Data

Many of the major search engines provide the option to search for people. In addition, several search engines on the Internet are specific to finding people. APNs can use these search engines to find a person's phone number or e-mail or postal address. Although most of these sites provide basic information such as address, phone number, and e-mail address for free, often their main goal is to sell personal information.

It is also possible to do a reverse lookup by entering a person's phone number and searching for the person's name. A list of these search engines for finding people is included in Box 8–3. These lists are sometimes referred to as the white pages. Each search engine accesses

Exhibit 8–2 A Description of an E-Mail Discussion List

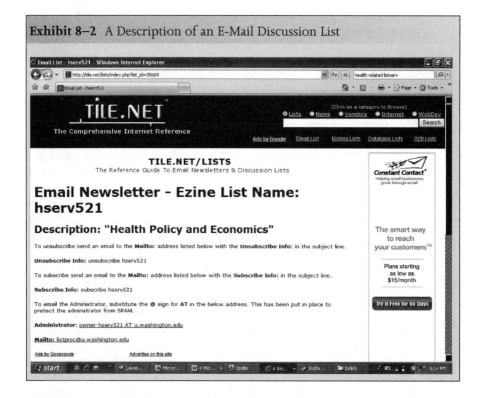

Box 8-3 Search Engines for Finding People

- http://people.yahoo.com/
- http://peoplesearch.lycos.com/
- http://www.anywho.com/
- http://www.bigfoot.com/
- http://www.peoplefinders.com

a different database; therefore, the search results will vary. If the person the nurse is looking for is not located on the first search engine site, another site might list it. Note that most educational institutions and government sites maintain a directory of individuals that are employed at that institution. However, these types of directories are much less common at healthcare institutions and commercial sites.

Health Sites

Search engine sites may also be topic-specific. Several are specific to health. Like general search engine sites, topic-specific sites can include a directory and a search engine. Lists of health-specific search engines can be located at the following URLs:

http://www.martindalecenter.com/

http://www.medexplorer.com/

Key Words in Searching for Health Policy–Related Resources

Healthcare policy is an interdisciplinary field. It is of interest to healthcare providers, administrators and consumers, employers who provide healthcare benefits, companies that provide healthcare services and products, elected and appointed government officials, and academic and not-for-profit institutions that study or fund the study of healthcare policy issues. These interested parties can focus on a specific health problem or they can focus on the delivery of healthcare services. Depending on the specific issue, a wide range of terms can be used to search for health policy data on the Internet. Regardless of the issues, there are some general terms that tend to locate health policy data, such as "administration," "economics," "law," "management," "policy," and "statistics" preceded by the terms "health" or "medical." How these words are combined can have a major impact on the results that are returned.

When doing a search, the most common problem is to have too many hits, many of which are not of interest. APNs can use several approaches to narrow the search, thereby making the search results much more specific. In the majority of search engines, enclosing the terms in quotation marks (e.g., "health law" or "medical economics") identifies the term as a phrase and results in more specific results. If the keywords are not in quotation marks, documents that include both or even either of the terms may be listed in the results.

Using the Boolean operator AND between terms can also narrow the search. For example, using "health law" AND children AND smoking as the search phrase will return documents that include all three of the terms/phrases. A document containing the terms children and smoking but missing the phrase "health law" would not be in the search results. A plus sign (+) in front of a term has the same effect as using AND between terms. This approach would appear as follows: "health law" + children + smoking. Some search engines allow the user to select the option "all of the terms" when entering search terms. This also functions as an AND operator. However, the use of a term in a document does not always mean that the document contains information on that term. For example, a document that includes the following: "This article focuses on health law and smoking as it applies to adults. Health law and smoking related to children is not discussed" would be included in the search results. The more terms that are used with the AND operator and the more specific the terms are the more likely the search will return the specific documents that are of interest.

Sometimes, though, the search results are too few. In such cases, it is necessary to expand the search. Decreasing the number of terms and phrases between the AND operator and using less-specific terms can increase the number of hits. Using the Boolean operator OR can also expand the results. For example, the search for children OR kids OR pediatric will return documents that include any of these terms. In other words, if one document discusses pediatric patients and smoking and a second document discusses children and smoking, both documents are returned in a search when the operator OR is used. Search engines often include the option "any of the terms" when entering a search. This option has the same effect as using the OR operator between each of the terms in the search string.

Evaluating Internet Resources and Information

As noted in this chapter, the Internet can provide almost unlimited access to information. However, access to information does not guarantee the quality or credibility of the information. The Internet is open to all. Anyone with a limited knowledge of HTML can design and post a Web page on the Internet. Anyone with access to e-mail can send a message to an e-mail discussion list group or post to a newsgroup. On the Internet, the information of the highest quality is mixed with the worst of misinformation. It is the responsibility of the user to evaluate the information and separate quality information from misinformation. Advanced practice nurses know the existence of misinformation is not unique to the Internet. The evaluation of health-related information is not a new process for the APN who has years of education and experience in this process.

Much of the background APNs have in evaluating information has been gained by assessing printed materials from a variety of sources as well as verbal data from colleagues and clients. These experiences have provided the APN with a set of informal criteria that are quickly used when new information is presented to the APN. For example, the advantages of a new treatment protocol are viewed differently if presented on a nightly news show rather than presented at a professional conference. Health-related information is frequently presented in vanity publications and advertising materials. The APN can be more confident about the accuracy of information on a topic if it is presented in a professional journal article.

However, on the Internet many of the cues used by APNs to judge the validity of information are missing or altered. For example, a publication from a major research university could be considered a reliable source. However, a Web page located at the same university domain address could be a very unreliable source because the Web page might be the personal homepage of a student who has no supervision, knowledge, or experience related to the topic. Therefore, the APN needs to apply criteria that are sensitive to Web-based issues. Two types of criteria can be identified. These are criteria that are effective in evaluating information in general and criteria that are effective for evaluating information specific to health.

With the growing emphasis on health literacy, a great deal of work has been done in developing and applying criteria for evaluating health information on the Internet. However, much of this work is directed at consumers of healthcare services. As a result, these evaluation criteria are often not very effective for evaluating health policy information.

Links vs Content

The Internet is organized by interlinking data. Many of the URLs presented in this chapter are "lists of lists." This means that most of the sites identified provide a list of pointers to other sites. The other sites contain primary source data as well as links to other related Web pages. Some links to other Web pages even point back to the URL included in this chapter. The URLs selected for this chapter were chosen because they are considered quality sites. However, this does not ensure the quality of the information at any linked site.

A site can decide what links or pointers to include on its Web page. However, a site does not have control over the content of or the links included at the linked site. In other words, the APN may start at a reliable site and, by following links, end up at a data source that is unreliable.

Many reliable sites provide an alert to warn users when they are about to leave the original Web site and access a different Web site. It is convenient to use the links to move around the Internet; however, APNs should apply Internet evaluation criteria as explained in the next subsection when they reach a primary data source.

Internet Evaluation Criteria

Initial information about the site can be identified by the URL. URLs are segmented into sections that are separated by dots (.). APNs can begin to gather information about a site by deciphering the URL segments. The initial segment, for example, http://, https://, or ftp://, describes the protocol used to transmit requests for information to and from the Web page. To the right of the two forward slashes (//) indicates the specific location of the Web page, whether it is on the World Wide Web or the Internet, for example, "www." To the right of that segment is the institution's name, usually in abbreviated format, such as "sru," which stands for Slippery Rock University. To the right of the institution name is the domain extension, which is used to represent the type of organization, for example: .edu for education, .com for commercial, .gov for government, and .org for organization. Any information to the right of the domain extension describes the location and content of a particular Web page on that organization's Web site. For example, the Slippery Rock University homepage URL is http://www.sru.edu.

Remember that the existence of a Web page at a site does not ensure that there is any oversight process related to individual Web pages. For example, universities rarely supervise faculty or student homepages. What can be even more confusing is that sometimes a URL is sold to a new organization that has a completely different mission from what the URL seems to represent. For example, the URL for the Computer Based Record Institute before it merged with the Health Information Management System Society (HIMSS) was http://www.cpri.org. After the merger, the URL was dropped by HIMSS and for a period of time it was a pornographic site. It is now a commercial site, but determining the owner of a site can be a challenge.

Many times, as in the previous example, it is important to learn more about the specific organization sponsoring the Web page. On the homepage, look for a link that uses the term "about us" or a similar term. This link should provide information about the organization's mission, funding, structure, leadership, and history. If this information is not available, be very careful about trusting information from that site. Always remember that someone is paying for a Web site and it is important to know the source of data.

Author. If the material being reviewed is a document, the first step is to determine the reliability of the author. Is the author of the information named? If the author is named, can the academic credentials, professional reputation, and person's affiliation be established? This information may be included on the Web page. There may even be a link to the author's curriculum vitae. However, the fact that author data are included does not ensure that the author data are accurate or current. Many universities, foundations, organizations, and government agencies include directories on their sites. APNs can access these directories to validate the author data. They can also use the search engines for people data presented in this chapter. From these sources, the APN can obtain the phone number and e-mail and/or postal address of the author. If the author of the document is not available, the Internet site may provide clues about the accuracy and reliability of the information.

Timeliness. Even good information can become outdated misinformation. If you have located a site using a search engine, you may have noticed a date in the search engine results. The date indicates the last time there was a physical change made to the Web page. It does not indicate that the information on the page was updated. Many Web pages include the date of the last update as well as the author of that update. Sometimes dates are included in the content on the Web page that can provide a clue as to the currency of the information. If there is no update date and no dates referenced in the content, it is impossible to know how old the information may be.

Content. Important parts of health policy information are opinions and viewpoints. Review the content to determine if it is presenting facts or opinions. Evaluate if the information presented is well written and easy to understand. Determine if the depth and breadth of the content are appropriate. If the information is accurate, it should be consistent with other sources. The APN should be able to validate Internet information by using information from other sources. If the Internet information is timely content from a reliable source and consistent with information from other sources, it can be useful in the process of developing health policy.

Internet Evaluation Criteria Sites

The Internet provides an overwhelming amount of information mixed with misinformation. As the need has grown for the user to determine what is quality information and what is misinformation, Internet sites related to this issue have evolved. Box 8–4 includes selected sites that include criteria and tools for evaluating all types of information on the Internet. Box 8–5 includes Web sites for evaluating healthcare information on the Internet.

Box 8-4 Sites Containing Criteria and Resources for Evaluating Information on the Internet

- http://www.lib.berkeley.edu/TeachingLib/Guides/Evaluation.html
- http://www.lib.washington.edu/subject/History/RUSA/
- http://www.library.georgetown.edu/internet/eval.htm
- http://www.bettycjung.net/Goodinfo.htm
- http://www.library.jhu.edu/researchhelp/general/evaluating/index.html
- http://www.library.ubc.ca/home/evaluating/
- http://school.discovery.com/schrockguide/eval.html

Key Health Policy–Related Sites on the Internet

Two questions guide the organization of key health policy sites on the Internet. The first question deals with who develops and who uses the sites. The answer to this question includes those interested in healthcare policy such as healthcare providers, administrators and consumers, employers who provide healthcare benefits, companies that provide healthcare services and products, elected and appointed government officials, and academic and not-for-profit institutions that study or fund the study of healthcare policy issues.

The second question deals with what type of data and information are used in studying or developing health policy. These data and information can be grouped into four areas: (1) data related to the regulatory and legislative process; (2) viewpoints and policy positions from interested groups, including businesses, health-related organizations and universities; (3) statistical and research results used in developing health policy; and (4) funding or granting agencies, including founda-

---

Box 8-5 Evaluating Health Information and Information Resources on the Internet

- http://www.genome.gov/11008303
- http://www.nlm.nih.gov/medlineplus/webeval/webeval.html
- http://www.uic.edu/depts/lib/lhsu/resources/guides/web-evaluation.shtml
- http://www.bettycjung.net/Quality.htm
- http://www.cancer.gov/cancertopics/factsheet/Information/internet
- http://www.hon.ch/HONcode/Conduct.html

tions, insurance agencies, and government. In selecting sites for inclusion in this section of the chapter, the author used three guidelines.

First, Internet sites appear and disappear with great frequency. The sites noted in this chapter are reliable sources and can be expected to be maintained over a period of time. It is important that the APN realizes that at least one URL referred to in this chapter may be nonfunctional by the time the chapter is printed. This is why the first part of this chapter that deals with information literacy is important. Because the Internet constantly changes, the reader must be able to find new and evolving sites.

The second guideline is to select sites that include access to large databases or well-developed lists of links to key sites. This helps to preserve the credibility of the data and increases the probability that the nurse can access additional data from many points. The third guideline involves selecting sites of general value to health policy and not limiting them to a specific issue in the field of health policy. In this way, the APN can take the broadest approach to finding information and begin to narrow the list, rather than become stymied if a first, narrow search is nonproductive.

Four general sites (government related, academic, health policy organizations, and health law resources) contain URLs to sites that can provide the APN with a wide range of information. Each is described briefly and common URLs are provided.

Government-Related Sites

Government-related sites include sites from the executive, legislative, and judicial branches of the federal government, state government sources, local government sources, and international government sources.

http://www.usa.gov This site is the U.S. government official Web portal. It contains links to all levels of government from federal to local and links to all branches of the federal government. The purpose of the site is to make it easy for the public to access government information and services. A variety of information access approaches are used to facilitate access, including searching the site, A-to-Z agency index, government services by topic, and tabs for different audiences. In addition, the site is organized for logical access. For example, clicking Federal Government provides a link to the executive, judicial, and legislative branches of the federal government.

http://www.access.gpo.gov GPO Access is a service of the U.S. Government Printing Office that provides access to a wide range of important information products distributed by the federal government. The Web site provides a large number of these products through free electronic access. The information provided is the official, published version. The information retrieved from GPO Access can be used without restriction, unless specifically noted. Four key approaches are used to provide access to the information. First, there are three prominent tabs across the top of the page: (1) Legislative Resources (i.e., Congressional bills, United States Code), (2) Executive Resources (i.e., Code of Federal Regulations), and (3) Judicial Resources (i.e., Supreme Court Web site). Second, an A-to-Z index provides a comprehensive list of all federal resources available through the GPO. Third, a quick index search is offered, and fourth, a Web site search engine is available. This site also offers a link to the online Government Bookstore, which is the official bookstore for the U.S. government. In most cases, electronic documents become available on the day of publication, exactly as they appear in print. These electronic documents, like the print version, are the official published version.

http://www.ntis.gov The National Technical Information Service is a branch of the U.S. Department of Commerce. It is the official resource for government-sponsored U.S. and worldwide scientific, technical, engineering, and business-related information. Covering more than 350 subject areas from more than 200 federal agencies, the National Technical Information Service is the largest central resource for government-funded scientific, technical, engineering, and business-related information available today.

http://www.who.ch This site is the homepage for the World Health Organization. It provides electronic access to numerous reports on international health programs. Two links on this site are of special importance to health policy researchers: first, the research tools located at http://www.who.int/research/en/. The page includes links to the following tools:

- WHO Library Information System (WHOLIS) is the World Health Organization library database available on the Web. Included here are indexes of all WHO publications from 1948 onward.
- WHO Statistical Information System (WHOSIS) is a guide to epidemiologic and statistical information available from WHO.

The second link is located at http://www.who.int/topics/health_ policy/en/ and provides links to international health policy initiatives.

http://www.ncsl.org/ and **http://www.ncsl.org/programs/health/ forum/forum.htm** The National Conference of State Legislators was founded in 1975 as a resource for lawmakers and staffs of the nation's 50 states. The Forum for State Health Policy Leadership was established in 1995 under the direction of the National Conference of State Legislators. In an effort to help state legislators and their staff stay current on healthcare policy issues, the Web site includes links to workshops, issue briefs, and newsletters.

http://www.naccho.org/ The National Association of City and County Health Officials (NACCHO) is a nonprofit membership organization serving local public health agencies (including city, county, metro, district, and Tribal agencies). NACCHO provides education, information, research, and technical assistance to local health departments and facilitates partnerships among local, state, and federal agencies to promote and strengthen public health. This site includes current information on health policy issues as well as links and tools for understanding the process of influencing health policy.

Academic Sites

A number of universities and research institutions have established health policy–related sites. These sites include links to a number of other government- and non-government-related sites.

http://www.hpolicy.duke.edu/resources/ This site provides a portal to two extensive sets of health policy links. The goal of the first portal (CyberExchange) is to "foster evidence-based health policy decisions by allowing users to get the right information to the right place at the right time. We hope that the Gateway ultimately improves the quality of health policy decisions made at all levels of government and the private sector, non-profit and for-profit" (Duke University, Center for Health Policy, 2006). The second portal provides links to (1) federal government, (2) private, nonprofit, nonpartisan health policy and research organizations, (3) professional associations, and (4) college or university-affiliated centers.

http://law.slu.edu/healthlaw/research/links/topical.html The Center for Health Law Studies at the Saint Louis University School of Law maintains an extensive list of links to Internet resources in health policy. Included are links to specific topics, such as aging and elder law, foundations, health financing, and public health laws.

http://www.healthpolicy.ucla.edu/ The University of California, Los Angeles (UCLA) Center for Health Policy Research focuses on understanding and advancing public health policies that can improve access to health care as well as promote good health among diverse populations in California and the nation. As part of its public service mission, the center maintains online access to its research data and results. These are made available through reports and policy briefs as well as through fact sheets at no cost to the public. In addition, this site maintains links to several other health policy resources at http://www.healthpolicy.ucla.edu/links.html.

http://muskie.usm.maine.edu/research/research_institutes_ihp.jsp The Muskie School's Institute for Health Policy conducts research and policy analysis to identify and promote solutions to complex healthcare challenges. Major areas of focus include children's health, healthcare finance and access, mental health, rural health, chronic illness, healthcare quality, and public health. The site contains a reference list of published papers and a list describing several funded research studies.

http://www.nhpf.org/ The National Health Policy Forum (NHPF) is housed at Georgetown University. The site is designed to support informed decision making and informal off-the-record communication on issues surrounding healthcare policy. It serves mainly senior staff in Congress, the executive branch, and congressional support agencies. The site provides access to a wide range of issue briefs, which are short, analytical reports on a wide range of health policy issues, information on site visits around the United States, and an extensive list of links to other Internet resources.

Health Policy Foundations and Organizations

http://www.academyhealth.org/index.htm AcademyHealth was established in June 2000 following a merger between the Alpha Center and the Association for Health Services Research (AHSR). The members are health services researchers, policy analysts, and practitioners. The mission of the society is to be a leading, nonpartisan resource for the best in health research and policy. "AcademyHealth promotes interaction across the health research and policy arenas by bringing together a broad spectrum of players to share their perspectives, learn from each other, and strengthen their working relationships."

http://www.nightingalepolicygroup.org The Nightingale Policy Group was established in 2006. The mission of the organization is to showcase the expertise of experienced policy nurses and thereby to effect positive change. The key resources offered by this site are the names, bios, and contact information for the founding members, all of whom offer consultation services.

http://www.kaisernetwork.org/ The Kaiser Family Foundation established KaiserNetwork.org in 2000 as an online resource for health policy news, debates, and discussion. The site is free and takes a multimedia approach to providing online information. Examples of this approach include live and archived Web casts of health policy events, podcasts, a searchable database of public opinion questions, and daily e-mail updates.

Health Law Resources

http://www.law.cornell.edu/ The Legal Information Institute at Cornell University offers one of the most extensive collections of legal information on the Web and links to a wide array of U.S. and international legal reference Web sites. It includes Internet-accessible sources of constitutions, statutes, judicial opinions, and regulations. For example, this site's archive contains all opinions of the U.S. Supreme Court handed down since 1992 as well as 600 earlier opinions selected for their historical importance.

http://www.findlaw.com This site is a legal site and not limited to health-related information. It includes an extensive directory of links to legal information and sites as well as a law-focused search engine. The site does require registration, which is free.

Impact of the Internet on the Process of Developing Health Policy

The Internet is making a major impact on healthcare policy by changing the process of health policy development in three primary ways. These are (1) improved access to health data and information, (2) improved communication between all stakeholders, and (3) improved opportunities for all citizens to participate in health policy development.

The following initiatives demonstrate the federal and state governments' efforts to improve communication and policy development in all areas including health care.

http://www.regulations.gov/ At this site, citizens can review and submit comments on federal regulations that are open for public comment and published in the Federal Register. The site makes it easy to determine which regulations are open for comment. Comments may be linked to the regulation or submitted to the appropriate agency.

http://aspe.hhs.gov/sp/nhii/FAQ.html The National Health Information Infrastructure (NHII) can be understood as a national electronic healthcare system. NHII infrastructure enables enterprise-wide integration of information among all sectors of the healthcare industry. It consists of three overlapping focus areas:

- Personal health: Includes a personal health record that is created and controlled by the individual or family
- Healthcare delivery: Includes information such as provider notes, clinical orders, decision-support programs, digital prescribing programs, and practice guidelines

■ Public health: Enables sharing of information to improve the clinical management of populations of patients such as vital statistics, population health risks, and disease registries

A fairly new approach to discussing healthcare policy issues is the use of **blogs.** The term blog is derived from the merger of the terms *Web* and *log.* A blog is an online journal in the sense that a diary is a journal. Interested readers can add comments, responses, and opinions to the ongoing journal. The focus and the nature of the discussions on a blog are strongly influenced by the owner of the blog, which can be anyone from an individual to a professional society. It is still unclear how blogs will affect the development of healthcare policy, but given their potential the APN should be aware of blogs focused on healthcare policy.

http://www.thehealthcareblog.com/ This blog was established in 2003 by Matthew Hold, a consultant and speaker in healthcare delivery. Several current healthcare policy issues are discussed and the blog can be searched using the Google search engine. The commercial nature of the site is obvious on the front page where sponsored links are sold. The site also includes several positive quotes from the *Wall Street Journal*, Web MD, and others.

http://www.healthpolitics.org/ Health Policies with Dr. Mike Magee is sponsored by the Pfizer Medical Humanities Initiative. In addition to the blog, the site provides podcasts, links, weekly e-mail and news articles along with other information services.

http://healthaffairs.org/blog/about-the-blog/ The Health Affairs blog was established by the journal *Health Affairs*. The journal is nonprofit and has been publishing for more than 25 years. This site provides a very clear description of the organization's policies, its procedures, and its goal: to offer a wide variety of views by providing posts from invited authors and comments from the general public.

Conclusion

This chapter has introduced a number of key health policy–related sites on the Internet. The first section prepared the reader for searching and locating new and interesting health policy sites. Each of the sites selected for inclusion includes links to a number of other important health policy sites. Because the Internet is a network and not a hierarchical structure, the links will interweave and overlap. In other words, users can reach any of the health policy resources included here from several different starting points or through much juxtaposition. The Internet and the various links on the Internet are constantly changing. The existence, location, and content of sites change frequently. The information-literate APN can use these sites to:

■ Access enormous amounts of data and information
■ Evaluate the quality of the data and the usefulness of the information
■ Use those data to influence current public policymakers effectively and thereby improve the health care of individuals, families, and communities

Discussion Points and Activities

1. Using the search terms "health policy" AND research AND nursing, conduct a search using the Google search engine located at http://www.google.com. Repeat the search using the same terms at the Lycos site located at http://www.lycos.com/. Compare the results from these two searches. Which search engine found the largest number of sites? Which search engine found the most useful list of sites? How does each site differ in presentation of information about the sites found? Both of these sites will let you do a more focused search. Look at the homepage for both search engines to determine how to conduct a more focused search. Conduct the searches on both search engines and then compare your results.

2. Use the e-mail discussion list search engines to search for a discussion group that is of interest to you. Find the directions for signing up. After you have signed on, you will begin to receive e-mail messages that contain information that was posted to the group. Select a topic that is being discussed by other subscribers to the list and conduct a literature search on this topic. You may find MEDLINE, CINAHL, and Lexis-Nexis useful resources for doing your literature search. Do the data that you found in your literature search support or contradict the point made by the e-mail discussion list participants? Why do you think this would occur?

3. Use the Internet to identify your elected representatives to both houses of the U.S. Congress. Locate the e-mail addresses for these representatives. Send an e-mail message to each of the representatives asking his or her position on third-party payment for advanced practice nurses. Look at who responded to your e-mail. Compare the responses. Was it the representative or one of his or her staff? Was the response individualized to your question or was it an e-mail version of a form letter? Did the representative or the staff person express an interest in your opinions about this issue?

4. Each state decided on prescriptive authority for advanced practice nurses. How can you use the Internet to locate individuals and organizations that support enhancing prescriptive authority in your state?

5. Both the U.S. House of Representative and the Senate maintain a homepage on the Internet. Locate these homepages. Both houses use a committee and subcommittee structure for the purpose of considering legislation,

conducting hearings and investigations, or carrying out other assignments. In both houses, health policy issues are considered in a number of different committees and subcommittees. Use the located homepages to identify the names of all committees and subcommittees that would consider health policy issues. You will also find the names of all committee members. Use these sites to identify which current health policy issues are being considered in the various subcommittees and which representatives are important contacts. If you are accessing the Internet from a computer that has the capability, find the C-SPAN link and attend a hearing.

6. Select a health policy topic that is of interest to you. For example, you might select smoking or access to health care for children. Locate the homepage for the Library of Congress. You may find the name Thomas Jefferson of help in your search (http://thomas.loc.gov). The Library of Congress has several different databases that you may search. Determine if either the House of Representatives or the Senate is considering any current bills related to your topic. Search the catalogs of the library to determine if there are related references in the collection. What other resources at this site provide you with information about your topic?

7. The U.S. House of Representatives Internet Law Library contains the text of current public laws enacted by Congress. This Internet site is searchable. Locate this site. Be sure to read the introduction to this site so that you know what codes are not located there. Using your topic from question 6, identify what current laws already exist. From this site can you find any state laws that apply to your topic?

8. Most current Supreme Court opinions are on the Internet. One of the most complete collections is maintained by the Cornell Law School. Find this site and determine the Supreme Court opinions related to your topic.

9. Another key resource for understanding laws and regulations that relate to your topic are the Executive Orders from the executive branch of the federal government. These can be found in the White House Virtual Library. Locate this site and then search the site for any executive orders related to your topic.

10. This chapter contained several sites focused on health policy research. Locate these sites and determine if there are any current or published research studies related to your topic. Are there any researchers interested in your topic?

11. Use the http://www.usa.gov site to determine if there are other federal or state documents pertinent to your topic that were not located on the sites you have already reviewed.

12. Access the three blogs listed in this chapter (or other similar blogs) for comments and information concerning the uninsured population. Contrast and compare the approaches suggested in these three different blogs.

References

Association of College and Research Libraries. (2000). *Information literacy competency standards for higher education.* Chicago: American Library Association.

Duke University, Center for Health Policy. (2006). *CyberExchange.* Retrieved July 17, 2007, from: http://www.hpolicy.duke.edu/resources

Internet Systems Consortium. (2007). *ISC domain survey FAQ.* Retrieved July 17, 2007, from: http://www.isc.org/index.pl?/ops/ds/faq.php

Policy Nurses Advance Policy Agendas in Many Arenas

Nancy J. Sharp, MSN, RN, FAAN

Key Terms

➤ **Advocacy training** All nursing organizations, either singly or in coalition style, have promoted 1- to 5-day advocacy workshops to educate nurses on the skills needed to be an advocate for patient and nursing issues. The courses offer either continuing education credits or academic credit.

➤ **Nursing specialty organizations** Nurses who work in clinical specialties and advanced practice nurses have organized into national specialty and subspecialty associations in which members receive continuing education in the clinical specialty, obtain journals, research programs and other benefits, and may seek certification. The largest clinical specialty organization is the American Association of Critical Care Nurses with about 65,000 members.

➤ **Policy nurses** Nurses employed in positions where public policy is developed in the legislative or executive branches of local, state, or federal government; or those employed in private entities where agenda setting, design of programs, implementation strategies, and evaluation are developed.

Introduction

I stand often in the company of dreamers: they tickle your common sense and believe you can achieve things which are impossible.

—Maryanne Radmacher-Hershey, 1998

Nurses working in public policy cannot only see the future of an improved healthcare system for the coming generations, but are in the middle of designing it through their daily work. The policy nurses of today are visionaries who are passionate in their desire to make positive change in healthcare delivery. They work in executive branches of state, local, and federal governments (e.g., Office of Secretary in the U.S. Department of Health and Human Services); in regulatory offices of state and federal government (e.g., Food and Drug Administration, Centers for Disease Control); state and federal legislative offices (e.g., U.S. Senate, House of Representatives); and in advocacy organizations for certain patient populations (e.g., AARP, Children's Defense Fund), various health conditions (e.g., American Diabetes Association, American Cancer Society), or in health professional societies (e.g., American Nurses Association, American College of Nurse Practitioners, Oncology Nursing Society). This chapter describes some of the growth and maturity in the number of policy nurses, but the bottom line is that we need many more nurses to look at nursing in the policy world as a rewarding career path.

Policy Nurses in Nursing Associations

The large, organized nursing organizations (American Nurses Association, National League for Nursing, American Association of Colleges of Nursing, and the National Student Nurses Association) had Washington, DC–based government relations staffs as early as the 1950s. These staff made regular visits to Capitol Hill to lobby for federal grants and scholarships to fund nursing education and research. In addition, they worked with federal agency staff to work out implementation of various legislative policies that had been passed.

In the late 1970s, the clinical specialty nursing organizations recognized the need to add their voices to these advocacy efforts and become more involved in lobbying for federal funds for nursing research and education, as well as for their specific clinical nursing issues. Some of the early efforts were made by advanced practice nursing organizations such as the American College of Nurse Midwives and the American Association of Nurse Anesthetists. These groups were joined later by other clinical **nursing specialty organizations** with members who worked in emergency departments and operating rooms, as well as nurses working in oncology and nephrology units.

In those early days, not all of the government relations (GR) staff of the large nursing organizations were pleased to have the specialty organization representatives join in these efforts. Specifically, in 1982, a staff member of one of the large organizations told a specialty association GR staff member to "Get the hell out of legislation!" (personal communication, 1982). Stunned and saddened by this interaction, it took the staff member 24 hours to report this to the director because the staffer needed time to process the interaction. Having been hired as the specialty organization's GR staff, it was certainly a slap in the face to the specialty organization that had decided to add GR staff to the Washington organization. It had seemed very reasonable to expect that the larger nursing community would be pleased that another nursing association staff member was joining the overall lobbying force for nursing.

Nurse in Washington Roundtable

Simultaneously, in the late 1970s, the nurses who worked in Congressional offices on Capitol Hill and in scattered offices of the various federal agencies in the Washington, DC, area needed a vehicle to meet and network with each other. They were fairly isolated in various offices across the Washington, DC, area. It was at this time that Thelma Schorr, then-editor of the American Journal of Nursing, and Sheila Burke, RN, BSN, who worked as a health legislative assistant to Senator Robert Dole (R-KS), decided to found the Nurse in Washington Roundtable (NIWR) and hold dinner meetings with a speaker to network among this early group of **policy nurses**. The NIWR started with a small group of a dozen or so and eventually grew into a group of several hundred. This group continued to function up until the early 2000s, when it became too large and unwieldy as a networking vehicle with volunteer organizers. An interesting dilemma!

Nursing Specialties Advocacy

The nursing specialty groups became much more active in the 1980s when it became necessary to coalesce to lobby for continued federal funding for nursing education and research. Nursing appropriations are in a constant state of danger of being eliminated. Late in 1984, a small coalition named the Nurses Coalition for Legislative Action was formed in the Washington, DC, community. The coalition leadership consisted of GR staff and volunteer representatives of the National Association of Pediatric Nurse Practitioners (NAPNAP), American College of Nurse Midwives (ACNM), Association of Women's Health, Obstetric, and Neonatal Nurses (AWHONN), American Nephrology

Nurses Association (ANNA), and the National Association of Orthopedic Nurses (NAON). The coalition expanded and was open to include membership from as many of the nursing specialty organizations as possible.

The NCLA focused on general nursing issues such as nursing education and research funding. It quickly became enlightened on the politics of nursing research, as it promoted legislation to establish the National Institute of Nursing Research (NINR), within the National Institutes of Health (NIH). It was eye-opening to view the disagreements when some nurses supported this effort to become an institute while others vehemently opposed it.

To assist with operations and communications of the NCLA, the leadership solicited $100 donations from the specialty organizations. With those funds, and using regular mail and faxes (this was pre-e-mail), the NCLA sent notices and information packets to all specialty nursing organizations to ask that their members step up to the plate and participate in influencing policymakers at the national level. In this coalition, it was interesting to note that the five co-leaders each evolved into specific roles: one prepared overall strategy, one acted as policy analyst, one was the legal eagle, one was street-savvy and could interpret nuances seen and heard on Capitol Hill, and one was the schmoozer and communicator, welcoming participants with a smile and a hug when they came to meetings.

In an effort to further educate their individual members, several of the specialty nursing organizations had begun to hold 1- to 3-day advocacy workshops for their specialty groups in Washington, DC. In this **advocacy training**, the nurses learned how to advocate for their own specialty issues, such as seat belt laws, increased dialysis reimbursement legislation, maternal-child health programs, and others.

Nurses in Washington Internship

The NCLA leaders learned from the previous experience that the nursing community needed to educate and mentor a much larger cadre of nurses who would become nurse policy activists of the future. It was then that the leadership of NCLA formed a committee to prepare a proposal to present to the National Federation for Specialty Nursing Organizations (NFSNO). The proposal envisioned establishing an annual 5-day Washington, DC, experience for 50 to 100 members of the specialty organizations to attend. The proposal was titled "Nurses in Washington Internship (NIWI)" and described that the faculty of the 5-day program would include members of Congress and staff, regulatory bureaus federal agency staff, association lobbyists and GR staff, and other experts from the Washington policy world. The goal was to demystify the legislative process for specialty nurses.

The attendees of those NFSNO meetings were the leaders of then approximately 50 nursing specialty groups. Upon presentation of the proposal, the presidents and executive directors were a bit skeptical. The arguments against the proposal were that clinical nurses would either not want to come to Washington, DC, to learn about policy; could not afford to take 5 to 6 days off work to learn about the policy process; and could not afford the expense of a week in Washington, DC.

At the end of the day, however, the NFSNO agreed to treat this launch of NIWI as a pilot study and allowed that in the first year the NIWI should aim for 20 participants. The event was held in 1985 with 20 participants and received rave reviews from those 20 nurses. The committee recommended that the following year the number be increased to 50. Those 50 arrived the next year, and the committee recommended the limit be raised to 100, which it has been achieving ever since.

The Nursing Organizations Alliance (NOA) became the new name for the NFSNO in 2002, and the NOA now administers the NIWI as an educational policy experience. It is still going strong, although the time frame for the program has been reduced to three and one-half days. Approximately 2200 nurses have attended this policy workshop since 1985. Information is available at http://www.nursing-alliance.org.

Advanced Practice Nurse Organizations' Advocacy

As described earlier, the advanced practice nurse (APN) groups began their advocacy and policy agendas before the specialty nursing organizations with AANA and ACNM leading the way in the late 1970s. In 1985, a professional-facilitated forum was held in Chicago as an effort to unite the multiple national nurse practitioner (NP) organizations into one entity, or at least develop a mechanism that would make it easier to work together on policy issues.

An outcome of the Chicago Forum was the establishment of a group called the National Alliance of Nurse Practitioners (NANP). The leadership of several national NP groups met twice a year to come to consensus on issues of mutual concern. The group expanded to include representatives of state NP organizations, and New York and California were two very active members. One individual NP came to represent the interests of all NPs who were not members of any NP organization. The NANP put forth an enormous effort to produce some very sophisticated public relations brochures to elaborate on what an NP is and does, and these were distributed on Capitol Hill. This group, despite outstanding, exceptional individual NP leadership, got stuck in place because of its need for a full consensus agreement on policy issues. Without agreement, a public position could not be taken. The NANP continued to meet for awhile, mainly as a vehicle for networking among the remaining representatives.

For NPs, the next significant event occurred in 1993 at the first National Nurse Practitioner Summit in Washington, DC. At that meeting, a loosely organized group formed and named itself the National Nurse Practitioner Coalition (NNPC). This coalition formed upon hearing a loud, clear call from those present that it was time to form a collective of all NP groups. It was time to unite efforts, including time, energy, and money, to produce one shared message to give national policymakers, after listening and reflecting on every NP group's perspectives.

In 1994, the coalition changed its name to the American College of Nurse Practitioners (ACNP), and today remains a solid coalition-model organization focused on public policy. Membership includes state and national NP groups, as well as individual NPs who are focused on public policy. ACNP has utilized its volunteer members to advocate for policy issues affecting NPs, but also has contracted with Drinker Biddle Reath Carton, a Washington, DC, law firm with health specialists, to provide representation. ACNP has made a total commitment to its long-standing mission to ensure a solid policy and regulatory foundation that enables nurse practitioners to continue providing accessible, high-quality health care. The ACNP is clearly focused full time on policy issues that improve the practice environment and healthcare system and that would allow NPs to practice at their fullest potential, without restrictions.

The ACNP has added another continuing education policy offering to the health professional community titled "Public Policy Institute for Health Professionals (PPI-HP)." This week-long educational program in Washington, DC, invites all advanced practice nurses, all advanced specialty nurses in administrative or managerial positions, and all nursing school faculty interested in updating their knowledge of the policy world to attend this expansive educational experience to hear from policymakers about how they frame the issues and debates on the latest policy issues. Information is available at http://www .acnpweb.org under the Conference tab.

The Nurse's Directory of Capitol Connections

In 1991, an idea sprang from two personal lists the author was keeping in her phone book. From this idea, a directory titled The Nurses Directory of Capitol Connections (Sharp, 1991–2000) was published (in five editions). The directory was a listing of nearly 500 positions and opportunities for nurse participation in health policy development in Washington, DC. It included nurses in (1) the legislative or congressional branch of government, including the three nurses elected to the House of Representatives; (2) the executive branch, or regulatory branch with the federal agencies, and, finally; (3) nurses in government relations positions in the private sector world, whether in a healthcare association, consulting firm, public relations firm, law firm, or a non-profit group or foundation. The objective was to locate all the nurses in any of these positions so that they could be invited to networking events and meet others who were also using their nursing backgrounds in different sorts of health policy and advocacy roles.

By the year 2000, five editions of the directory had been published. When an agency or association or congressional office called looking for a nurse with a particular expertise, the directory was used to find such nurses. This directory was one component of the cosmic glue that connected these policy nurses together.

University Policy Courses

At the same time, there has been steady growth in the development of health policy or public policy courses and majors in universities. These courses can be a powerful motivator for students to start a career path toward work in the public policy sphere. However, more recently, a concern has surfaced that as the clinical and administrative faculty shortage grows, so does the faculty for teaching health policy in the nursing school curriculum.

As computer technology advances, there has been a further movement to put more and more courses online so that students can access the course and participate using their own computer remotely. Students and graduates can take a number of health policy courses, workshops, seminars for continuing education. Also, there are the concentrated 5-, 7-, and 10-day courses where graduate students can earn university credits. These students may be required to attend 35 to 40 hours of class, with reading assignments to be completed before the policy courses start, and preparation of a 10- to 15-page policy analysis at the conclusion of the course. George Mason University School of Nursing and Health Sciences began such a course in 1993. This is called the Washington Health Policy Institute (WHPI), and further information on this excellent course is found at http://www.gmu.edu.

Nightingale Policy Institute

In 2007, we both fear and embrace these changing times, but change always offers opportunities for visionaries. One phenomenon is the presence of the Internet and the fact that it is now mainstream. Nearly all nurse leaders either have their own personal computers in their own homes or have access to a computer and the Internet in a community-based setting. The Internet is no longer an odd phenomenon, and a group of nurses in Washington, DC, and beyond began to think about how we could use the Internet to expand nursing's reach into the policy world, as well as how we could use the Internet to continue to grow this cadre of policy nurses.

In 2006, a group of five nurses with a variety of solid policy experience gathered to collectively establish a new sense of direction and focus for the future in regard to nurses and public policy. Originally conceived as the Nightingale Policy Group, the name soon was changed to the Nightingale Policy Institute (NPI). One of the goals is to move what had been pen and paper formats in the past to an electronic format on the Internet, moving it into cyberspace. The NPI Web site (http://www.nightingalepolicygroup.org) can serve as a space where policy nurses can debate critical issues affecting the healthcare system and nurses in that system.

The previously mentioned Nurse's Directory of Capitol Connections had been a useful publication, but even with five editions it was time-consuming and difficult to keep updated as nurses move from position to position and others fill new positions. If the publication were digitized and posted on the Internet, the entire world of nurses, as well as other healthcare professionals, could access it to find a policy nurse with expertise in a certain area. Finding such a specific policy nurse could be important if you have been asked to name a nurse for an important commission or advisory council.

The intent is to develop a virtual organization for policy nurses that would not be chapter-bound, state border-bound, or bound by any of the other constraints that hold an organization down. This organization would be open to all nurses, either working in public policy or aspiring to learn more and wanting to acquire the skills needed to become policy nurses.

The Nightingale Policy Institute's Founding Five members envision that the membership of NPI will grow and establish itself as an unparalleled vehicle for national and international interaction among policy nurses. We will write policy and make policy; inform other policymakers of our work; educate new, aspiring policy nurses; and present policy solutions to the transition into a evolutionary new healthcare system led by nurse professionals at every level of government. We are involved in the reformation of the current healthcare system and are working to develop the system into a more caring, humanistic, safe, and vital environment.

The Founding Five of NPI and their contact information are as follows:

- Sharon A. Brigner, MS, RN, sbrigner@phrma.org
- Pat Ford-Roegner, MSW, RN, FAAN, pfordroegner@aannet.org
- Carole P. Jennings, PhD, RN, FAAN, jennjournal@aol.com
- Jeri Milstead, PhD, RN, FAAN, jmilstead@bex.net
- Nancy J. Sharp, MSN, RN, FAAN, NurseSharp@aol.com

Conclusion

The community of policy nurses will continue to grow. The nation needs more nurses with policy expertise and passion. We encourage all nurses who have an interest in policy work to contact any of the Founding Five, or to follow any of the links mentioned to obtain more information about a particular program.

Discussion Points and Activities

1. Convene a group of nurses to discuss how to motivate and inspire nurses toward involvement in the policy process.
2. Attend NIWI and write a brief article about your experience.
3. Discuss a local, state, or national health issue with nurse colleagues and propose a solution to the agency responsible for the issue.
4. Analyze the impact of nurse advocacy for a specific health issue.

Reference

Sharp, N. J. (1991–2000). *The nurses directory of capitol connections* (1st–5th eds.). Bethesda, MD: Sharp Legislative Resources.

Suggested Readings

Kalisch, B. J., & Kalisch, P. A. (1982). *Politics of nursing.* Philadelphia: Lippincott.

Longest, B. (2002). *Policymaking in the United States.* Chicago: Health Administration Press.

Mason, D. J., Leavitt, J., & Chaffee, M. (2007). *Policy and politics in nursing and health care* (5th ed.). St. Louis, MO: Saunders.

Redman, E. (1973). *The dance of legislation.* New York: Simon & Schuster.

Reese, S. (2006). Nurses as policy makers. *Nursing Spectrum.* Retrieved July 17, 2007, from: http://community.nursingspectrum.com/MagazineArticles/article.cfm?AID= 22637

Applied Healthcare Economics for the Noneconomics Major

Nancy Munn Short, DrPH, MBA, RN

Other people, including the politicians who make economic policy, know even less about economics than economists do.

—Herbert Stein, *Washington Bedtime Stories*

Key Terms

➤ **Adverse selection** A situation in which, as a result of private information, the insured are more likely to suffer a loss than the uninsured. A form of information asymmetry.

➤ **Externalities** The effects that the acts of consumers or producers have on each other; may be positive or negative.

➤ **Information asymmetry** Occurs when some parties to business transactions may have an information advantage over others.

➤ **Microeconomics** A branch of economics that studies how individuals, households, and firms make decisions to allocate limited resources.

➤ **Moral hazard** The change in peoples' behavior as a result of a perceived reduction in the costs of misfortune (health insurance changes the costs of becoming ill or injured).

> ➤ **Opportunity costs** The value of the next best choice that one gives up when making a decision. Also called *economic costs.*

> ➤ **Rationality** A choice taken from competing options yields anticipated net benefits that exceed the opportunity cost.

> ➤ **Utility** An economic term indicating a measure of happiness or satisfaction gained by consuming goods and services. Economists assume that all people seek to maximize utility.

Introduction

Economics is not widely considered to be one of the sexier sciences. The annual Nobel Prize winner in economics never receives as much publicity as his or her compatriots in peace, literature, health, or physics. Economics is an art that consists of ascertaining the immediate effects of any act or policy (personal, institutional, or political) while also looking at the long-term effects. The science of economics may indicate a direction to take to achieve the greatest **utility** from an act or decision, but the art of economics requires tracing the consequences (both intended and unintended) of that action not merely for one group but for all groups.

This is especially true for healthcare economics: If you were to line up 10 economists and ask them to recommend how to implement universal health care in the United States, you would likely have 10 different answers spanning from classical economic theories to Keynesian and beyond. This chapter introduces the reader to a broad understanding of applied economic principles that explain the complexities of the U.S. health system in a health policy context.

How Do Markets Work and What Is the Healthcare Market?

Market competition represents the core concept of what is known as **microeconomics**. In a free-market economy such as that in the United States, individual choices generally determine the course of our lives. Simultaneously, as voters and citizens, we make decisions that determine regulations and policies that govern our choices.

We base our choices on what economists refer to as utility. Theories of demand and supply are derived from this concept of utility. Consumer preferences are based on the perceived utility of a good or a service: As people's tastes change for some reason, they may want more of one good and less of another. Depending on the demand for a good or a service, supply theory tells us that firms will adjust production (and prices) to meet the demand unless some sort of constraint on production exists.

For example, a constraint on the "production" of registered nurses is the number of open slots for admission to nursing schools. To some extent, the federal government's policies for funding nursing education programs and student scholarships or loans affects the number of schools of nursing and available slots for admission. So, you can see that the government can create incentives or disincentives for increasing or decreasing the nursing workforce. One purpose of government is to properly align incentives and disincentives to meet goals for a healthy population. However, in the course of aligning these forces, unintended consequences may occur.

Nurse Shortages

Economic definitions of worker shortages are based on considerations of how characteristics of a given market for professionals differ from the ideal, highly competitive market. An economic definition of a labor shortage is the excess of the quantity demanded over the quantity supplied at market prices. Nursing shortages have been cyclical for more than 30 years—have wages risen to an "equilibrium" where supply of nurses equals demand?

In reality, we depend on reported percentages of unfilled, budgeted nursing positions to describe excess or shortage. In healthcare markets, large employers such as hospitals may want to recruit more nurses but not incur additional costs to "lure" additional nurses. Recruiting new nurses at a higher wage results (theoretically) in adjusting all nurses' wages upward. If the cost of adding one more nurse (her wage plus adjusted wages) exceeds the revenue that adding the nurse will provide, the hospital will not hire another nurse.

This scenario gets even trickier in the case of nurse staffing because hospital revenues are not often attributed to nurses and nursing care: (1) most hospitals account for nursing care as a cost center and roll the labor costs into room rates, and (2) hospital administrators are often schooled without a basic understanding of nursing's contributions to patient outcomes.

There is a seemingly endless supply of capable nurses in the global market. For example, the Philippines have developed their nurse education system to be an export market for registered nurses. Nurses from many impoverished nations are eager to better their lives as well as the lives of their families and are willing to move to accomplish this. When considering the healthcare workforce market, the global market for nurses is a hot-button political and moral issue. However, the economics of this market are based on rational behavior.

Economic Rationality

People generally demand those things that put them at the highest level of welfare, given the resources available. This is true to some extent in the healthcare markets. Individual choices exhibit **rationality** in the sense that the individual gains something of importance (to him/her) by a specific choice. Individuals may find maximum utility in choices that appear irrational to healthcare providers: The choice to smoke is the best example. Suppose a person smokes but knows that smoking is harmful and dangerous to his or her health. The pleasure or relief of smoking has higher utility than quitting. But what if the smoker does not have complete information about the dangers of smoking? Exhibit 10–1 describes a game of rational choice when incomplete information is known.

Information Economics

Asymmetrical information is the term used by economists to point out that healthcare consumption differs from purchasing other goods and services because of the inability of patients, providers, or payers to possess all of the information needed for completely rational decision making. Optimal rational decision making requires "perfect information" where consumers are just as knowledgeable as sellers.

Think about when you buy a car. You gather all of the information that you can to eliminate any advantage the car seller may have in terms of the worth of this particular car. Being newly informed, you may choose to go to several dealerships before you find a seller that meets your expectations (or utility). Now think about your typical healthcare experience. You go to your primary care provider for your annual physical and the physician finds an abnormality and refers you to a specialist. Depending on your level of information, you will blindly trust the specialist or you may "shop around." You may be very hard-pressed to learn about the quality or performance of either your primary care provider or the specialist. If you are referred to a hospital, you are probably unable to learn the nurse-to-patient ratio even though evidence shows that this is critical to your well-being. There is **information asymmetry**.

Healthcare professionals generally know what is "best" for patients, right? The problem of asymmetric information differs from a simple information problem in that one party possesses knowledge needed to enable rational decision making that the other party lacks. In health care, the patient delegates much decision making to the healthcare professional (and sometimes even to the insurer). However, the healthcare professional and the insurer have a potential conflict of interest because of the

Exhibit 10–1 The Prisoner's Dilemma

The Prisoner's Dilemma

A classic economic "game" that explores rational choice is known as the Prisoner's Dilemma. In the game, two suspects, A and B, are arrested by the police. The police have insufficient evidence for a conviction, and, having separated both prisoners, visit each of them to offer the same deal: If one testifies for the prosecution against the other and the other remains silent, the betrayer goes free and the silent accomplice receives the full 10-year sentence. If both stay silent, both prisoners are sentenced to only 6 months in jail for a minor charge. If each betrays the other, each receives a 2-year sentence. Each prisoner must make the choice of whether to betray the other or to remain silent. However, neither prisoner knows for sure what choice the other prisoner will make. So, this dilemma poses the question: How should the prisoners act? The dilemma can be summarized using a two-by-two table:

	Prisoner B Stays Silent	Prisoner B Betrays
Prisoner A Stays Silent	Both serve 6 months	Prisoner A serves 10 years Prisoner B goes free
Prisoner A Betrays	Prisoner A goes free Prisoner B serves 10 years	Both serve 2 years

The dilemma arises when one assumes that both prisoners only care about minimizing their own jail terms. Each prisoner has two options: to cooperate with his accomplice and stay quiet, or to defect from their implied pact and betray his accomplice in return for a lighter sentence. The outcome of each choice depends on the choice of the accomplice, but each prisoner must choose without knowing what his accomplice has chosen to do.

Such a distribution of losses and gains seems natural for many situations because the cooperator whose action is not returned will lose resources to the defector, without either of them being able to collect the additional gain coming from the "synergy" of their cooperation. For simplicity, we might consider the Prisoner's Dilemma as zero-sum insofar as there is no mutual cooperation: Each gets 0 when both defect.

The problem with the Prisoner's Dilemma is that if both decision makers were purely rational, they would never cooperate. Rational decision making means that you make the decision that is best for you whatever the other actor chooses. Suppose the other one would defect; then, it is rational to defect yourself: You won't gain anything, but if you do not defect you will be stuck with a loss. Suppose the other one would cooperate; then, you will gain anyway, but you will gain more if you do not cooperate, so here too the rational choice is to defect. The problem is that if both actors are rational, both will decide to defect, and none of them will gain anything.

A common view is that the puzzle illustrates a conflict between individual and group rationality. A group whose members pursue rational self-interest may all end up worse off than a group whose members act contrary to rational self-interest. More generally, if the payoffs are not assumed to represent self-interest, a group whose members rationally pursue any goals may all meet less success than if they had not rationally pursued their goals individually. You can see that the Prisoner's Dilemma can relate to individual versus group healthcare decisions, especially in light of scarce resources.

exchange of money. Benefiting monetarily from a decision may affect the decision-making process.

Asymmetric information also affects healthcare professionals when patients conceal lifestyle information or state that they are compliant with a treatment when they are not. A patient's caregiver may also withhold or distort information that would be helpful to the provider. Insurers also face information asymmetry: Clients (buyers of insurance like you and me) know much more about the state of their health and their future plans than an insurer knows.

Adverse Selection and Moral Hazard

Economists use two terms to describe the situation insurers face when consumers have greater information: (1) **adverse selection** occurs when a person selects a health plan based solely on the likelihood that they will have higher than usual health expenses (e.g., planning to get pregnant), and (2) **moral hazard** occurs when a health plan member uses more health services than that person ordinarily would because he or she is insured (e.g., a person with orthodontic coverage gets braces on his teeth for cosmetic purposes only).

Insurers may also lack sufficient information regarding the choices and decisions of providers and may be unable to ascertain if a procedure is medically necessary or not. "The patient, who does not pay the bill, demands as much care as possible; . . . the insurance company maximizes profits by paying for as little as possible; and . . . it is very costly for either the patient or the insurance company to prove the 'right' course of treatment. In short, information makes health care different from the rest of the economy" (Wheelan, 2002, p. 86).

Economics is amoral—that is, it is neither a moral science nor an immoral science. The science of health economics can suggest what makes a person, a population, a region, or a nation better off, but philosophy and ethics must be debated elsewhere and are represented by political tradeoffs when policy is made. Similarly, the health market as viewed by economists is amoral: When confronted with finite resources, there will be losers and winners. This is a tough concept for nurses to swallow.

Externalities

Economists analyze the consequences of economic decisions and economic policies by identifying positive and negative externalities. An **externality** is the gap between the private cost and the social cost of a behavior. Almost every activity generates an externality at some level. A tongue-in-cheek example of externalities is my husband's decision to buy and drive an SUV: The private costs of his decision are different from the social costs. My husband's private costs of driving the SUV are extra gas costs, higher car payments, more expensive tires, higher emissions, and social disdain from an environmentally conscious wife. The public costs may include aggravating asthmatic children, melting the polar ice caps, and perhaps driving up insurance rates for tiny sport cars in his path. These potential social costs are not paid by my husband. Governments often deal with externalities by taxing or regulating the behavior. Examples include emissions standards testing, cigarette taxes, and motorcycle helmet laws.

Opportunity Costs

There is no such thing as a free lunch: For every opportunity taken and for every option discarded there are tradeoff costs. When you purchased the Saturn, you did not purchase the Honda wagon. You also did not take a vacation, buy a new wardrobe, or pay off your college debt. Not acquiring the Honda, the vacation, the new wardrobe or eliminating your debt are the **opportunity costs** of purchasing the Saturn.

Opportunity costs may also be described in terms of time spent on an activity (researching the safety of the Saturn) and other indirect measures or intangibles. An example of opportunity costs related to health policy is the current Medicare policy: 90% of Medicare funds are used for 10% of the beneficiaries. Most Medicare dollars are expended in the final events of a person's life. Because there are finite funds available, deciding to pay for an elderly person's last weeks of life represent an opportunity cost. For example, the funds could also be used for preventive care of 30-somethings, more school nurses, or health research. These are hard choices and are the core of perennial political debates at the federal, state, and local levels.

The economic consequences of a policy may last for years and may be argued equally eloquently by economists who fall on both sides of an issue. Because poverty (socioeconomic status) is the main determinant of poor health, shouldn't the government raise the minimum wage to fix this? This is an important example because it gets at the heart of a larger issue: Is the role that government plays in the United States economy too big, too small, or just right? If you lined up 10 economists, you would get 10 different answers. Economists disagree and present competing research findings over the consequences (intended and unintended) of raising the minimum wage. So, if you are a policymaker wanting to improve the health of Americans, what do you do?

What Makes the U.S. Healthcare System and Economy Strong?

The basis of a strong economy is good government. Good government makes markets possible by setting rules, regulating commerce and quality of essential products, protecting property rights, providing secure transportation and distribution systems, punishing those whose behavior endangers free trade (such as fraud or embezzling), keeping the peace, providing a strong banking system (the Federal Reserve banks), maintaining policies that strengthen the currency, educating the workforce, and maintaining basic sanitation for health. Much of the blame for poverty in the world can be placed on bad government. The primary reason for American ascendancy in pharmaceutical research and development is the protection of property rights—patents protect the investments of individuals and firms who develop new drugs.

Government can also wreak havoc on markets through overregulation or counterproductive policies. Economics may assist us in finding the right balance between growing the economy and providing for social programs.

Nurses must have a basic understanding of economics, especially the economics of provider practice. If advanced practice registered nurses want a bigger piece of the primary care pie, if schools of nursing want government support to fund building new facilities, they must know and provide the economic outcomes of these proposals. Conservative governments and groups advocate strongly that markets should be allowed to adjust themselves to reach equilibrium: market theory holding that wages will rise or fall to nudge the supply of nurses toward equilibrium with demand. However, from the overview you have just read, you know that information asymmetry, externalities, government regulation, and other forces contribute to, or interfere with, healthcare markets. To promote "good" health policy, nurses need to participate in discussion, debate, and hold their own in terms of general health economics.

Web Sites of Interest

A Student's Guide to *Freakonomics: A Rogue Economist Explores the Hidden Side of Everything* at http://www.freakonomics.com/pdf/StudentFREAKONOMICS.pdf

America's Health Insurance Plans at http://www.ahip.org

Economic history at http://www.frbsf.org/publications/education/unfrmd.great/greattimes.html

Elias, R. (2006). Financing long term care at http://www.kaiseredu.org/tutorials/longtermcare/longtermcare.html

Gladwell, M. (2005). The myth of moral hazard. *The New Yorker* at http://www.newyorker.com/printables/fact/050829fa_fact

Health Economics Information Resources: A Self-Study Course at http://www.nlm
.nih.gov/nichsr/edu/healthecon/

Westmoreland, T. (2006, February). Health Policy and the Federal Budget Process at
http://www.kaiseredu.org/tutorials/federalbudget/HPandFederalBudget.html

National Library of Medicine at http://www.nlm.nih.gov/nichsr/corelib/hecon.html

Alliance for Health Care Reform. Covering Health Issues 2006 at http://www
.allhealth.org/sourcebook2006/toc.asp

The Need for a National Focus on Health Care Productivity at http://content.health
affairs.org/cgi/reprint/9/1/107.pdf

Discussion Points and Activities

1. Discuss the role of economists in healthcare policy. Using Gail Wilensky, PhD, as a model of a health economist, watch clips of her presentations at http://www.gailwilensky.com/. Note that although she is not a clinician, she is a commissioner on the World Health Organization (WHO) Commission on the Social Determinants of Health. Why are economists so influential in health policy?

2. Read several issues of the journal *Health Affairs*. Access the blog at http://www.healthaffairs.org/blog/ and search keyword "economics" for the latest articles about healthcare economics. Discuss the gross national product in terms of healthcare expenditures.

3. Walter Williams is a Libertarian economist on the faculty at George Mason University. Discover his point of view on public health issues such as the ban on trans fats. How does his economic view reveal a Libertarian ideology?

4. What is a think tank and how do these organizations affect health policy and nurses? Explore the Council on Economics and Health Care Policy membership. Identify at least four think tanks and research (a) their political philosophy; (b) whom they influence; and (c) how they obtain information about nursing.

5. Read about the Medicare Part D "donut hole" and consider if this policy is based on sound economic theory.

6. Discuss the role of research in nursing. What has been the focus over the past decade? To what extent has nursing research had an influence on healthcare economics?

7. Read about the birth of health services research. Are nurses performing health services research? Provide examples.

8. Identify policies advocated by the American Nurses Association that reflect an influence on healthcare economic policies of the federal government.

9. Identify policies advocated by your state nurses association or specialty organization that have influenced healthcare economic policies in your state.

10. Construct a list of ways nurses can become more knowledgeable about health economics and influence policy.

11. Read about social capital. A good Web site is http://www.socialcapital gateway. org/.

12. Read about cost shifting in health care. Identify policies that use this method. Argue the benefits and losses of cost shifting.
13. Examine two economic indicators that you have never understood before. Look for these indicators in newspaper articles and analyze how they apply to health care.
14. Watch videos by experts on healthcare systems at http://www.kaiseredu .org/picks/documentary_search.aspx. Most of these videos include economic or cost information. Discuss with your colleagues the impact on health care.
15. What are the economics of decriminalizing marijuana for use as a medicine? Trace the history of this debate in terms of economics. Argue the benefits and harm in economic terms.
16. Who finances long-term care in the United States? Take a poll of your colleagues prior to researching this question. Are nurses well informed about this economic issue and does this meet your expectation?

Case Study: The Economics of End-Stage Renal Disease

(This case is provided in conjunction with Dr. John D. Sullivan.[1])

End-stage renal disease (ESRD) is defined as permanent kidney failure and is generally covered by Medicare for the usual beneficiaries and for individuals younger than 65. Students are often baffled that other serious, chronic illnesses such as cancer are not covered by Medicare (for people less than 65 years old) while ESRD is. The 1972 policy decision to cover ESRD was spurred by both politics and economic forecasts, including the belief that transplant was soon to become routine and would replace dialysis. In 1972, federal costs for ESRD beneficiaries were expected to be manageable because transplant technology would ensure that patients would receive transplants; however, in 2006 there were 65,000 covered individuals waiting for a kidney transplant and the expectation was not met.

---

[1]Dr. Sullivan is presently an associate professor at Boston University teaching mergers and acquisitions, and healthcare strategy. Prior to Boston University, Dr. Sullivan worked for Fresenius Medical Care and W. R. Grace providing the analysis for and constructing the acquisitions and joint ventures of almost $4 billion in healthcare companies throughout the United States, Latin America, and Asia. While at Fresenius Medical Care, Dr. Sullivan laid plans for a new transplant business and participated in the divestiture of two non-core lines of business. An active consultant, Dr. Sullivan has assisted in the valuation of several healthcare businesses and served as an expert witness in several lawsuits concerning business valuation. Dr. Sullivan holds a BA from Regis University in Denver, Colorado, an MBA from Northeastern University, an AM from Harvard University, and a PhD from Northeastern University.

Two basic forces govern the economics of ESRD treatment: (1) patient and provider choice of treatment option; and (2) government reimbursement policies. With reimbursement assured, in the 1970s the dialysis industry's challenge was to meet the demand and provide access to services. In the 1980s, the industry focused on cost containment and improving quality of care. In the 1990s, there was a movement toward consolidation of so-called Mom and Pop treatment centers to mega providers with large chains of treatment centers (see Figure 10–1). For example, with at least 27% of the market, in 2007 Fresenius National Medical Care (FNMS) is North America's largest provider of dialysis treatments. It provides these services to 85,500 patients with ESRD in North America (and a total of 124,400 worldwide). In North America alone, FNMS provides care at 1,130 dialysis centers where in 2004 it provided 12,908,788 dialysis treatments. In this role, it has been in an enviable position to negotiate with payers and vendors. Although the majority of its revenue comes from Medicare and Medicaid, which offer just so much leeway in negotiating payments for ESRD treatments, FNMS also has third-party payers. Its size also gives it some market clout in negotiating with vendors such as Amgen the sole provider of erythropoietin, which is essential to ESRD patients.

In the 2000s, reimbursement is the challenge: The Medicare Modernization Act of 2003 provided the first change in reimbursement for dialysis since 1973. The dialysis industry is considered to have a strong U.S. market growth potential of 5–6% annually.

Figure 10-1

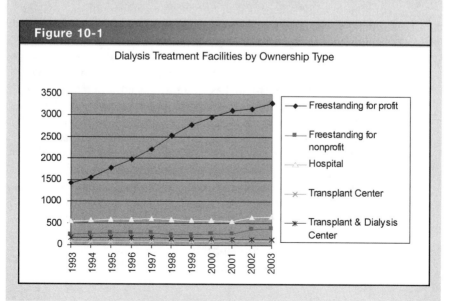

Dialysis Treatment Facilities by Ownership Type

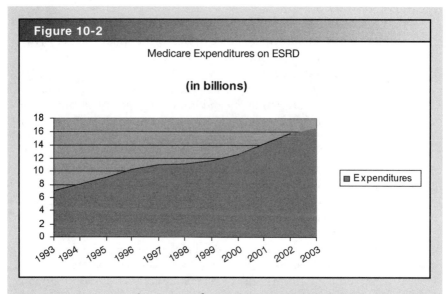

Figure 10-2

Medicare Expenditures on ESRD

(in billions)

Despite the Centers for Medicare and Medicaid Services (CMS) close monitoring of ESRD expenditures, costs for the program increased to more than $18 billion in 2005, consuming a higher and higher percentage of the budget ($500 billion total budget for federal Medicare and Medicaid expenditures) while covering fewer and fewer of the Medicare beneficiary population (see Figure 10–2). Expenditures will continue to rise as a result of the new technology and drugs, aging population, increasing survival on dialysis, the growth of minority populations, increasing incidence of obesity and diabetes as well as hypertension. To control costs, the federal government has historically eroded the payment structure through inflation and continuously revising and delaying the ESRD coverage for patients not previously of Medicare age. This strategy, known as *cost shifting*, will continue to reduce government expenditures on a per-treatment basis so long as commercial carriers continue to bear the financial burden not covered by the federal government.

Treatment options for ESRD include hemodialysis, peritoneal dialysis, and kidney transplant. To provide treatments in outpatient clinics requires a high initial capital investment and a high capacity and volume of patients to break even or be profitable (and remain open). Treatment of ESRD with peritoneal dialysis requires low investment but also has high variable costs. The government reimbursement rate for dialysis has remained unchanged since 1973, which has resulted in cost shifting.

Prior to the Medicare Modernization Act of 2003, reimbursement provided bundled rates for treatments (example of a bundle: dialysis, EPO, Vitamin D, disease management). CMS's goal is to drive toward breakeven where reimbursement rates equal the cost of providing the services. Earnings before interest, taxes, depreciation, and amortization (EBITDA) is a standard financial indicator of a firm's success. Currently, the range of EBITDA facility breakeven is from $199.45 per treatment, assuming three patient shifts per week and no patients holding commercial insurance, to $138.99 based on 15% of the patients holding commercial insurance. Publicly held companies (i.e., has stockholders) usually seek an EBITDA of approximately 15%. If CMS accomplishes its policy goal of reaching breakeven, there may be unintended consequences such as loss of investment in the industry, facility closings (especially for smaller competitors in the industry), and decreased quality. If this is the result, we could be back to the challenge of the 1970s: providing access to treatment.

Reference

Wheelan, C. (2002). *Naked economics: Undressing the dismal science.* New York: W. W. Norton.

Suggested Readings

Blank, R. M. (2000). Fighting poverty: Lessons from recent U.S. history, *Journal of Economic Perspectives, 14,* 2.

Cogan, J., Hubbard, G., & Kessler, D. (2005). *Healthy, wealthy, and wise.* Washington, DC: American Enterprise Institute Press.

Gwartney, J., Stroup, R., & Lee, D. (2005). *Common sense economics: What everyone should know about wealth and prosperity.* New York: St. Martin's Press.

Hazlitt, H. (1979). *Economics in one lesson: The shortest and surest way to understand basic economics.* New York: Three Rivers Press.

Landsburg, S. (1995). *Armchair economist: Economics and everyday experience.* New York: Free Press.

Leavitt, S., & Dubner, S. (2005). *Freakonomics: A rogue economist explores the hidden side of everything.* New York: William Morrow & Sons.

Poundstone, W. (1992). *Prisoner's dilemma.* New York: Doubleday.

Rice, T. (2003). *The economics of health reconsidered* (2nd ed.). Chicago: Health Administration Press.

Sowell, T. (2003). *Applied economics: Thinking beyond stage one.* New York: Basic Books.

Tu, H. T., & May, J. H. (2007). Self-pay markets in health care: Nirvana or caveat emptor. *Health Affairs Web Exclusive.* Retrieved July 17, 2007, from: http://content.healthaffairs.org/cgi/reprint/hlthaff.26.2.w208v1?ijkey=s0E2UwIIzuJa2&keytype=ref&siteid=healthaff

Global Connections

Jeri A. Milstead, PhD, RN, FAAN

Key Terms

> ➤ **Grassroots response** Spontaneous reply to a social problem, often in contrast to a planned answer prepared by a formal organization.

> ➤ **Problem fading** A tendency for interest in a current problem to diminish. Declining attention can occur as a result of inaction, replacement by a more important issue, or lack of mobilization of resources.

> ➤ **Softening up** A political process in which ideas are discussed in an attempt to gain acceptance. Alternative solutions are considered in a variety of situations, opposition is identified, and counterarguments are developed.

> ➤ **Storefront program** A social program situated in a building.

> ➤ **Street program** A social program that is operated, literally, on the street. For example, workers in a needle-exchange program conduct the trading on the sidewalk rather than in a building.

Introduction

McLuhan and Fiore (1968) described the world as a global village in which each person is affected by and affects all inhabitants. Although the majority of this book assumes a federal or state focus, this chapter considers the global reality of health care today. A brief presentation of health issues that have emerged around the world may stimulate the reader to consider how policy (or lack of policy) in one country is linked to policy in other countries. This chapter also explains the comparative approach to research and presents a model for the study of nursing and health policy at an international level. A case study of a comparative analysis of two needle-exchange programs in the United States and one in the Netherlands offers an example of how the model can be used.

Global Issues

Although few doubt that official health policy affects the provision of care in a country, has anyone considered how the health status of individuals or populations affects policymaking in a country? Certainly, the presence of conditions and illnesses such as HIV/AIDS, infectious diseases (e.g., tuberculosis, malaria, influenza), environmental health concerns, and abuse (e.g., addictions and violence) direct how a nation allocates resources for attending to those health problems. In contrast, consider how a government's philosophy of social justice, ethics, personal responsibility, and political will can influence the management of epidemics, disasters, and healthcare delivery. Although the U.S. policy is to fund research on treatment options for those with HIV/AIDS, our government is unable to convince some African governments to even acknowledge how HIV is contracted and spread.

A policy that sends mixed messages to our own citizens and to those of other countries is the funding of millions of dollars for education to prevent sexually transmitted disease (STDs). The U.S. policy releases funds only if the focus is on sexual abstinence, a policy that some perceive as promulgating conservative and religious bias, not education.

An advanced practice nurse (APN) must think about the relationship between what she or he sees in the clinic, school, or other practice sites and the incidence, prevalence, and treatment options available in other parts of the world. With the movement of people across continents and oceans quickly and often, APNs must be alert to the possibility of vectors that transmit pathogens to humans and the possibility of contagion. Seasoned travelers know the dangers of being in a foreign environment. Even traveling from one developed country to another can wreak havoc on one's digestive system as food that is different or prepared differently with spices or condiments not usually found at home can affect the traveler's immediate health. When a traveler journeys to a country that is more or less developed than the home country, the likelihood of illness is even greater.

One cannot write about global health issues without acknowledging the nurse shortage and the nurse faculty shortage. The Expert Panel on Global Nursing and Health of the American Academy of Nursing presented a white paper at the 6th International Conference on Priorities in Health Care in Toronto, Ontario, Canada, in 2006. "The mission [of the Academy] is to serve the public and nursing profession by advancing health policy and practice through generation, synthesis, and dissemination of nursing knowledge" (American Academy of Nursing, 2007). Members of the global panel addressed the nurse shortage in the international arena through factors that included stressful work environment, aging nurse population, decreasing school enrollments, increased career opportunities for women, inadequate salaries, and an increased demand for nursing services, especially in leadership and advanced practice (American Nurses Association, 2006, p. 1).

To what extent have nurses been involved in influencing governmental policies that affect health, the delivery of care, and nursing practice? Nurses in Thailand who focus on elderly clients worked with policymakers to create mechanisms that are leading to recommendations for reform of the health insurance system for the elderly and the delivery of care (Sritanyarat, Aroonsang, Charoenchai, Limumnoilap, & Patanasri, 2004). Collaboration among nurses and other stakeholders in 14 countries in east, central, and southern Africa (ECSA) resulted in the creation of ECSACON, a professional advisory group that has adopted primary care as the official governmental approach to health care in those countries. ECSA is an example of nurses, as the largest group of professional healthcare providers, banding together to assess the status of health and health care, identify major problems, prioritize the high burden of disease in the region, and begin to change the system of healthcare delivery. The goal of the group was to assure quality care (Ndlovu, Phiri, Munjanja, Kibuka, & Fitzpatrick, 2003). Similarly, nurses in Western Australia worked with the Chief Nursing Officer to produce legislation that permits nurse practitioners to practice in that part of the country (Adams & Della, 2005).

Not all nurses have been successful in their efforts. Ferreira (2004) writes that despite making great strides forward in getting technology incorporated into health care and attempts to improve access to care, Brazilian nurses were not able to bring together enough political and ideological power to accomplish a municipalization project in the district. A similar finding occurred in Botswana. Phaladze (2003) reports a study that described a lack of nurses in that country who participated in the process of developing healthcare public policy or resource allocation. The researcher notes that the "minimal participation . . .

resulted in implementation problems, thus compromising a service provision" (p. 22).

However, it is the responsibility of nurses to seek leadership positions in government and quasi-government institutions. Beverly Malone, PhD, RN, FAAN, is former American Nurses Association (ANA) president, deputy assistant secretary for U.S. Department of Health and Human Services, immediate past executive secretary of the Royal College of Nursing of England, Scotland, and Northern Ireland, and most recent chief executive officer for the National League for Nursing. She notes that most countries do not have nurse contacts in government (personal communication, April 10, 2007). This situation means that health-related grants, information, and policy ideas that are considered in various offices are never seen by a nurse. Dr. Malone agrees that nurses are always available to provide care, but are not at the policy table. She suggests that nurses in countries such as the United States who are in government positions must advocate at the World Health Assembly for access to care issues. Malone also urges nurses to exert leadership to assume positions that are recognized by governments and to pressure officials (minister-to-minister) to appoint nurses to important government stations so that nurses can become policymakers.

To emphasize the importance of developing expertise in public policy, the American Association of Colleges of Nursing designed a Doctor of Nursing Practice (DNP) degree that not only prepares practitioners at the highest level of direct care competence, but also offers a focus on executive administration and on public policy (American Association of Colleges of Nursing, 2006). Harrington, Crider, Benner, and Malone (2005) assert that nurses must have a very sophisticated comprehension of the policy process. These leaders urge that formal education is necessary to supplement any tangential experience nurses may have had. To this end, the authors describe a new program at the master's and doctoral levels that offers specialization in health policy for advanced practice nurses at the University of California San Francisco School of Nursing. Policy courses will provide content on the process of policy development and the political processes needed to work in a public governmental system. Nurses throughout the world need to know how to maneuver through whatever political system is operating in their countries. Academic programs with the policy option of the DNP may attract nurses who come to the United States from other countries to obtain doctorates in nursing. Most countries outside the United States have set the standard for professional nursing at the baccalaureate level but have not yet developed doctoral programs. Nurses with master's degrees frequently come to the United States to earn their doctorates. For example, the late King Hussein of Jordan, a land-locked, oil-poor country in the Middle East, determined that his country would be known for its exceptional educational system. The current King

Abdullah II continues his father's legacy and has directed the construction of universities throughout the country. The Ministry of Education supports master's-prepared academics in all fields to obtain doctorates in other countries. As these well-prepared educators return to Jordan, they will accomplish the goals of their country of conflict resolution, economic development, and education.

Policymakers are redefining time and space as the process of economic development—especially the logistics of moving goods and services—is computerized through global positioning programs on satellites that circle the earth. Intermodal transportation is redefining the way in which people and cargo are delivered. Supply chain managers and logistics professionals constantly seek methods to increase the efficient flow and cost effectiveness of intermodal and other cargo types moving in international commerce. New routes are being developed to avoid overburdened hubs such as Chicago. For example, Toledo, Ohio, where 40% of the U.S. population and 40% of Canadian population can be reached within a 6-hour transportation day and where all transportation modes converge, has few rivals and is viewed with considerable interest as an ideal center for distribution. Loads can be dispatched from any continent to this Lake Erie port and sent by ship, air, rail, or road to their destinations quickly and efficiently (J. Hartung, personal communication, April 4, 2007). Cruise ships are increasing their business in the Great Lakes as they discover new markets for people with leisure time. States are pondering a different system of government regulation of seaports, airports, roadways, and rail vis-à-vis economic development and regional responsibility. Nurses who serve on Port Authority boards can offer a perspective of organizational change and critical thinking through the lens of a healthcare expert.

Many nursing and health policy issues are international issues. For example, bioterrorism, communicable disease and immunization, family planning, and acquired immune deficiency syndrome (AIDS) are health concerns that all countries must address. Nurses work with vulnerable populations of all types—abused, poor, and disenfranchised. Nurses are conducting research in international settings and developing models for cultural competence (Campinha-Bacote, 2002; Villarruel, Gallegos, Cherry, & Refugio de Duran, 2003; Ross, 2002). One group of researchers has translated and validated a French version of a tool to permit cross-cultural research in perinatal health (Goulet, Polomeno, Laizner, Marcil, & Lang, 2003). International health issues have economic, political, and sociocultural dimensions. The allocation of resources is at least a political decision. Today, advanced practice nurses (APNs) must have a deep knowledge of health, illness, and wellness plus an understanding of the broader social and political context in which these conditions exist. Issues of social justice, the relief of health disparities, and support for those with stigmatized disease or disability are integral to APNs' practices. Research is needed to help nurses and policymakers understand the extent of health problems, cultural and other variables that affect treatment, and political systems and players. There have been no comprehensive models for studying nursing and health policy from an international perspective. One approach to the study of systems from different countries is known as comparative analysis.

Case Study: Implementation of Three Needle-Exchange Programs

Comparing issues and problems between and among countries can be an antidote to ethnocentrism, especially if the researcher is someone who is an outsider or who does not live in the situation. Commonly accepted values in one country are not necessarily universal, even though the country may be quite large or the values deeply ingrained. Comparative analysis searches for differences and diversity in addition to commonalities. Experimentation that is possible in a controlled laboratory is not possible in a human environment. "The comparative method was perceived by John Stuart Mill, Auguste Comte, and Emile Durkheim as the best substitute for the experimental method in the social sciences" (Dogan & Pelassy, 1984, p. 13).

The Milstead Model was developed to guide researchers in analysis of complex health issues in an international framework (Milstead, 1993). Essential components of the model include selecting the international setting, identifying the problem or policy, analyzing the sociocultural system, specifying the economic and political systems, and evaluating the specific health system. The Milstead Model provides a comprehensive approach to the study of nursing and health policy issues across countries and cultures and integrates the policy components of political science with the roles of the nurse in advanced practice.

International Setting

The choice of country for one's personal research can be guided by previous travel, a possible health crisis occurring in that country, a particular population, or something unique to the country that is worth studying. The researcher should ascertain for purposes of context if the country is a developed democracy, second world or communist (or former communist) country, or third world or developing country. The investigator should describe the general governmental structure of the country. The choice of the national, provincial, regional, state, or local level may involve defining each of those terms to understand the scope of the study.

The Policy Process

A policy or program must be selected for study. Policy can be thought of as both directives and processes. There are four major components to the policy process: agenda setting, government response, program/policy implementation, and program/policy evaluation. Even though the components of the policy process do not follow a linear sequence and many times blend with each other, APNs can choose a component for the purpose of analysis.

Sociocultural Systems

The researcher should examine elements of the social and cultural systems to place the policy or program in a realistic context (Pye & Verba, 1965). Policies that are studied without regard to the human systems in which they function have little relevance. One must start by identifying the values of those who affect and are affected by the policy. The researcher can identify music, dance, clothing, art, language, food, and work. It is important to discern the general attitudes of the population. Are the people healthy? How do they demonstrate feelings? Are they clean (according to what standards)? Is there a clear system of patriarchy or matriarchy? Does family hold special meaning? Is the family a nuclear unit or an extended family? What is the degree of spirituality of the population? What is the underlying philosophy about health, and how is it manifested in public policy? How do people access the system? How does one's level of health relate to other segments of life, such as work and relationships with others? Assuming the researcher is studying health policy, how is the policy or program influenced by other governmental policies such as education and transportation?

A competent scholar will identify ethnic groups and minorities within the general population. What is the history of the majority and minority groups? What strategies does the scholar use to account for cultural bias on the part of the target population and the scholar? What is the relevant history of the area? What is the geography of the immediate area? In what way have the history and geography contributed to the problem that is being studied?

Economic Political Systems

The researcher who is studying an issue regarding health care or nursing must place the issue in a framework that includes economic and political factors. Is there economic stability? Is an economic crisis occurring that has major impact on the issue? The researcher uses economic indicators to place the policy in a relevant economic perspective. The nurse also must describe the political ideologies and their influence on the policy or program under study. Legal structures, interest groups, the role of the media, and the relationship between public and private enterprise are areas of investigation for the researcher.

The Health System

The nurse researcher should describe the healthcare system being studied. Is there a national healthcare delivery system? Is there national health insurance? Is there access to health care for all residents or citizens? What are the similarities between or among the systems being studied? If the healthcare systems are significantly diverse, what indicators will be used for comparison?

Often a researchable problem surfaces as an "irritation" or concern that has been encountered by the researcher. For example, in the United States, tobacco use is becoming regulated through government bans on smoking in public buildings or whole cities. Violence in schools, homes, and on the street is becoming commonplace in many countries and can be studied as a health problem. Getting a problem to government is one thing; avoiding **problem fading** is another. On the global scene, nurses will have to be especially vigilant and well organized to maintain the attention of government officials.

A focus on cure, disease prevention, or a holistic approach to health may be evident. Analysis of healthcare workers is a fertile field for the nurse policy analyst. Who provides health care can be an indicator of sociocultural, economic, and political interweavings. Nurses, physicians, feldshers, *curanderas*, Chinese barefoot doctors, and folk healers all reflect the philosophy and values as translated into public policies related to health care. The education of healthcare providers is broad and inconsistent among and within countries.

Programs may be centered on formal structures such as community health, home health, hospice, long-term care, hospital acute care, maternity centers, information centers, and nurse- or physician-managed health clinics. Programs also may be situated in informal or spontaneous circumstances. The researcher must be attentive to the names that programs are given in different countries. Community-based programs are not necessarily the same as community programs. Clinics in other countries may provide services and carry connotations different from those in the United States. The scholar should describe the extent to which technology is used in the unit of investigation. A discussion of the adequacy of infrastructure and technical support, training, and maintenance can shed light on some health problems.

Case Study: Implementation of Three Needle-Exchange Programs through Application of the Milstead Model

Implementation of three needle-exchange programs will be examined vis-à-vis the Milstead Model in an effort to demonstrate the utility of the model for the nurse researcher. The model is not complete, but models are representations of reality that evolve as situations change. This study was conducted to discover how needle-exchange programs (NEPs) were implemented. NEPs are defined as organizational arrangements in which sterile (also known as clean) medical supply hypodermic needles and syringes are exchanged for those that have been used at least once and, thus, are considered contaminated or "dirty."

Research Questions

A major health problem at the beginning of the 21st century is human immunodeficiency virus (HIV) and AIDS. In the early 1990s, drug users who shared needles and syringes (hereafter referred to as needles) to inject drugs intravenously had the highest proportion of HIV/AIDS of any group (Grund, Kaplan, & Adriaans, 1991; Inciardi, 1990; New York State AIDS, 1988).

Needle-exchange programs are one response to reduce the spread of HIV/AIDS. Early research found that NEPs do no harm, reduce the spread of HIV, and are cost effective (Ginzburg, 1989;

Joseph & Des Jarlais, 1989; Needle swap program, 1991; Tacoma supports, 1989). In the mid-1990s, NEPs were illegal in the United States, although they were an accepted, legal component of drug programs in other countries (e.g., the Netherlands). Because NEPs were not considered legal programs in the United States, how did they develop? What was the motivation to disobey the law and to create controversial programs? Two sites in Tacoma, Washington, two sites in New York City (in the Bronx and Harlem), and several sites in Rotterdam, the Netherlands, were selected for investigation.

The research questions addressed included the following: What are the barriers and facilitators to implementing needle-exchange programs, and what program design is most effective? A qualitative cross-cultural approach was used to study the three NEPs. The researcher interviewed 41 policymakers and service providers using elite interview techniques (Dexter, 1970) and limited participant observation at NEP sites. Informants were protected through standard procedures for the protection of human subjects. The researcher did not speak Dutch, but most Dutch people speak English well and there was an interpreter available at each site.

International Setting and Level of Analysis

The United States and the Netherlands are developed democracies, although with different political structures. Three cities were selected, each a large, urban center. The study was comparative in that NEPs in the three cities were examined in relation to each other. Policy decisions in one country may affect or be affected by decisions in another. Lessons learned in one country might be applicable to another (Rose, 1991). The possibility of examining a health program in another country could explicate similar or different cultural and political values and highlight tools that may be transferable.

The Netherlands is a constitutional monarchy with a bicameral parliamentary system (Upper and Lower Chambers). The U.S. system is a democratic republic. The focus of this study was at the local level in three cities. However, state levels of government became involved. The three programs are described briefly.

Rotterdam

The Netherlands has a national health insurance plan that is funded by the central government and administered through private and government programs (Brasker, 1989; Buning & Verheijen, 1990;

Fact sheet, 1989).The Dutch NEP was supported legally from its beginning in 1986 as a response to a hepatitis-B epidemic. The Rotterdam NEPs exist in a variety of settings such as **street programs**, **storefront programs**, and community organizations. Contrary to popular belief, drug use is not legal in Holland.

Tacoma

The Tacoma, Washington, NEP was selected for the sample for several reasons. First, it is one of the first programs in the United States and was started in 1988 (King, 1988). In 1990, the program came under the direction of the joint city-county health department, which agreed to provide funding even though the legality of the program was questionable (Tacoma supports, 1989). In February 1991, the program was "approved" for operation through a court ruling (Shatzkin, 1990a), although the paraphernalia law remained unchanged. The process of creating a covert program and moving it to legal status was important to investigate.

Second, the program was developed by one person with his own money and objectives. This singular grassroots effort at policymaking prompted investigation.

Third, this program is primarily a street program; that is, service workers park a van at a regular site on a city street, and clients exchange needles at the van. However, a "delivery service" also was available, in which requests for clean needles were made to the cellular phone in the van and needles delivered to an arranged site (Maples, 1991). A small exchange also was available at the health department pharmacy. The structure, variety, and innovation were important to investigate to determine what kinds of structures are effective.

Fourth, the target group is varied. Tacoma-Pierce County was composed of African Americans, Asians, Hispanics, indigenous people (mostly Native American and some Aleuts from nearby Alaska), and Caucasians. Members of all groups participated in the program.

New York City

The New York City program was included in the sample because of the scope of the drug problem in the city. According to interview data and media reports, drug availability and use was pervasive in New York City (Gonzalez, 1992). In many families, all family members used drugs. In many neighborhoods, an individual was considered "abnormal" or "deviant" if he or she did not "do drugs" ("The world," 1992). To use IV drugs has status, not stigma, in this subculture.

Originally begun by AIDS activists as an underground transaction in 1988, the needle-exchange program became quasi-legal as a pilot program under the aegis of the New York State Health Department from November 1988 through February 1990. After this program closed, a clandestine program was operated by Rod Sorge and six to eight other activists until June 1, 1992, when a waiver was granted by the state commissioner of health for official approval of a second attempt at an authorized program. This study addressed the program as it evolved prior to that waiver.

The Policy Process

The component of the policy process on which this study focused was implementation. Because the NEPs in the United States were outside the aegis of government, actually in opposition to current laws, these programs were examined from the perspective of those who actually initiated and implemented the programs.

Doomed New York City Pilot Program

The New York program began as a **grassroots response** of the gay community to a growing belief that the government was not responding to this emergency as it has to other public health emergencies.

Although the state, not the city, would fund the program, political support for the program from both state and city officials was crucial. The governor and state assembly Republican minority, the New York City chief of police and his staff, all five New York City district attorneys, the Manhattan borough president, and the former special narcotics prosecutor were vigorous opponents of the program (Elovich & Sorge, 1991; New York State Assembly's, 1988; New York State Health Commissioner, 1988; Private Drug Abuse Agency, 1988). They feared an increase in drug traffic, drug use, crime, and violence. National political figures became extremely vocal. The U.S. Surgeon General and the Secretary of Health and Human Services supported the concept (Dr. Louis Sullivan, 1989; Evans, 1988). The head of the Bush administration's antidrug program adamantly opposed federal plans to support needle exchange ("Aides to William Bennett," 1989), as did U.S. Congressman Charles Rangel from Harlem.

A legal loophole was found in the law that criminalizes needle sale or possession. The law allowed the state health commissioner to exempt organizations or individuals (Elovich & Sorge,

1991) and the commissioner issued a limited waiver to allow the pilot program. The original program sample of 6,000 was whittled to 400 and a budget of $240,000 was appropriated. The press reported that the program would be based in a neighborhood, but because several neighborhoods complained loudly to city hall that they did not want it there, a health department was selected as the site. However, the New York City mayor surprised public health officials and declared that there would be no exchange within 1000 feet of a school, so the department could not be used as a site. An abandoned former X-ray clinic in downtown Manhattan was selected. This site was distant from where most drug addicts lived and most intravenous drug users (IDUs) did not have money for transportation.

The building was next door to "the tombs," the municipal building that housed the city jail and the courtroom in which drug addicts were tried. Clients would be asked to come to an area in which police and prosecuting attorneys would be present in large numbers. Because the state code of laws made it illegal to possess or sell drugs or drug equipment, it was probable that clients would be in possession of illegal substances or supplies, which would put them at great risk for arrest. A plan to provide identification cards marking clients as participants in the pilot study did little to encourage attendance.

Policies limited eligibility to those on (long) wait lists for drug treatment programs. Treatment programs mailed invitations to IDUs, many of whom were homeless and had no address. Outreach programs conducted by other service and research groups such as Association for Drug Abuse, Prevention, and Treatment (ADAPT) became the primary source of clients. This meant that an IDU had to be signed up in a local neighborhood on a waiting list for treatment and driven by a volunteer to the program site in Manhattan where the IDU had to fill out many forms regarding informed consent and treatment options. After lengthy processing, the exchange was limited to only one needle and syringe per client per trip.

The pilot program was doomed to failure because of a mismatch between bureaucrats' and program administrators' definitions of benefits and needs. In distinct contrast to Tacoma and Rotterdam, opposition was intense, polarized, and vocal. In the political stream, there was much confusion among politicians, bureaucrats, and the public about AIDS and how HIV was spread. The program was started the day after George H. W. Bush was elected president in the hope that the story would get lost amid the big political news. The program ran for 14 months, and less than 300 people participated. The program was a grassroots effort, developed by AIDS activists who put their grave concern about the epidemic into action, selected two sites in drug-active neighborhoods, and showed up every Saturday morning, snow or shine, to distribute needles, brochures about AIDS, condoms, and material to clean IV "works": clean water, bleach, and cotton balls. Workers met in a narrow cellar lit with a single bare bulb on Friday nights to fill two-ounce containers with bleach or water, place cotton balls in bags, and fill grocery sacks with their materials, which they took to the sites by car or on the subway.

Tacoma

The Tacoma NEP had the quiet knowledge of many city officials. The originator, Dave Purchase, a former drug counselor who had strong ties with many service workers and agency heads, had become convinced that AIDS was going to be a huge health crisis. He read articles about HIV and IDUs and a brief report about the Dutch needle-exchange program and decided that, regardless of the lack of compelling outcomes at the time, the program made intuitive sense as a means to reduce the transmission of HIV. Purchase started with his own money. Kingdon (1995) speaks of needing visibility to propel a concern to problem status. Purchase determined that he would allow himself to become the visible catalyst to get attention for his cause.

Implementation Tools and Games

Bardach (1977) wrote of games played by public officials and interest groups during implementation. Purchase was described by himself and many others as a ham, a glib SOB, spacey, a lone bandit who is offensive and crude and gets away with it, and a true hero who believes needle exchange is saving lives. In a twist to the "Reputation" game (in which players seek to enhance their chances of reelection, promotion, or deference), Purchase used his adeptness with colorful phrases to get his ideas into the media. Rather than promoting his own reputation for personal good, he risked his reputation to bring the issue of needle exchange to the political agenda. He acknowledged a shrewd political sense that he used to get things done.

Policy tools are mechanisms that are used to plan the structure and functions of a policy or program (Schneider & Ingram, 1990). Tools are classified as (1) authority that carry the force of government (e.g., incentives such as tax breaks, subsidies, grants and loans, fines, and sanctions; (2) capacity (information and training); (3) symbolic (link policy preferences to personal values); (4) learning (used in uncertain situations); and (5) innovative (e.g., use of language).

To educate the Tacoma board of health members, Purchase used street language, such as *cookers* and *works*, to defuse discomfort upon hearing them. Metaphors were used to combat metaphors. Activists developed sound bites that often became a 10-second clip on the evening news. Sunglasses, foot powder, and soap were distributed at the exchange site. New York City informants discussed personal incentives for implementing programs. Some found work in which they excel. They developed skills in management, assertiveness and other communication techniques, media relations, and business. They learned how to maneuver through the legislative and court systems and the bureaucracy.

Education is a tool that was used by the policy entrepreneur in Tacoma. Purchase taught himself and a small cadre of colleagues about HIV/AIDS and NEPs, and these people became a core committed to teaching the board of directors of the health department. Formal study sessions were held prior to board meetings in which workers discussed myths and their own fears about the disease in an open forum. Another education tool included public hearings and speeches to service organizations and initiation of North American Syringe Exchange Conferences. Kingdon (1995) describes a "primeval policy soup" (p. 122) as a process in which problems and solutions connect and disconnect as they are discussed among bureaucrats, elected officials, and interest groups. Policy windows are opportunities for action in which problems and solutions join. Rather than wait for a window of opportunity, Sorge and his colleagues forced open a window of opportunity in New York City. The window already was open in Rotterdam because the NEP was being implemented, although for a different problem. There was no **softening-up** period in Rotterdam; top administrators believed the program would work, so they implemented it without fanfare.

Sociocultural Systems Values

A strong value was expressed by all informants: the moral certainty in the rightness of what they were doing. All informants (except one in Tacoma) felt an ethical and moral responsibility to oppose the law and to implement NEPs for the greater good of reducing the spread of HIV.

There are no laws in the Netherlands that criminalize possession or sale of drug paraphernalia and small amounts of marijuana
for personal use are tolerated by the police and courts. Risk was a
value that was expressed often by U.S. informants as a willingness
to take significant personal chances. An NEP was considered outside the letter of the law. Courage, in the form of support for the
program, was a value expressed by nearly all respondents. In
Tacoma, informants stated that there is danger in opportunity and
that the program was a make-or-break issue.

A concept of imagery emerged and American opponents to
NEPs feared a pied-piper effect where neighborhoods would be
overrun with sellers and users. In contrast, prevention teams were
established in Rotterdam that patrolled their own neighborhoods
for discarded dirty needles. Neighborhoods became environmentally cleaner and safer.

Drug Treatment Philosophy

The value of acceptance of personal differences and personal responsibility for one's own behavior was evident in relation to two
opposing philosophies about drug treatment. Dutch informants
expressed amazement over American "rigidity" and "puritanical"
approach to drugs. They either smiled or shook their heads when
discussing the U.S. "war on drugs" policy. Several Dutch informants commented that the "war" seemed directed at the "victims"
(users) rather than the drugs (dealers and importers). The Dutch
espouse the philosophy of harm reduction that was formalized as
a policy within the Dutch drug and alcohol rehabilitation community of policy specialists. The concept of personal responsibility was supported by both major Dutch political parties and served
as the cornerstone of health services. This idea accepts that people
may choose behaviors that others perceive as dangerous or dam-
aging to one's health. The Dutch believe the role of the provider of
health services is to support the personal choices of the individual
and to help the person live in such as way as to reduce the harm
that may be a consequence of the behavior. For example, even
though drugs can be harmful, proponents of this philosophy believe that a person cannot be forced to give up drugs and will not
be successful in treatment if the person does not have a commitment to the program. Harm reduction directs that injectors should
be taught safe injection techniques, how to recognize and obtain
treatment for abscesses, and how to clean IV works and not share

them. An extension of this philosophy is seen in the free provision of condoms and literature on how to clean IV works, the dangers of sharing works with others, and how to avoid transmitting HIV.

In contrast, the official American policy for drug treatment is abstinence as espoused by Narcotics Anonymous and similar programs. Most American respondents agree with harm reduction, although many believe that abstinence should be tried first. In New York City, if a person is in a methadone treatment program and a random drug test shows positive for any drug (not just heroin), the person is terminated from the program. The concept of harm reduction, in which drug use is tolerated, is not accepted by the political community.

Economic-Political Systems

The Netherlands operates as a free market economic system in the European Union. The unit of currency is the euro. Thirty-three percent of European Union goods that are transported by sea are loaded or unloaded in Dutch ports, mainly in Rotterdam (Buning & Verheijen, 1990), which is the largest port in the world. After having been bombed nearly to extinction during World War II, major portions of Rotterdam were rebuilt.

Data indicate that concern over budgets does not lessen during the implementation phase and may intensify after programs get started because money must be appropriated for program continuation or expansion. The Rotterdam program was added to existing comprehensive drug rehabilitation programs in which support was offered and treatment was not required. Program officials reported that funding was a continuous problem. The overwhelming failure of the New York City pilot program did little to encourage funding for current needle exchanges. In contrast, much money and effort were expended to oppose these programs.

One of the most significant political events came in the form of a court decision relevant to the NEP in New York City. Nearly all respondents spoke of the 1991 arrests of eight people for possessing needles at the exchange program; some informants had been defendants. All of those arrested were acquitted of criminal charges. Manhattan Criminal Court Judge Laura Drager considered testimony from many individuals and organizations. Activists solicited testimony from local drug users whose personal stories were compelling in their intensity and their pleas for help to seek treatment and prevent HIV transmission. Manhattan Borough President Ruth

Messinger confessed to being against the program originally but admitted she had changed her opinion after having gone personally to an exchange site. Researchers in the field of drugs and HIV/AIDS marshaled their political forces and educated the court on the incidence, prevalence, and transmission of the virus.

In a landmark decision on June 25, 1991, Manhattan Criminal Court Judge Drager ruled that the defendants' possession of needles was a "medical necessity" that was intended to prevent a greater societal harm, AIDS (Judge acquits, 1991; Manhattan Criminal Court, 1991). She held that the AIDS epidemic is a "grave medical emergency" that justifies illegal conduct. She distinguished between death by dirty needles versus drug addiction by clean needles and determined that in this age of the AIDS crisis "the defendants' actions sought to avoid the greater harm" (*Decision and order*, 1991). The finding of the court did not provide legal action to allow exchange programs. However, after much political activism, a waiver was granted by the state health commissioner for the two programs in the Bronx and Harlem, effective June 1, 1992.

The history of most respondents in Tacoma included social and political action. Several talked about having marched together in civil rights actions in the South in the 1960s and having worked together for local political issues. The inbred quality of the policy community in Tacoma was reflected in the language that used the same phrases and terms, such as *bridge to treatment* and *drug user* rather than *addicts*. Another noted that "people know each other, they get their arms around each other" and talk together. Kingdon (1995) notes that familiarity can spawn stability and a common outlook, but even he did not describe as tight a network as observed in Tacoma.

The mood in Tacoma did not involve antagonism about political issues but about a legal one. Concern continued that the needle exchange was patently illegal. Respondents spoke of considering ways to get the issue before the court without making it a criminal case as in New York City. Purchase and his friends reasoned that they might have a clearer decision if the case were heard in civil court. After much thought, they convinced the health department to ask the state's attorney general for an opinion on the legality of NEPs. The response was that the programs were illegal, based on the drug paraphernalia law. The city of Tacoma then agreed to withhold its part of the funding designated for the needle exchange from a joint city-county budget until the legality of the program was established. This allowed the health department to sue to recover the funds. By organizing the political forces in this way, the case would be heard in a civil, not a criminal, court where criminality would not be at issue. Many respondents commented on the courage of the director of the health department in permitting this idea to go forward. The judge ruled that although it is illegal to distribute needles and syringes without a prescription, health department workers were exempt because, as municipal officers, they were carrying out their legal duty to prevent the spread of disease (Shatzkin, 1990b). The exemption allowed the local health officer broad powers to take extraordinary measures to stop an epidemic. Most respondents confided that the term *officer* had been thought of in the past as the police. It was a matter of reframing the definition to accommodate the health officer.

Health Systems

Dutch health care essentially is publicly funded and privately administered. With few exceptions, everyone who lives in the Netherlands is covered by health insurance (Brasker, 1989). Those who earn more than a base salary must purchase their own insurance from a plethora of private insurance companies. All employees contribute a percentage of their salaries toward the national health insurance plan. A basic package of health care consists of a choice of family physician, certain specialists, dental care, medicines, and hospital nursing care plus long-term care and unemployment benefits to those who cannot work as a result of sickness, disability, or accident (Buning & Verheijen, 1990). Health care consists of curative care (a two-tier system of family physician and hospital specialist) and preventive care. Hospitals mostly are proprietary organizations that are administered with public funds in a competitive market atmosphere. Regional planning by means of boards and councils regulates the types of services offered.

Drug assistance occurs in four cities: Amsterdam, Rotterdam, The Hague, and Utrecht (Odyssee Information, 1992). The cities are making their own policies and planning their own programs independently. Committees, with representation from their prescribed geographic areas, develop local policy, plan specific programs, and draft budgets that are approved by the central government.

Many of Rotterdam's residents are immigrants, predominantly from Surinam, Turkey, Morocco, and the Antilles. Many of them are Moslem, a religion that has a strong taboo against injecting foreign substances into the body, including drugs and tattoos. Because of cultural practice, those immigrants with drug problems tend to smoke rather than inject. However, interviewees stated that migrants from northern France and Belgium have easy access to pills in their countries and bring them to Holland to sell so that they can buy heroin to take back to their countries for resale or use.

In Rotterdam, unlike Tacoma or New York City, the site of the drug problem is not on the street as much as in houses. Groups may "shoot up" together as a type of ritual behavior. This is done in "shooting galleries" (rooms or buildings appropriated for this activity) or at home. Because of this, street models for needle exchange are not popular. Most programs are within community health organizations.

Conclusion

This chapter introduces several global health issues. The importance of the role of the APN in the formation of public policy, especially health policy, cannot be emphasized enough. Linking nursing expertise in health care and in policy design, implementation, and evaluation will affect the health of individuals and populations around the earth. There is a powerful need for nurses to become involved with policymakers and stakeholders to eradicate pestilence and disease and to improve the quality of life of the earth's inhabitants.

This chapter presents a model for analyzing nursing and health policy. The model is comprehensive and can serve as a framework for conceptualizing and implementing the process of inquiry into policy issues between and among countries. Advanced practice nurses are encouraged to cultivate an expansive intellect and consider all local health and nursing interests in the context of a global perspective. APNs should use the model, evaluate the components, and validate the model's utility or improve it.

There is a dearth of policy research on nursing at the global level, and little comparative research has been done by nurses. The policy field is appropriate for APNs who have integrated the multiple roles of the professional nurse into their practices. Nurses have an obligation to extend scientific inquiry beyond national borders and can serve as role models for those who are beginning an interest in a broader arena. Nurses are mentors and experts who are accountable to clients and consumers of health care, to nurse colleagues for authoring (Kennedy & Charles, 1997), and to other health professionals and policymakers for leadership in providing intelligent, insightful health care. The potential for contributing to knowledge of health, nursing, and public policy is unlimited.

Discussion Points and Activities

1. State three reasons for conducting a comparative study of health problems.
2. Describe the type of government and general governmental structure in two countries in which you note a serious health problem. Identify where you could obtain information about each country. At what level would your focus be most beneficial?
3. Compare the values of family, language, and food in two countries. What are the implications of your analysis in planning for health care in each country?
4. How might not including minorities of a country in a research study bias or skew the results of that study?
5. What resources does a researcher use in a country in which he or she does not know the language? What are the advantages and disadvantages of conducting a study under these circumstances?
6. In studying two countries with differing economic systems, what common indicators may be used to reduce variance?
7. In studying two countries with differing political systems, what common indicators may be used to reduce variance?
8. What indicators are useful in comparing two different healthcare systems?

References

Adams, E., & Della, P. (2005). Development of nurse practitioner roles in Western Australia. *Transplant Nurses' Journal*, 14(1), 21–24.

Aides to William Bennett, head of the Bush Administration's anti-drug program protest health and human services department plan to support needle exchange. (1989). *New York Times*, 10 March, pp. 1–4.

American Academy of Nursing. (2007). *Mission statement*. Washington, DC: Author.

American Association of Colleges of Nursing. (2006). *The essentials of education for advanced practice nursing*. Washington, DC: Author.

American Nurses Association. (2006). *White paper on global nursing and health*. Washington, DC: Author.

Bardach, E. (1977). *The implementation game: What happens after a bill becomes a law*. Cambridge, MA: MIT Press.

Brasker, H. M. (1989). *Health insurance in the Netherlands*. Rijswijk: Ministry of Welfare, Health and Cultural Affairs.

Buning, A. de C., & Verheijen, L. (1990). *The Netherlands in brief*. The Hague: Foreign Information Service, Ministry of Foreign Affairs.

Campinha-Bacote, J. (2002). The process of cultural competence in the delivery of health care services: A model of care. *Journal of Transcultural Nursing*, 13(3), 181–184.

Decision and order, People of the State of New York v. Bordowitz et al. Docket No. 90N0248423, June 25, 1991.

Dexter, L. A. (1970). *Elite and specialized interviewing*. Evanston, IL: Northwestern University Press.

Dogan, M., & Pelassy, D. (1984). *How to compare nations.* Chatham, NJ: Chatham House Publishers.

Dr. Louis Sullivan, Secretary of HHS, endorses needle exchange program. (1989, March 9). *New York Times*, p. 9.

Elovich, R., & Sorge, R. (1991). Toward a community-based needle exchange for New York City. *AIDS & Public Policy Journal*, 6(4), 165, 172.

Evans, H. (1988, December 28). Needle exchange program is still mostly in vain. *New York Daily News*, p. A-1.

Fact sheet on the Netherlands. (1989). Rijswijk: Ministry of Welfare, Health and Cultural Affairs.

Ferreira, J. M. (2004). The health municipalization process from the perspective of the human being—nursing worker in the basic health network. *Revista Latino-Americana de Enfermagem*, 12(2), 212–220.

Ginzburg, H. M. (1989). Needle exchange programs: A medical or a policy dilemma? *American Journal of Public Health*, 79(10), 1350, 1351.

Gonzalez, D. (1992, December 20). Where children live in fear: Life in Red Hook, Brooklyn. *New York Times*, p. 16.

Goulet, C., Polomeno, V., Laizner, A. M., Marcil, I., & Lang, A. (2003). Translation and validation of a French version of Brown's support behaviors inventory in perinatal health. *Western Journal of Nursing Research*, 25(5), 561–582.

Grund, J. C., Kaplan, C. D., & Adriaans, N. F. P. (1991). Needle sharing in the Netherlands: An ethnographic analysis. *American Journal of Public Health*, 8(12), 1602–1607.

Harrington, C., Crider, M. C., Benner, P. E., & Malone, R. E. (2005). Advanced nurse training in health policy: Designing and implementing a new program. *Policy, Politics, & Nursing Practice*, 6(2), 99–108.

Inciardi, J. A. (1990). AIDS, a strange disease of uncertain origins. *American Behavioral Scientist*, 33(4), 397–407.

Joseph, S. C., & Des Jarlais, D. C. (1989). Update. *AIDS Updates*, 2(5), 1, 8.

Judge acquits 4. (1991, November 8). *New York Times*, p. 7.

Kennedy, E., & Charles, S. C. (1997). *Authority.* New York: Simon & Schuster.

King, W. (1988, August 10). Making a point. *Seattle Times*, p. F-8.

Kingdon, J. W. (1995). *Agendas, alternatives, and public policies* (2nd ed.). Boston: Little, Brown.

Leininger, M. M. (Ed.). (1991). *Culture care diversity and universality: A theory of nursing.* New York: National League for Nursing Press.

Manhattan Criminal Court Judge Laura E. Drager. (1991, June 26). *New York Times*, p. 1.

Maples, P. (1991, August 18). Needle exchange gains backing in AIDS fight. *Dallas Morning News*, p. E-13.

McLuhan, M., & Fiore, Q. (1968). *War and peace in the global village.* New York: McGraw-Hill.

Milstead, J. A. (1993). *The advancement of policy implementation theory: An analysis of three needle exchange programs* (Doctoral dissertation). University of Georgia, Athens.

Ndlovu, R., Phiri, M. L., Munjanja, O. K., Kibuka, S., & Fitzpatrick, J. J. (2003). The East, Central, and Southern African college of nursing: A collaborative endeavor for health policy and nursing practice. *Policy, Politics, & Nursing Practice*, 4(3), 221–226.

Needle swap program gaining favor. (1991, October 30). *New York Times*, p. 16.

New York State AIDS official Dr. Don C. Des Jarlais. (1988, June 6). *New York Times*, p. 3.

New York State Assembly's Republican minority. (1988, February 18). *New York Times*, p. 1.

New York State Health Commissioner Dr. David Axelrod says. (1988, March 15). *New York Times*, p. 5.

Odyssee Information. (1992). *Drugs and relief operations in Rotterdam*. Amsterdam: ROTOR Offsetdruk BV.

Phaladze, N. S. (2003). The role of nurses in the human immunodeficiency virus/ acquired immune deficiency syndrome policy process in Botswana. *International Nursing Review, 50,* 22–33.

Private Drug Abuse Agency. (1988, January 8). *New York Times,* p. 1.

Pye, L., & Verba, S. (Eds.). (1965). Political culture and political development. Princeton, NJ: Princeton University Press.

Rose, R. (1991). What is lesson-drawing? *Journal of Public Policy,* 11(1), 3–30.

Ross, C. A. (2002). Building bridges to promote globalization in nursing: The development of a Hermanamiento. *Journal of Transcultural Nursing,* 11(1), 64–67.

Schneider, A., & Ingram, H. (1990). Behavioral assumptions of policy tools. *Journal of Politics,* 52(2), 510–529.

Shatzkin, K. (1990a, October 12). A coming of age for needle exchange. *Seattle Times.* Accessed NewsBank, Health, 1990, fiche 111, grid A9.

Shatzkin, K. (1990b, February 17). Tacoma needle exchanges ruled legal. *Seattle Times,* pp. A1, A5.

Sritanyarat, W., Aroonsang, P., Charoenchai, A., Limumnoilap, S., & Patanasri, K. (2004). Health service system and health insurance for the elderly in Thailand: A knowledge synthesis. *Thai Journal of Nursing Research,* 8(2), 159–172.

Tacoma supports needle exchange to combat AIDS. (1989, January 5). *Seattle Independent,* p. 1.

The world of a drug bazaar. (1992, October 1). *New York Times,* p. 1.

Villarruel, A. M., Gallegos, E. C., Cherry, C. J., & Refugio de Duran, M. (2003). La uniendo de fronteras: Collaboration to develop HIV prevention strategies for Mexican and Latino youth. *Journal of Transcultural Nursing,* 14(3), 193–206.

Index

A

AACN (American Association of
Colleges of Nursing), 122
AAG (assistant attorney general), 103
academic Web sites, 213–214
AcademyHealth organization, 214
access, addressing with policy
initiatives, 81–82
accountability. *See also* credentialing,
methods of
for decision making, 97
ethical. *See* ethics
program evaluation, 179–181
accreditation, program evaluation and,
181
ACNP (American College of Nurse
Practitioners), 226
activism, 5, 7, 32
getting heard, 22, 86. *See also* agenda
setting

global health issues, 246–250
PACs (political action committees),
5, 74
participation in government
programs, 129, 135
participation in policymaking,
152
policy nurses, 221–229
reform in health professions
regulation, 120
RN Activist Tool Kit, 116
serving on boards of nursing, 107
actors in policy process, 19
communicating with, 83–85,
114–115
legislative process, 66–78
policy implementation, 159–161
stability of, 57
administration (government). *See also*
boards of nursing

execution and enforcement of law, 102

impact of policy implementation, 159

role in agenda setting, 49

administration (nursing), 29

Administrative Procedures Act (APA), federal, 19, 109–110

administrative procedures acts (APAs), state, 94, 104

administrator of program, as its evaluator, 185

advanced practice nurses. *See* APNs

Advanced Practice Task Force, NCSBN, 100–101

advantaged (target population), 58

adverse selection, 231, 236

advocacy for nursing specialties, 223–224, 225–226

advocacy training, 221, 224

agencies, administrative. *See* administration (government)

Agency for Healthcare Research and Quality, 9

agenda setting, 19, 22, 41–61, 132–133

case studies

National Center for Nursing Research Amendment, 46–47

Nebraska Humane Care Amendment, 43–46

defined, 42

healthcare reform (1990s), 30

models for, 48–60

contextual dimensions, 52–58

Kingdon model, 48–52

Schneider and Ingram model, 58–60

nursing's agenda for health, 1, 30

social issues, 130

AHCPR (Agency for Healthcare Research and Quality), 9

AIDS (acquired immune deficiency syndrome), 22

alternatives, policy, 137

ambiguity in policymaking, 134

amendments, 93, 116

American College of Nurse Practitioners, 226

American Nurses Association. *See* ANA

ANA (American Nurses Association), 5–6, 31

NCNR, influence on, 54

pain management, 162

policy nurses, 222–223

political action committee of (ANA-PAC), 74

analyzing regulations, 105–106

AND searches (Internet), 206

anxiety over program evaluation, 182, 189, 190–191

"any willing provider" laws, 106

APA (Administrative Procedures Act), federal, 19, 109–110

APAs (administrative procedures acts), state, 94, 104

APNs (advanced practice nurses), 2

defined, 1

as important constituents, 76

interstate mobility of, 120

as legislative assistants, 72

letters of support for, 107

nursing research and, 9

organizations advocacy, 225–226

pain management (implementation case study), 161–162

regulation of, 95–97, 100–101, 121–124. *See also* regulation

reviewing regulations for promulgation, 105–106

roles of nurses, 4–5, 25–32

political, 5–8

shortage of, 123–124

applied healthcare economics, 231–238. *See also* cost issues

end-stage renal disease (case study), 240–243

global issues, 252, 261–263

appointments to boards and commissions, 107

appropriations committees, 79–80
APRNs, prescriptive authority of, 162
ASPMN (American Society for Pain
        Management Nursing),
        162
assertiveness training, 3–4
assistant attorney general, 103
associations. *See* organized nursing
asymmetrical information, 231,
        234–236
attendance at meetings, 116
Aunt Mary Network, 115
authority policy tools, 138
authorizing committees, 79, 80
authors of online content, 208–209
autonomy for decision making, 97.
        See also credentialing,
        methods of

B
bachelor of science degrees in nursing,
        2. *See also* nursing education
    policy courses, 227
    political education in, 26
Back to Sleep Campaign (BTS),
        164–168
Balanced Budget Act of 1997, 173
behavior and motivation, 139–141
    policy tools, 138–139
    role of policy in, 130
    societal costs, 236–237
belief systems, program evaluation and,
        187
Betts, Virginia Trotter, 6
bills (proposed legislation), 78, 93
bipartisan support, 53
blogs, 197, 216
blood lead screening (case study),
        163–164
boards of nursing, 91, 93, 96, 102
    composition, 102
    joint regulation with boards of
        medicine, 96
    mandatory reporting, 103–104
    meetings, 103, 116

official recognition from, 92, 95, 99
    serving on, 107
    as sole regulators of APNs, 122
bookmarks (Internet), 197, 201
Boolean operators, 206
browsers (Internet), 197, 200
    bookmarks (Internet), 197, 201
BSNE programs, 2. *See also* nursing
        education
    policy courses, 227
    political education in, 26
BTS (Back to Sleep Campaign),
        164–168
Burke, Sheila, 6
business cards, 84

C
capacity-building policy tools,
        138–139, 140
case management, 14
caucuses, 66, 69
causation, 188
Center for Health Law Studies (St. Louis),
        213
Center for Health Policy Research
        (UCLA), 213–214
certification, 91, 99. *See also* licensure
    multiple educational pathways to,
        121
    of nurses, national agencies for,
        100–101
CFR (Code of Federal Regulations), 111
child health
    policy tools and, 140–141
        case study, 141–153
    SIDS prevention campaigns,
        164–168
clinical nursing research, 9. *See also*
        research in nursing
clinical problems, 27
closed meetings, boards of nursing,
        103
CMS (Centers for Medicare and
        Medicaid Services), 108
coalitions between interest groups, 74

Code of Federal Regulations (CFR), 111
codes of ethics. *See* ethics
collaboration, 11, 15
college education in nursing. *See*
    nursing education
commenting on proposed regulations,
    114
Commerce Clause (U.S. Constitution),
    109
committees to review and approve
    regulations, 104–105, 107
  meeting attendance, 116
  staff of, 72–73. *See also* congressional
    committees
communicating effectively to policy-
    makers, 83–85
communication during program
    evaluation, 186–187, 190
  sharing findings, 192–193
competency assessments, 94, 100
  certification and, 99
  licensing boards and, 102
  licensure and, 98
  professional self-regulation and, 100
  recruitment of foreign nurses, 124
  registration and, 98
compliance with policy rules, 160–161
  blood lead screening (case study),
    163–164
  oversight, 164, 208
  oversight committees, 78–79
compromises, 87
condition vs. problem, 50
conference committees, 23
confidence, 86–87
conflict in evaluation. *See* ethics, in
    program evaluation
Congress, members of, 67–69
  congressional staff, 69–72. *See also*
    congressional committees
  role in policy formation, 49
congressional classes, 55
congressional committees, 77–78,
    78–79
  staff of, 72–73

working with personal office staff,
    72–73
Congressional Nursing Caucus, 32
congressional staff, 69–72. *See also*
    congressional committees
constituents, 66, 76
  communicating to, 76
  interest groups and, 73–74
Constitution (U.S.), 109
containment of healthcare costs,
    12–13, 107–108, 140,
    174
contenders (target population), 58
content quality, online, 206–210
contextual dimensions for agenda
    setting, 41, 52–58
continuing competency regulations, 94
continuing education. *See also* nursing
    education
  licensing boards and, 102
  professional self-regulation and, 100
  regulations on, 94
control, in policy implementation,
    160–161
Cornell University, 215
coronary care, 3
correspondence to policymakers,
    83–84
cost issues. *See also* economics of applied
    health care
  addressing with policy initiatives,
    81–82
  containment of healthcare costs,
    12–13, 107–108, 140,
    174
  fiscal impact statements, 104–105
  opportunity costs, 232, 237
  societal costs, 236–237
court system, role of, 18
credential review. *See* registration
credentialing, methods of, 97–101,
    121–122
"crippled at birth" (policies), 134, 135
crisp charges, 129, 136
CyberExchange portal, 213

D

Davis, Carolyne, 6
debate, learning, 30
decision making, responsibility for. *See*
        credentialing, methods of
deflection of goals in policy implemen-
        tation, 160
demand-and-supply theories, 232–233
dependents (target populations), 58
design of program evaluations, 172,
        188–190
    potential for ethical conflict, 182–183
    to reduce ethical dilemmas, 186–188
design of programs, 23, 129–153. *See
        also* implementation of
        policy; policy process
    behavioral dimensions, 139–141
    case study, 141–153
    control of, by policy actors, 57
    instruments of policy, 136–138
    link between design and implemen-
        tation, 134–136
    link between design and outcome,
        129, 133–134
    policy design model, 138–139
    review of policy research, 131–134
deviants (target population), 58
dialysis industry (economics case
        study), 240–243
director of Capitol connections,
        226–227
directories, online
    of content, 200–201
    of people, 205
directory of Capitol connections, 228
disciplinary action, 98
dissipation of energy game, 160
divisiveness within the profession, 116
DNP programs. *See* doctoral programs
        in nursing
doctoral programs in nursing, 4, 122,
        248
    funding for, 28
    policy courses, 227
    political education in, 26

documenting program outcomes,
        178–179
doing nothing, 174
Drager, Laura, 261–262
drug treatment philosophy
        (case study), 260–261
Dutch needle-exchange programs
        (case study), 254–255,
        260–261, 263–264
Dutch prenatal care (case study),
        141–153

E

e-mail communications to policymakers,
        83–84
earmarking legislation, 68
EBITDA value, 243
economics of applied health care,
        231–238. *See also* cost issues
    end-stage renal disease (case study),
        240–243
    global issues, 252, 261–263
ECSACON advisory group, 247
education. *See* nursing education
education as policy tool, 138–139, 259
elected officials, role in agenda setting,
        49
elections, interest groups and, 74
emergency regulations, 110
end-stage renal disease (case study),
        240–243
environmental factors
    policy evaluation and, 187–190
    policy implementation, 131–132,
        157, 159
    program design, 135
ESRD (end-stage renal disease) case
        study, 240–243
ethics
    lobbying, 115
    mandatory reporting, 103–104
    moral hazards, 231, 236
    professional self-regulation, 100
    in program evaluation, 171,
        182–188

evaluating online resources and
information, 206–210
evaluation of programs, 19, 24,
171–193
accountability in, 179–181
defined, 171
defining "good enough", 160–161
design options, 172, 188–190
ethics issues, 182–188
process of, 176–179
reporting on evaluations, 171,
184–185
sharing results of, 190–193
understanding public policy and
social programs, 173–176
using theory in, 172, 181–182
evaluation theory, 181–182
execution of policy. *See* implementation
of policy
executive branch of government,
18–19, 75
executive sessions, 103
experience gains, importance of, 86
expertise, 87–88
extent of problems, determining, 177
externalities, 231, 236–237

F

faculty shortages in nursing, 28
family planning, 151
fear of program evaluation, 182, 189,
190–191
federal court system, role of, 18
federal funding. *See* funding
Federal Register, 91, 109–110, 111, 114,
215
federal regulatory process, 107–110
Federal Trade Commission (FTC), 23
feedback on program interventions. *See*
outcome evaluations
fellows in congressional offices, 70
findlaw.com Web site, 215
fire alarms (in policy), 129, 132
fiscal impact statements, 104–105
fiscal year, 79

FNMS (Fresenius National Medical
Care), 241
foreign nurse recruitment, 124, 233
formality of board meetings, 103
Forum for State Health Policy
Leadership, 212–213
free-market economy, 232–233
"freedom of choice" laws, 106
FTC (Federal Trade Commission), 23
funding, 28–29. *See also* cost issues;
economics of applied
health care
appropriations committees, 79–80
program evaluation and, 179–180
future roles of nurses, 25–32
fuzzy charges, 129, 136

G

game playing in policy implementation,
132
garbage can metaphor (policymaking),
133
Gebbie, Kristine, 6
Georgetown University, 214
getting heard, 22, 86. *See also* agenda
setting
global issues, 245–264
goal deflection during policy
implementation, 160
"good enough" compliance, 160–161
Governance Performance and Results
Act of 1993, 176
government administration. *See also*
boards of nursing
execution and enforcement of law,
102
impact of policy implementation, 159
role in agenda setting, 49
government-related Web sites,
211–213
government response to public
problems. *See* laws and
legislation; regulation
government (U.S.), Web site for, 211
GPO Access, 211–212

GPRA (Governance Performance and
    Results Act), 176
graduate education in nursing, 4, 122,
    248
  funding for, 28
  policy courses, 227
  political education in, 26
grants. *See* funding
graphical reports on program
    evaluation, 191
grassroots campaigns, 74, 106, 115
grassroots response to programs, 245,
    256–258

H
harm, protection from, 183–184, 186
HCFA (Health Care Financing
    Administration), 108
Health Affairs blog, 216
health LAs, 70–72
health law resources (online), 215
Health Policies blog, 216
health policy foundations and
    organizations, 214
Health Research Extension Act of 1983,
    46
health sites (Internet), 205
health systems, international, 252–253,
    263–264
healthcare economics, 231–238. *See also*
    cost issues
  end-stage renal disease (case study),
    240–243
  global issues, 252, 261–263
healthcare paradigm, 12–16
hearings, public, 92, 114
High Risk Channeling Project, 150
Hinshaw, Ada Sue, 53
HIPAA (Health Insurance Portability
    and Accountability Act),
    183
Hold, Matthew, 216
homepage (Internet), 197, 200
honor, 86–87
hortatory policy tools, 138–139

hospital systems, 12–16
  mergers and partnerships, 14–15
host, computer, 197, 199
Humane Care Amendment (Nebraska),
    43–46
hyperlinks, 198, 200, 207–208

I
icebreakers in communication, 87
identifying problems, 27
implementation games, 157, 160,
    258–259
implementation of policy, 19, 24,
    131–132, 157–168. *See also*
    program design
  case studies
    Back to Sleep Campaign (BTS),
      164–168
    lead poisoning in children,
      163–164
    pain management, 161–162
  defined, 157
  documenting intent of policy, 134
  international (global) effects,
    245–264
  people involved in, 159–161
INA (Illinois Nurse's Association), 161
incentive policy tools, 138
incrementalism, 7
Indian Health Services, 109
infant mortality rate, 140–141
  case study, 141–153
  SIDS prevention campaigns,
    164–168
information asymmetry, 231, 234–236
information literacy, 199, 207
information requests, answering,
    180–181
Institute for Health Policy
    (Muskie School), 214
instruments of policy, 136–139
  how to choose, 139–141
  needle-exchange programs
    (case study), 258–259
intensive care, 3

intent of policy, 134
interdisciplinary education, 14
interest groups, 22, 45, 49–50, 66,
    73–75
    ethical conflict in program
        evaluation, 182–183,
        184–185, 187, 188
    national nursing groups, influence
        of, 46–47
    NCNR example, 53–54, 56, 57
international health issues, 245–264
international political relations, 56
Internet-based legislative information
    services, 111–113
Internet for obtaining policy
    information, 197–217
    evaluating resources and information,
        206–210
    impact on policy development,
        215–216
    information literacy, 199, 207
    key sites for health policy, 210–215
    key words for searching, 205–206
Internet sites. See Web pages
internship programs in politics, 7,
    224–225
    in congressional offices, 70
interpretation of policy and regulation,
    18, 117, 129, 133–134
interstate compact, 91, 120–121
interstate mobility of nurses, 120
interventions. See also program design
    revising, 180
    unintended effects, 181
investment in nursing research, 29
inviting policymakers to events, 85
involvement, creating, 86
iron triangle, 41
issue specialists, 66, 81

J

jargon in program evaluation reports,
    191
joint regulation, 96. See also regulation
judicial interpretation. See interpretation
    of policy and regulation

K

Kaiser Family Foundation, 214
key words for Internet searches, 205–206
Kingdon model (agenda setting), 48–52
knowledge
    documenting program outcomes,
        178–179. See also outcome
        evaluations
    education as policy tool, 138–139,
        259
    importance of, 86
    obtaining and sharing, 87–88

L

LAs (legislative assistants), 66, 70–72
laws and legislation, 19, 23, 65–88. See
        also legislative process
    from bills to laws, 78–80, 93
    health law resources (online), 215
    as policy initiative, 18
    regulation vs. legislation, 92–94
    that govern nursing, 4–5
    tracking, 111–113
lead poisoning (implementation case
        study), 163–164
Leapfrog Group, 15
learning policy tools, 138–139
Legal Information Institute (Cornell),
    215
legislative assistants, 66, 70–72
legislative commissions, 104–105
legislative directors, 70
legislative process, 7, 21, 93. See also
        laws and legislation; policy
        process
    agenda. See agenda setting
    from bills to law, 78–80, 93
    effective communication, 83–85
    NCNR legislation (example), 51,
        53–58, 59–60
    nursing research in, 81
    people of, 66–78
    putting issues in context, 81–82
    recommendations from lessons
        learned, 85–88
    visibility of nurses' views, 82–83

legislative recognition, 92, 95, 99
letter writing, 83–84
letters of support for APNs, 107
levels of program design, 135
licensure, 91, 97–98, 121–122. *See also*
        regulation
    current issues in, 117–121
    duties for licensing boards, 102
    mandatory licensure laws, creation
        of, 96
    mandatory reporting, 103–104
    nurse shortage and, 123–124
    purpose, in health processions,
        94–97
life expectancy, 130
links (Internet), 198, 200, 207–208
lobbyists, 73–75, 91, 115–116. *See also*
        interest groups
    PACs (political action committees),
        5, 74
    pushing for regulation, 106
    relationships with members of
        Congress, 68

M
Madigan's NIN amendment. *See* NCNR,
        understanding legislative
        process of
Magee, Mike, 216
mail, sent to policymakers, 83–84
mailing lists, online, 203
Malone, Beverly, 6, 248
managed care contracts, 123
mandatory overtime legislation,
        123–124
mandatory reporting, 103–104
    lobbying efforts, 115
    negative effects of programs, 186,
        192
    program evaluations, 171, 184–185
    program outcomes, 178–179
market competition, 232–233
master's degrees. *See* graduate education
        in nursing
media, role in legislative process,
        77–78

Medicaid program, 107–108
Medicare program, 12, 106, 174
    dialysis industry (case study),
        241–243
    reimbursement policy, 107–108
meetings, boards of nursing, 103, 116
members of Congress, 67–69
    congressional staff, 69–72. *See also*
        congressional committees
    role in policy formation, 49
mergers, hospital, 14–15
Messinger, Ruth, 261–262
meta-search sites, 202
microeconomics, 231, 232–233
Milstead Model, 250, 253
misinterpretation of regulations, 117
monitoring program operations, 178
monitoring state regulations, 105–106
moral hazards, 231, 236
motivation. *See* behavior and motivation
multistate licensure, 104
multistate regulation, 91, 109, 120–121
Muskie School, 214
mutual recognition, 92, 120–121

N
N-STAT (Nurses Strategic Action Team),
        6
NACCHO (National Association of City
        and County Health
        Officials), 213
NANP (National Alliance of Nurse
        Practitioners), 225–226
National Alliance of Nurse
        Practitioners, 225–226
National Association of City and
        County Health Officials,
        213
National Center for Nursing Research.
        See NINR (National
        Institute of Nursing
        Research)
National Center for Nursing Research
        Amendment, 46–47
National Conference of State
        Legislators, 212–213

National Council of State Boards of
Nursing. *See* NCSBN
National Federation of Nursing
Specialty Organizations,
224
National Health Information
Infrastructure, 215–216
National Mental Health Act of 1946, 28
National Nurse Practitioner Coalition,
226
National Performance Review, 176
National Technical Information Service,
212
NCLA (Nurses Coalition for Legislative
Action), 223–224
NCNR (National Center for Nursing
Research), 46–47. *See also*
NINR
understanding legislative process of,
51, 53–58, 59–60
NCSBN (National Council of State
Boards of Nursing),
100–101, 102, 122
NCSL (National Conference of State
Legislators), 212–213
Nebraska Humane Care Amendment,
43–46
needle-exchange programs
(case study), 250–264
negative effects of programs, reporting,
186, 192
negative public policies, 174
negatively viewed target populations,
58–60
negotiating compromises, 87
NEPs (needle-exchange programs),
250–264
Netherlands
needle-exchange programs
(case study), 254–255,
260–261, 263–264
prenatal care in (case study),
141–153
networking, 85, 87, 115
new organizational paradigm, 1, 2,
10–12

New York City NEP (case study), 255,
256–258, 261–262
news stories and newspapers. *See*
media, role in legislative
process
NFSNO (National Federation for
Specialty Nursing
Organizations), 224–225
NHII (National Health Information
Infrastructure), 215–216
NHPF (National Health Policy Forum),
214
Nightingale Policy Initiative, 214,
227–228
NIH bill. *See* NCNR, understanding
legislative process of
NIN amendment. *See* NCNR, understand-
ing legislative process of
NINR (National Institute of Nursing
Research), 29, 46
amendment, 46–47
NIWI (Nurses in Washington
Internship), 224
NIWR (Nurse in Washington
Roundtable), 223
NNPC (National Nurse Practitioner
Coalition), 226
NOA (Nursing Organizations Alliance),
225
nongovernmental actors in agenda
setting, 49
Nothing But Baby campaign, 165
notice of proposed rulemaking (NPR),
109–110
NPAs (nurse practice acts), 94, 96,
103–104
NPI (Nightingale Policy Initiative),
214, 227–228
NPR (notice of proposed rulemaking),
109–110
N-STAT (Nurses Strategic Action Team),
6
NTIS (National Technical Information
Service), 212
numbers, communicating, 77, 84,
85–86

Nurse Education Act, 79
Nurse in Washington Roundtable, 223
nurse practice acts (NPAs), 94, 96,
    103–104
nurse practitioners, 3–4. *See also* APNs
Nurse Reinvestment Act, 31
nurse shortage, 123–124, 233
Nurse Training Acts (NTAs), 28
nurses. *See* APNs
Nurses Coalition for Legislative Action,
    223–224
The Nurse's Directory of Capital
    Connections, 226–227,
    228
Nurses in Washington Internship,
    224–225
Nurses Strategic Action Team, 6
nursing, organized. *See* organized
    nursing
nursing administration funding, 29
nursing associations. *See* organized
    nursing
nursing education, 8
    about political process, 6, 26–27,
        227
    advocacy training, 221, 224
    approval of educational programs,
        102
    bachelor of science degrees, 2
        political education in, 26
    continuing education, 94, 100, 102
    doctoral programs, 4, 122, 248
        funding for, 28
        political education in, 26
    funding for, 28
    interdisciplinary, 14
    learning how to debate, 30
    proliferation of, 121, 124
    regulation of, 122
Nursing Organizations Alliance, 31,
    225
nursing practices, changes in, 2–5
nursing research, 8–10
    funding for, 29
    policy implications of, 81
nursing science programs, 3

nursing specialty organizations, 221,
    222
    advocacy for, 223–224
nursing theories, 8–10
nursing's agenda for health, 1, 30

O
objective program evaluation,
    185–186, 190
official recognition, 92, 95, 99
OMB (Office of Management and
    Budget), 55
online educational programs, 227
online legislative information services,
    111–113. *See also* Internet
    for obtaining policy
    information
online mailing lists, 203
open meetings, boards of nursing,
    103
opportunity costs, 232, 237
oral communication to policymakers
    comments on proposed regulations,
        114–115
    suggestions for, 83–84
organizational paradigm of 21st century.
    See new organizational
    paradigm
organized nursing, 5–6, 30–32
    lobbying, 115. *See also* lobbyists
    nursing specialty organizations, 221,
        222
        advocacy for, 223–224
    policy nurses in, 222–223
    professional self-regulation, 92,
        99–100
outcome evaluations, 171, 175,
    178–179
    accountability for, 179–181
    explanation of unexpected outcomes,
        192
    objectivity in, 185–186, 190
outdated information, online, 209
oversight, 164, 208
oversight committees, 78–79
overtime legislation, 123–124

P

PACs (political action committees), 5, 74

pain management (implementation case study), 161–162

paradigm for 21st-century organizations. *See* new organizational paradigm

paradigm for health care, 12–16

participation. *See also* political activism
communicating effectively to policy-makers, 83–85
in government programs, 129, 135
meeting attendance, 116
in policymaking, 152

Partnership for a Health Generation, 150

partnerships between interest groups, 74

people data, locating online, 204–205

people involved. *See* actors in policy process

perfect information, 234

periodic evaluation of social programs, 179. *See also* evaluation of programs

permission to act. *See* credentialing, methods of

permissive regulation of nurses, 95–96

personal data, locating online, 204–205

personal office staff, 69–72. *See also* congressional committees
working with committee staff, 72–73

Pew Health Professionals Commission, 117–118

Pew Task Force on Health Care Workforce Regulations, 118

Pfizer Medical Humanities initiative, 216

philosophical foundation of nursing, 8–10

phone numbers, Internet searches for, 204

physical examinations, 3–4

plus sign (+) in Internet searches, 206

policy, defined, 171, 173

policy analysts, 66, 81

policy design. *See* program design

policy entrepreneurs, 50–51, 193

policy evaluation. *See* evaluation of programs

policy formation models, 48–60
contextual dimensions, 52–58
Kingdon model, 48–52
Schneider and Ingram model, 58–60

policy foundations and organizations, 214

policy implementation. *See* implementation of policy

policy interpretation, 18, 117, 129, 133–134

policy links, 129, 133–134

policy nurses, 221–229
defined, 221

policy process, 1, 7, 21–25, 131
agenda. *See* agenda setting
communicating effectively to policy-makers, 83–85
costs. *See* cost issues
design. *See* program design
evaluation. *See* evaluation of programs
government response. *See* laws and legislation; regulation
implementation. *See* implementation of policy
NCNR legislation (example), 51, 53–58, 59–60
research on, 131–134

policy reform, 20–21, 120

policy streams, 48, 50
NCNR amendment (example), 51

policy structure, 157, 159

policy tools, 136–139
how to choose, 139–141
needle-exchange programs (case study), 258–259

policy vs. public policy, 17

policy windows. *See* window of opportunity

political activism, 5, 7, 32
    getting heard, 22, 86. *See also* agenda
        setting
    global health issues, 246–250
    PACs (political action committees),
        5, 74
    participation in government
        programs, 129, 135
    participation in policymaking, 152
    policy nurses, 221–229
    reform in health professions
        regulation, 120
    RN Activist Tool Kit, 116
    serving on boards of nursing, 107
political contextual influence. *See*
        contextual dimensions
political roles of nurses, 5–8
political streams, 48, 51
    NCNR amendment (example), 51
positive public policies, 174
positively viewed target populations,
        58–60
PPI-HP (Public Policy Institute for
        Health Professions), 226
practice acts, 94, 96, 103–104
practice of nursing, changes in, 2–5
prenatal care, 140–141
    case study, 141–153
prescriptive authority, 92, 95, 97
    pain management, 162
press releases, 76
pride, 86–87
Prisoner's Dilemma, 235
problem, condition vs., 50
problem fading, 245
problem identification and
        interpretation, 27, 177
problem response at grassroots level,
        245, 256–258
problem streams, 48, 50–51. *See also*
        streams of policy process
    NCNR amendment (example), 51
process, policy as, 19–20. *See also* policy
        process
professional self-regulation, 92,
        99–100

program administrator, as its evaluator,
        185
program design, 23, 129–153. *See also*
        implementation of policy;
        policy process
    behavioral dimensions, 139–141
    case study, 141–153
    control of, by policy actors, 57
    instruments of policy, 136–138
    link between design and implemen-
        tation, 134–136
    link between design and outcome,
        129, 133–134
    policy design model, 138–139
    review of policy research, 131–134
program evaluation. *See* evaluation of
        programs
program evaluation design, 172,
        188–190
    potential for ethical conflict,
        182–183
    to reduce ethical dilemmas,
        186–188
program implementation. *See* imple-
        mentation of policy
program selection, 177
promulgating regulations
    emergency regulations, 110
    federal regulations, 109–110
    state regulations, 104–105
proposed legislation (bills), 78, 93
proposed regulations
    publications of, 111
    reviewing, 104–107, 109–110
protection from harm, 183–184, 186
protocol, Web, 208
public hearings, 92, 114
public policy, 15–21, 173–174
    defined, 1, 172
    as entity, 17–19
    evaluating. *See* evaluation of programs
    as process, 19–20. *See also* policy
        process
    reform. *See* policy reform
Public Policy Institute for Health
        Professions, 226

publications of proposed regulations,
111
purse-string committees. *See* appropriations committees

Q
qualitative evaluation design, 172,
188–189
quality of care
addressing with policy initiatives,
81–82
calculating value of, 13
quality of online resources, evaluating,
206–210
quantitative evaluation design, 172,
188

R
rationality (economics), 232, 234, 235
recognition, official, 92, 95, 99
recruitment of foreign nurses, 124,
233
reengineering organizational systems,
11, 14
reform, 20–21, 120
Register. See Federal Register
registration, 92, 98–99
creation of RN title, 95, 99
regulation, 19, 23, 91–125. *See also*
licensure
of APNs, 95–97, 100–101,
121–124
credentialing methods, 97–101
current issues in, 117–121
defined, 92
definitions and purpose, 94–95
emergency regulations, 110
federal regulatory process, 107–110
finding information about, 111–113
future of APN regulation, 121–124
of health professions, history of,
95–97
interpretation of policy, 18, 117,
129, 133–134
legislation vs., 92–94

lobbying for, 115–116. *See also*
lobbyists
nurse shortage and, 123–124
as policy initiative, 18–19
promulgating, 104–105, 109–110
providing public comment on,
114–115
purpose, in health processions,
94–97
of self. *See* professional self-regulation
state regulatory process, 101–107
strengths and weaknesses, 116–117
regulations.gov Web site, 215
Rehabilitation Act of 1973, 18
reimbursement
dialysis industry (case study),
241–243
for Medicare, 107–108
regulations on, 106, 122–123
relationships, maintaining, 85, 87, 115
within policy implementation, 132
renal disease (economics case study),
240–243
"reporting out" bills, 80
reporting requirements, 103–104
lobbying efforts, 115
negative effects of programs, 186,
192
program evaluations, 171, 184–185
program outcomes, 178–179
representatives (U.S.). *See* members of
Congress
requests for information, answering,
180–181
research in nursing, 8–10
funding for, 29
policy implications of, 81
responsibility. *See* accountability
restrictive regulation, 97
results of programs. *See* outcome
evaluations
reverse phone number lookups, 204
review of credentials. *See* registration
reviewing regulations for promulgation,
105–106

revising program interventions, 180
RN Activist Tool Kit, 116
RN title, creation of, 95, 99
role conflict in program evaluations,
184–185
roles of nurses, 4–5, 25–32
political, 5–8
Rotterdam. *See* Netherlands
rules and regulations, 93
compliance with, 160
defined, 92. *See also* regulation

S

Saint Louis University School of Law,
213
saliency of an issue. *See* streams of
policy process
Schiavo, Terri. *See* Nebraska Humane
Care Amendment
Schneider and Ingram model (agenda
setting), 58–60, 138
scholarship funding, 28
Schorr, Thelma, 223
scientific approach to nursing education,
3
scope of policies, 17–18
scope of practice, defining, 95, 96–97,
106, 117–118
proliferation of APN educational
programs, 121
search engines, 198, 200–201
key words for, 205–206
locating, 201–203
selecting specific programs, 177
self-regulation, 92, 99–100
senators. *See* members of Congress
"server down" messages, 201–202
settings for nursing, 4
severity of problems, determining, 177
sexually transmitted diseases, 246
needle-exchange programs
(case study), 250–264
shortage of nurses
economics of, 233
policy impact of, 123–124

SIDS (sudden infant death syndrome),
164–168
signature files, 198, 203
slogans as policy tool, 139
social construction of target populations,
58–60
social programs, 175–176
defined, 172
effectiveness of, 129–130. *See also*
program design
evaluating. *See* evaluation of programs
monitoring, 178–179
results of. *See* outcome evaluations
selecting among, 177
storefront programs, 245, 255
street programs, 245, 255
Social Security Act of 1935, 28
societal cost of behavior, 236–237
sociocultural systems, 251, 259–260
softening up, 245
sound bites, 22
South Carolina prenatal care
(case study), 141–153
speaking to policymakers
comments on proposed regulations,
114–115
suggestions for, 83–84
special care, 3
special-interest groups. *See* interest
groups
specialty nursing organizations, 221,
222
advocacy for, 223–224
sponsors. *See* funding
stability of policy actors, 57
staffing ratios, 124, 233
stakeholders, 41. *See also* interest groups
ethical conflict in program evaluation,
182–183, 184–185, 187,
188
standards of practice, 100, 104
state attorney general's representative,
103
state boards of nursing. *See* boards of
nursing

state court system, role of, 18
State Register (State Bulletin), 111
state regulatory process, 101–107
    monitoring regulations, 105–106
    promulgating regulations, 104,
        109–110
    serving on boards, 107
statutes. *See* laws and legislation
STDs (sexually transmitted diseases),
        246
    needle-exchange programs
        (case study), 250–264
Stevenson, Joanne, 56
storefront programs, 245, 255
strategic thinking, 137
streams of policy process, 41, 43,
        48–51, 133
    NCNR amendment (example), 51
street-level bureaucrats, 159
street programs, 245, 255
strength of U.S. systems, 238
subjectivity of program evaluation,
        185–186
success of policy, key elements in,
        158–159
Sullivan, John D., 240
supply-and-demand theories, 232–233
Supremacy Clause (U.S. Constitution),
        109
sustainability of programs, 179
symbolic policy tools, 138–139
systems thinking, 11

T

Tacoma needle-exchange program
        (case study), 255, 258,
        259, 262–263
tailoring program evaluations to
        audience, 189, 191–192
target populations
    behavior of. *See* behavior and
        motivation
    participation in policymaking, 129,
        135, 152
    social construction of, 58–60

technology, impact on healthcare
        delivery, 109, 120–121
telemedicine services, 120
testimony on proposed legislation, 80
theories of nursing, 8–10
theory as program evaluation tool,
        172, 181–182
Third House of Congress, 23
timeliness of online content, 209
timing, importance of, 116. *See also*
        window of opportunity
title protection, 98, 99
tools of policy, 136–139
    how to choose, 139–141
    needle-exchange programs
        (case study), 258–259
tracking legislation, 111–113
tracking program operations, 178
tractability, 157, 164
training. *See* nursing education
Tuskegee experiment, 25

U

UAPs (unlicensed assistive personnel),
        123
UCLA Center for Health Policy
        Research, 213–214
unavailable Web pages, 201–202
Uniform Requirements for
        Licensure/Authority to
        Practice, 101, 121
uniform resource locators (URLs),
        198, 199–200, 208
unintended effects of programs, 181
unity within the profession, 116
University of California, Los Angeles,
        213–214
university policy courses, 227
unlicensed assistive personnel (UAPs),
        123
URLs (uniform resource locators),
        198, 199–200, 208
U.S. Congress. *See* members of Congress
U.S. Constitution, 109
U.S. government, Web site for, 211

usa.gov (Web site), 211
user interface, 198, 201
utility (economics), 232

V
vagueness in policymaking, 134
Veterans Administration hospitals, 109
veto points, 132
virtual groups, 203
virtual hosting, 199
visibility of nurses' views, 82–83
voluntary regulation of nurses, 95–96.
      See also professional self-
      regulation
voters. *See* constituents
voting, boards of nursing, 103
voting on proposed legislation, 80

W
Wakefield, Mary, 6
Waxman's NIH bill. *See* NCNR, under-
      standing legislative process
      of
Web-based legislative information
      services, 111–113. *See also*
      Internet for obtaining
      policy information
Web pages, 198, 200
  blogs, 197, 216

evaluating quality of, 206–210
key sites for health policy, 210–215
where to get information, 197–217
  evaluating resources and
    information, 206–210
  impact on policy development,
    215–216
  information literacy, 199, 207
  key sites for health policy,
    210–215
  key words for searching, 205–206
Wennberg, John, 50
white pages, online, 204–205
WHO (World Health Organization),
    212
who you know, 85
window of opportunity, 41, 48, 51
  importance of timing, 116
  reform in health professions
    regulation, 120
  regulation development input, 114
word bites, 22
workforce regulation, 118–119
World Health Organization, 212
World Wide Web, about, 199–206
written communication to policymakers,
    83–84
  comments on proposed regulations,
    114–115